SAUNDERS

Manual of Medical Office Management

ALICE ANNE ANDRESS

Health Care Consultant
Chief Executive Officer
Lehigh Valley Orthopedics
Allentown, Pennsylvania

S A U N D E R S
Manual of
Medical Office
Management

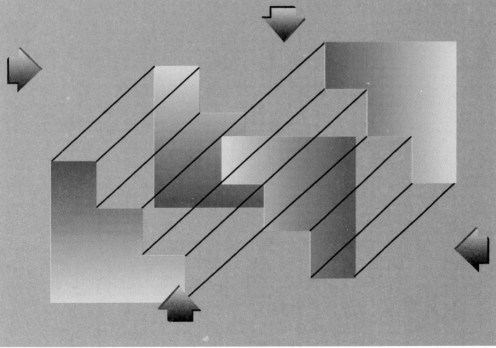

W.B. SAUNDERS COMPANY
A Division of Harcourt Brace & Company

Philadelphia   London   Toronto   Montreal   Sydney   Tokyo

W.B. SAUNDERS COMPANY
A Division of Harcourt Brace & Company

The Curtis Center
Independence Square West
Philadelphia, Pennsylvania 19106

Library of Congress Cataloging-in-Publication Data

Andress, Alice Anne.
    Saunders manual of medical office management/Alice Anne Andress.
    —1st ed.
        p.   cm.

    Includes index.

    ISBN 0–7216–4820–7

    1. Medical offices—Management.   I. W.B. Saunders Company
    II. Title.

    R728.8.A56   1996

    651'.961--dc20   95-4642

Saunders Manual of Medical Office Management   ISBN 0–7216–4820–7

Printed in the United States of America.

Last digit is the print number: 9   8   7   6   5   4   3   2   1

I dedicate this book to my husband and parents,
who make my life whole

Preface

Saunders Manual of Medical Office Management is a summary of 24 years of varied experience in health care. In the preparation of this text I have attempted to convey my commitment to the professionalism and overall high standards of health care. It is my firm belief that today, more than ever, medical office managers need to broaden their organizational, technical, personal, and leadership skills. Ongoing continuing education, both formal and informal, coupled with innovative philosophies, is critical for a successful office manager in today's environment. With this foundation, the committed office manager will be able to thrive and excel in his or her chosen managerial career.

Among the most important features throughout this text are the special insights contained in **From the Author's Notebook*. These insights, obtained through years of practical experience, are intended to assist in daily decision-making. There are other special sections throughout the text labeled **Manager's Alert!*. These sections have been placed strategically throughout the book to caution the office manager about preventable difficulties.

This book was designed to provide a medical office manager with instant necessary information for immediate use. I have presented this information in a logical format that can be incorporated into the daily activities of a medical office manager. It is my belief that this book will assist the reader to obtain a greater understanding of the function of a medical office and the expertise necessary to be successful.

Alice Anne Andress

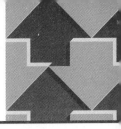

Acknowledgments

A special thanks must first be extended to Margaret Biblis, Senior Acquisitions Editor at the W.B. Saunders Company, who from our first meeting shared in the excitement of this project and whose continued support as my editor made it all happen. I wish to extend my gratitude and appreciation to many friends and co-workers who helped in the development of this text; Ann, Carolyn, Debbie, Chris, John, and Gilly. I would like to express appreciation to my mother, father, and other family members, who supported me throughout the birth and life of this text, and ate a lot of pizza during its conception. A tender thanks is extended to my husband, Joe, who stood beside me, encouraged me, and understood my commitment to this project.

An acknowledgment must be extended to the following people who contributed to the development of this text: Dr. Robert Hale, for his continued support; Larry Conklin, for his typesetting and design abilities; Keystone Computer Systems, for contributing information; Versyss Computer Systems, for their contributions; Kevcor Ltd., for sharing their new product with me; Bill Goralski, for his photography; Gastrointestinal Specialists, Inc. and their staff, for their contributions; and the office staff of Dr. Gene Levin.

Alice Anne Andress

Contents

Appendices

1

The Health Care Profession

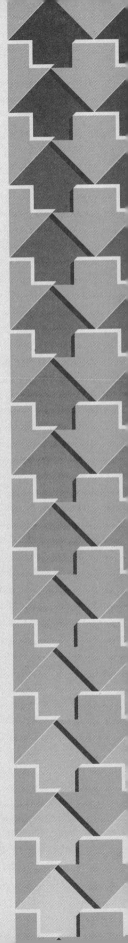

If we look in the dictionary under the word *profession,* we find:

1 "an act of declaring a belief, faith, or opinion"
2 "a calling requiring special knowledge and often long and intensive academic preparation"
3 "a principal calling, vocation, or employment"

If we look in the dictionary under the word *professional,* we find:

1 "relating to or characteristic of a profession"
2 "characterized by a conforming to the technical or ethical standards of a profession"

Now, if we page through our thesaurus to the word *professional,* we find such synonyms as *highly skilled, competent, knowledgeable, specialist, expert, experienced, well-trained.*

These honorable words describe well the health care profession and its members. Individuals are often urged to become more "professional" and to take a "professional" approach to their work. Professional standing cannot exist without training, practice administration, and recognition by qualified, state-approved agencies and governing bodies. Professionalism can be thought of as a distinctive way of providing a service that has its own science of reasoning and practice. Many people confuse the term *occupation* with the term *profession,* but there is a slight difference. Professionals must have formal training, certification, or licensure and must demonstrate a high level of skill in the services they offer. Individuals who are holding an occupation are providing either a product or a service and are making a living in today's market with this skill. The individuals involved in a profession are different from those in other types of occupations, because their use of judgment in their work and their years of education and training differ.

Some experts feel that to be a professional, a person must possess the following traits:

- Commitment
- Education
- Service orientation
- Autonomy of judgment

The health care profession is committed to dealing with the problems of human functioning. Health care professionals deal with life-and-death matters and also aid individuals by helping them solve problems and counseling them. They strive to maintain the dignity of all patients while advising them and their families in medical decision making. A bond forms between the health care professional and the patient. This bond is based on trust. Health care professionals have a duty to provide each and every patient with the information that is needed for decision making, and they must strive to protect the bond between themselves and their patients.

The term *medical care* encompasses the care an individual receives from physicians, technicians, dentists, nurses, medical office managers, and other health care professionals. People who lived many centuries ago were not blessed with having physicians and medicine, and, as a result, many died of diseases and conditions that are virtually nonexistent today. Progress and technology have no limits in the medical field as we know it now, and dramatic achievements are being made on an almost daily basis. Because of this, it is vitally important that medical office managers be well trained in running a practice. The physician, busy with "change," is free to concentrate on medicine while leaving the business side of medicine in the hands of a competent medical office manager.

THE HEALTH CARE SYSTEM

The United States has one of the best health care systems in the world. The physicians in the United States, unlike in some other countries, have the latest technology, medications, and training available to them. Because of this technological innovation, the health care profession is expected to provide better and more effective health care for all patients. Yet technological innovation is expensive and is resulting in pressures being placed on the physician that trickle down to the medical office manager. The pressures of cost containment, professional liability, continuing medical education, and federal intervention become the nightmares of not only the physician, but also the office manager. The office manager can monitor expenses, negotiate lower malpractice premiums, and ensure that staff are continually attending continuing education courses to keep abreast of the many changes. This process of continuous learning is necessary not only for the physician, but also for the office staff. The office manager must realize that staff education is important to provide the physician with the support that is needed.

A type of "social contract" exists between the physician, the office staff, and the patient. This contract is a bond based on the patient's trust that the medical office will provide top-quality care in a compassionate manner. As the U.S. population continues to grow, more and more pressure is being placed on physicians for their services. The health care profession is constantly striving to provide better health care at an affordable price.

THE PATIENT AND THE HEALTH CARE PROFESSIONAL

The health care system must serve people. Nothing is more human and more personal than health. Many health care providers know a great deal about disease and illness but, if asked, cannot define the word *health*. The World Health Organization defines *health* as a state of complete physical, mental, and social well-being and not merely the absence of disease or infirmity. An individual is not only a statistic, but also a complex system of needs. It is important that the staff of a medical office realize this and approach the treatment of patients in a way that reflects this realization. A well-trained medical office staff, at the direction of the office manager, understands and meets the needs of each patient as an individual. This, in addition to the medical treatment provided by the physician, provides each patient with total quality care.

Even though people are responsible for their own health, human nature is such that people are many times in need of others to help them accomplish or maintain good health. The true profession is basically a practice that doesn't produce anything, yet becomes a service directly to individuals. The job of a medical professional is to deal with problems at the psychological and biological levels of individual functioning. Individuals are not qualified to make decisions regarding their health unless they have the proper information. This is the job of the health care professional . . . this is the job of the medical office manager.

THE SPECIALIST

The American Medical Association projects that the specialty practices that will grow the fastest are

- Emergency medicine
- Medical subspecialty groups
- Anesthesiology

Office managers in these specialties must be prepared to face the growth that is predicted. The streamlining of office procedures and processes coupled with efficient and caring medical office staff will help the office manager prepare the physician practice for this growth.

The specialties that are projected to grow at a slower rate are

- General surgery
- Pathology
- Family medicine

With all the knowledge and technology available in the medical field today, it is becoming more and more difficult for physicians to be experts in all areas of medicine. This has caused the birth of the *specialist,* that is, a physician who is an expert in one particular field of medicine and confines her or his practice of medicine to the treatment and diagnosis of all disease falling under that specialty. Below is an overview of some of the *specialists* prevalent in the medical field today.

INTERNISTS

The *internist* is generally known as the "general specialist." Internists treat and diagnose internal diseases through nonsurgical methods. Often, they refer their patients to another specialist or to a subspecialist for treatment of a particular illness. This frequently occurs after the internist has made the diagnosis of the disease. A *subspecialist* is an internist who confines his specialty to a particular organ or area of the human body. Some of the areas of medicine that are specialties of internists are also specialties of surgeons (discussed later).

Allergists

Allergists, for example, are internists whose subspecialty is the diagnosis and treatment of allergies. One of their major roles is to determine the cause of patients' allergic reactions to certain substances. These substances can be anything from medicine to foods, plants, pollens, animals, trees, and so on. People may be allergic to certain types of soap, clothing, or the stuffing in pillows and mattresses. People may also be allergic to certain inhalants, such as perfumes, hair sprays, and chemicals that are spread on lawns.

Cardiologists

Cardiology is another subspecialty of internal medicine. *Cardiologists* are experts in the diagnosis and treatment of the heart and the cardiovascular system. These specialists treat such conditions as heart attacks, irregularities of the heart muscle, defects in the vessels and valves of the heart, arrhythmias, and general cardiac dysfunctions. They order electrocardiograms, which are graphic tracings of electrical impulses given off by the heart. These tracings tell the cardiologist what might have happened to the heart in the past and what is happening to the heart at the present time. Technologies have permitted the replacing of clogged valves and even heart transplants.

Dermatologists

Dermatologists are internists who specialize in diseases of the skin. They receive surgical training as well as training in internal medicine in this area. They diagnose and treat a wide variety of conditions, ranging from a simple wart to skin cancer. They have treatments for wrinkles and can perform face-lifts and almost any type of cosmetic surgery a person might desire. They can make lips full and eyelids thin. Through the use of medications and surgery, they can slow down the effects of aging on a person's face. With the continual depletion of the ozone layer, there is a high risk of skin cancer, and the dermatologist is continually explaining the hazards of the sun to his patients.

Gastroenterologists

Gastroenterologists are internists whose subspecialty is the diagnosis and treatment of any abnormal conditions of the gastrointestinal tract. This specialty covers a broad spectrum of the anatomy, including the esophagus, stomach, pancreas, gallbladder, liver, colon, and rectum. *Gastroenterologists* treat ulcers, excise polyps from the colon, remove food that is lodged in a person's esophagus, and diagnose and treat hepatitis.

Gerontologists

Because Americans are living longer than they ever have, *gerontology* is an up and coming subspecialty of internal medicine. The *gerontologist* specializes in the treatment and diagnosis of diseases specific to the elderly. Alzheimer's disease, dry skin, insomnia, dizziness, and many other conditions that are most prominent in our aging population are treated by gerontologists. In addition to understanding how the aging process affects people's minds and bodies, the gerontologist must understand how the aging of a person affects her or his family members and caregivers.

Gynecologists

A *gynecologist* is an internist who attends to the particular concerns and illnesses of women. A gyne-

cologist is also trained in surgery, even though she or he is considered a subspecialist in internal medicine. The treatment provided by a gynecologist can range from simple preventative medicine, such as Pap smears and breast exams, to major surgeries, such as hysterectomies and mastectomies. The gynecologist also helps keep in balance women's complex hormonal system.

Neurologists

Neurologists specialize in the diagnosis and treatment of the nervous system. Their patients can present with symptoms ranging from a headache to dizziness. They also monitor the epileptic patient and treat diseases involving motor function.

Ophthalmologists

An *ophthalmologist* attends to the diagnosis and treatment of the eye and ocular system. This specialty is found in both internal (that is, nonsurgical) and surgical medicine. Patients may seek the services of an *ophthalmologist* for a simple eye exam, for cataract surgery, or for many other conditions related to the eye and ocular system. A patient with an abrasion of the eye as a result of a contact lens may seek out the expertise of this physician, as would a patient with glaucoma. This specialty has advanced to the replacement of the lens of the eye, so that after cataract surgery, the patient is able to regain vision in the affected eye.

Obstetricians

Obstetricians are physicians who attend to the needs of women during pregnancy and childbirth. Physicians generally specialize in both gynecology and obstetrics, so as to be able to handle all aspects of care related to women's reproductive system. Monitoring of the fetus and the mother during pregnancy is a very important function of this specialty. We are even able to obtain information on the unborn child through medical advancement in this field. We can know in advance whether the baby has a genetic abnormality and whether it is a boy or a girl. More and more women are starting their families late as a result of having careers. With the advancements in this field, older women are able to produce healthy babies with little risk to themselves.

Orthopedists

Orthopedists are specialists who diagnose and treat conditions of the musculoskeletal system. They treat patients with ailments ranging from the sprained ankle to the herniated disk. This is also a surgical and a nonsurgical specialty. Athletic injuries of the muscle, bone, and tendon are treated by this specialist.

Pediatricians

Pediatricians specialize in the diagnosis and treatment of children's diseases. Their practice generally spans birth to adolescence. They attend to the prevention of childhood diseases by vaccinating babies with vaccines for polio, measles, tetanus, mumps, etc. They diagnose and treat such common ailments as tonsillitis, earaches, measles, chickenpox, mumps, etc. They also attend to children who have buried an eraser in their ear or pushed a raisin up their nose. They advise new mothers on how to care for their infants, when and what to feed them, and how to deal with diaper rash.

Physiatrists

A *physiatrist* specializes in the diagnosis of musculoskeletal conditions and their treatment by use of physical means. Treatments such as hydrotherapy, heat, massage, exercise, and electricity are commonly used in this specialty. This specialty is needed more and more as our aging population becomes plagued with the conditions associated with aging, such as arthritis.

Psychiatrists

Psychiatrists are specialists who diagnose and treat patients suffering from emotional and mental disorders. Their patients range from the depressed patient to the patient with more severe diseases of mental and emotional climates. Counseling plays an important role in their work, and their ability to listen is one of their biggest assets.

Radiologists

Radiologists specialize in the diagnosis and therapeutic treatment of patients through the use of x-rays, magnetic resonance imaging, computed tomography (CT) scans, and radioactive materials. They monitor the activities of the technicians doing the tests and advise of any problems with patient positioning and film developing. They study the results of the tests performed and report to the referring physician both normal and abnormal findings. The referring physician then uses these findings to diagnose and treat the patient. Some

patients require treatment with radioactive substances, which is also done by the *radiologist*.

Urologists

Urologists diagnose and treat diseases of the urinary system of the female and the genitourinary tract of the male. An examination of the bladder, called a *cystoscopy,* is done so that the physician can look directly into the bladder to check for abnormalities. Patients may consult a *urologist* for a urinary tract infection or for problems encompassing the testes or prostate.

SPECIALISTS BASED AT HOSPITALS

There are other specialties that are practiced by physicians based at hospitals. These physicians work only in the hospital setting.

Anesthesiologists

Anesthesiologists are physicians who administer all types of anesthesia necessary in the hospital setting. This can be as simple as a local anesthetic or as complex as general anesthesia.

Pathologists

Pathologists supervise the clinical laboratory located in the hospital. Their laboratory may include specialists in hematology, chemistry, bacteriology, serology, cytology, pathology, and urinalysis. It is the pathologist who examines *frozen sections* of tissue removed during certain surgical procedures to determine whether the tissues are malignant or benign. Pathologists may operate private laboratories outside the hospital also.

Surgeons

Surgeons limit their practice to the diagnosis and treatment of diseases requiring surgery. They may confine their specialty to a certain area of the body, such as the chest, brain, or cardiovascular system. These surgical subspecialties are along the same lines as the subspecialties in internal medicine. Often, a surgeon's patients have already been diagnosed by another physician and are referred to the surgeon primarily for the surgery. A typical surgeon's day may include the following surgeries: removal of a gallbladder, removal of a benign or malignant growth, removal of a gangrenous limb, or repair required after a traumatic event.

THE LIFE CYCLE OF A MEDICAL SERVICE

Because of the economic restraints put on health care in the twentieth century, it has become increasingly important for the medical office manager and the physician to seek out and use any management tools they feel will increase their practice's effectiveness. In 1960, Kotler and Levitt devised a method to forecast a product's life cycle. It has since been taught in all management and marketing courses as the most crucial way to monitor the growth of a product. The method identifies the various stages in the life cycle of a product in the market:

Stage 1: Introduction
Stage 2: Growth
Stage 3: Maturity
Stage 4: Decline
Stage 5: Revitalization

Dole and Gombeski, from the Cleveland Clinic Foundation, showed that this product life cycle could be applied to physician services. Physicians have since used this method to find out how their specialization has been affected by the competition's practices. They can also figure out what they can realistically expect in terms of volume of patients and total revenues. The method also allows a medical office to plot the time period before a new associate must be added and identify what ancillary personnel are needed. It can aid in practice decisions. Medical office managers can also use the product life cycle concept. Once the demographics regarding the practice have been collected and the philosophy of the established physician(s) is known, this cycle has allowed medical office managers to better understand the needs of the practice at which they work.

FORMS OF MEDICAL PRACTICE OWNERSHIP

There are three types of medical practices: sole proprietorship (solo), partnership, and corporation (Figure 1–1). A solo practice is a medical practice consisting of one physician only (Figure 1–2). A partnership practice consists of two or more physicians practicing as a group. A corporation can be one physician or two or more physicians practicing as a group. Each form of medical business ownership has advantages and disadvantages.

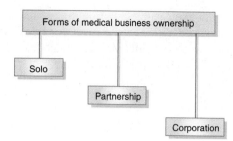

FIGURE 1–1. Three types of medical business organizations.

SOLE PROPRIETORSHIP

The advantages of a sole proprietorship are as follows:

1 It is easy to form.
2 The physician has a certain independence.
3 There is flexibility in the organization and management of the practice.
4 There is a certain amount of privacy in a solo practice.
5 There are tax advantages: the physician pays taxes only on personal income from the practice.

The disadvantages of a sole proprietorship are:

1 There is limited potential for profit.
2 There can be management problems.
3 There can be financial problems.
4 There exists *unlimited liability,* which means that any damages or debt incurred by the business can also be attached to the owner of the practice.
5 The life of the practice is limited; when the physician dies, the practice ends.

PARTNERSHIP

The advantages of a partnership are as follows:

1 There is the potential to create more profit than can be obtained from a solo practice.
2 There are incentives for talented employees.
3 There are legal and financial advantages.

The disadvantages of a partnership are as follows:

1 There is *unlimited liability,* just as in a solo practice.
2 There can be interpersonal problems between partners in the practice.
3 There can be management problems related to business expertise.
4 The life of the practice can be limited; when the last partner dies, so does the practice.

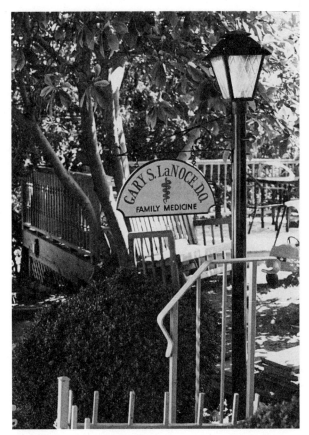

FIGURE 1–2. Signpost for the office of a sole practitioner. (Courtesy of Gary LaNoce, D.O.)

CORPORATION

The advantages of a corporation are as follows:

1 There is *limited liability;* damages/debt can be applied only to the practice, not to the physician.
2 The practice can easily raise cash by issuing stock.
3 The life span of the practice is unlimited.

The disadvantages of a corporation are as follows:

1 The practice must publicly disclose its finances and operations.
2 It is expensive to incorporate.
3 There are high taxes associated with corporations.

There are several types of corporations; however, in the medical field, generally only a few are found. An *open corporation* is a corporation that makes a profit for the owners and has shareholders. It is a public corporation. A *closed corporation* is also a profit-making business but has only a few owners and does not have an open market for shares of stock. *Nonprofit corporations* are service institutions that are incorporated mainly for the advantage of limited liability. A *single-person corpora-*

tion is an individual who incorporates to avoid paying high personal income taxes.

TYPES OF MEDICAL PRACTICE

There are two types of medical practice: solo and group. Group practices are further broken down into single-specialty and multispecialty groups and small and large groups.

A solo practice is a one-physician practice. A group practice consists of two or more physicians in practice together. A single-specialty medical office is a group practice that is limited to one specialty (for example, surgery or internal medicine). A multispecialty medical office contains physicians with different specialties practicing together; an example is an office with a cardiologist, a hemotologist, and a gastroenterologist, as shown in Figure 1–3.

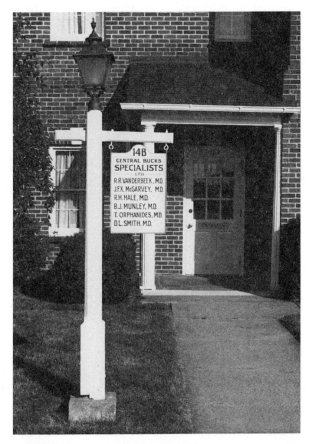

FIGURE 1–3. It is often more profitable for a group of specialists to form a partnership than for one specialist to go into business alone. (Courtesy of Central Bucks Specialists.)

The small group practice has the following advantages:

1 Physician coverage of the practice is available when needed.
2 Other physicians are available for consultation and assistance if needed.
3 Revenues may be enhanced.
4 It is easier to take vacations and sick days.

The disadvantages of the small group practice are as follows:

1 The physician cannot always take off when desired; there are others to consider.
2 Large amounts of capital are sometimes necessary for investment, and then cannot easily be retrieved (not liquid).

The large group practice has the following advantages:

1 It offers more free time.
2 Consultations with colleagues are readily available.
3 Some physicians may not want to be in charge of daily operations, in charge of investments, in charge of marketing and practice growth, etc.; other physicians can take over and assign tasks in these areas.

The disadvantages of the large group practice are as follows:

1 The physicians must conform to the rules of the practice and lose some of their independence.
2 It can take time to become a full partner in a partnership or corporation.

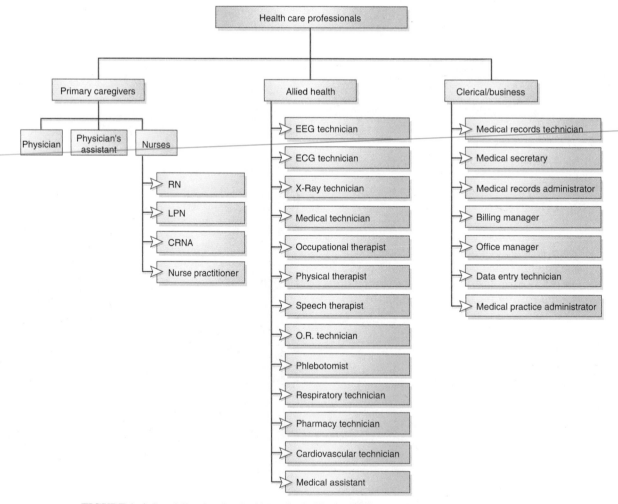

FIGURE 1–4. Specialists involved with medical office staff. RN = registered nurse; LPN = licensed practical nurse; CRNA = certified registered nurse anesthetist; EEG = electroencephalogram; ECG = electrocardiogram; OR = operating room.

TYPES OF HEALTH CARE PROFESSIONALS

In the past 50 years, many new health care professions have been born. For economic reasons, the health care field has been going through a change. This change has brought about a switch from hospital medicine to medical offices or free-standing clinics. More and more certification programs are available to individuals interested in working in various fields of health care. Various physician specialties were described earlier in this chapter. Other specialists in various health care areas can be directly involved with the medical office staff (Figure 1–4). The following is a partial list of some of the other health care professionals with whom the medical office manager will come in contact.

Cardiovascular technician—performs electrocardiograms on patients.

Electroencephalogram (EEG) technician—performs EEGs on patients.

Licensed practical nurse—aids physicians in the treatment of patients in the office or hospital setting.

Medical assistant—aids physicians to a limited extent in the treatment of patients in the office.

Medical laboratory technician—draws blood and performs laboratory tests on patients.

Medical records administrator—maintains the medical records department.

Medical record technician—maintains and transcribes patients' medical records.

Medical secretary—is trained in medical terminology to handle telephones and correspondence for physicians.

Medical technologist—performs the same function as the medical laboratory technician but has more education.

Medical transcriptionist—types all of a physician's dictation.

Nurse anesthetist—performs anesthesia services under the direction of the anesthesiologist.

Nurse practitioner—has education in addition to a nursing degree that enables her or him to perform specific duties under the direct supervision of the physician.

Occupational therapist—assists patients when needed in re-learning such daily activities as tying shoes, brushing teeth, and buttoning clothing.

Phlebotomist—draws blood from patients when tests have been ordered.

Physical therapist—teaches standing and walking and provides therapy to injured and diseased areas through the use of hot and cold packs, whirlpool treatments, paraffin baths, etc.

Physician's assistant—assists the physician by examining, diagnosing, and treating specific ailments of patients under the direct supervision of the physician.

Radiologic technician—performs x-ray examinations on patients.

Registered nurse—performs nursing procedures, such as injections or wound care, that the physician has ordered for the patient.

Respiratory technician—performs pulmonary function studies and treatments on patients.

Speech therapist—helps patients regain speech patterns after they have suffered strokes or some other event that has affected speech.

Surgery technician—assists the surgeon with operations, both major and minor.

Many of these professions have a direct line of communication with the physician's office. Everyone who is employed in a medical office finds herself or himself to be just a part of the big picture and recognizes the importance of teamwork. Many of the professionals listed above can be found on a daily basis working hand in hand with physicians to provide the best medical care possible.

References

Clarkson, K. W., Miller, R. L., & Jentz, G.A. *West's Business Law.* New York: West Publishing Company, 1986.

Wilson, F. A., & Neuhauser, D. *Health Services in the United States.* Cambridge: Ballinger Publishing Company, 1985.

2

Personnel Management

Understanding Employees' Personalities

Because we are all human, we share certain characteristics. Yet, each of us has a distinct personality and unique life experiences. There are several categories of employee operating styles, each with its assets and detriments. Having an understanding of these personality styles helps the office manager manage more effectively and efficiently. There are

- Rational employees
- Intuitive employees
- Feelers
- Doers
- Pragmatists
- Conservators
- Controllers

Rational employees think logically. They live their life in an orderly fashion and expect right or wrong, yes or no answers. Rational people tend to be skeptical and perfectionistic. They are not interested in experimentation, preferring to have a good plan, which they will show the determination to follow through to the end. They may be uncomfortable delegating responsibility and, because of this, often end up with excess amounts of paperwork and tend to burn out quickly.

Intuitive employees rely on their instincts and are somewhat introverted. They may appear to be lazy and ineffective; however, this is their work style. An office manager cannot measure an intuitive worker by partial accomplishments, only by final results. Their partial work may appear fragmented, but the final result is usually thorough and complete. They are process oriented, enjoying each procedural step without particular concern for the final goal. They are likely to question each step along the way. They must be treated with care, because they tend to try to read between the lines and misconstrue what you are telling them. Their demeanor is sometimes misunderstood by other workers as rebellious and arrogant. They do their best work when given assignments. They are not practical and do not like to deal with the bottom line.

Feelers are people who are adept at nonverbal communication with others. They listen intently and empathize with others. Because of their extroverted nature, they prefer personal involvement and like to be helpful. They tend to focus on other people's strengths, rather than on their faults, thus lowering workplace anxiety. They are tolerant of mistakes and are not critical. One disadvantage of the feelers' work style is impulsiveness, and frequently their first idea becomes their final one. They are very effective in solving personal problems and often impress others with their warmth and understanding.

Doers are action oriented and refuse to be confined or obligated. They are impulsive and do what they want to do when they want to do it. They live for the here and now. They have been known to cause crises just to liven things up. Doers have an "easy come, easy go" attitude and wander off when bored. They generally do not develop solid, in-depth friendships and feel that values are not important. They can be of real help during a crisis, because the situation allows them to direct their energies and really get into the thick of things. These individuals have the energy to get things done; however, they need the constant attention of the office manager for guidance.

Pragmatists are task-oriented individuals who direct their action to an immediate goal. They are known for their belief in the trial-and-error method and take calculated risks when necessary. They often act on principle and are excellent negotiators. Pragmatists have a real need for achievement and are assertive and controlling. Their co-workers often perceive them as manipulative and exploitative. Pragmatists usually do not work well with others and seem to have great difficulty with interpersonal relationships.

Conservators are traditionalists. Generally, they follow a set of rules and regulations to the letter and are stable, reliable, and organized. They look for respect and recognition and value status and position. They can be preoccupied with a personal problem (for example, a sick child or financial problems), but they can still maintain excellent quality control in the workplace and look to the past, many times, for direction.

Controllers want power and control. They crave responsibility and structure and are strong willed, decisive, and always interested in the bottom line. As goal-driven people, they are seen by other workers as tough skinned and will make decisions on an impersonal basis. Controllers pride themselves on being objective and look for well-ordered, scheduled plans. Controllers are apt to seek power over other workers as a way of controlling their working environment. Often, they will make rigid plans that do not fit into the scheme of things.

Once the office manager realizes the differences among work styles, she or he can integrate employees into an effective, innovative office staff.

Sizing Up the Medical Office Staff

"Hiring and training are costly, but it is definitely more costly to have a marginal employee."
—Gordon Wheeling, Beckman & Whitley

Having the proper personnel is the biggest asset the office manager can have. Therefore, one important duty of the office manager is to size up the staff on a regular basis and identify the employees who will help the practice achieve the physician's goals. The office manager must understand how each employee functions in her or his job and must then identify the strengths and weaknesses of each employee. Sizing up the employees can be done by simply talking to them, meeting with them on a regular basis, helping them set their goals, observing them on a daily basis, and holding regularly scheduled performance reviews to assess their efficiency and workload. Most employees will be on their best behavior if they think they are being observed.

Judgment regarding an employee's suitability for the office should be withheld until much time has gone by; this is not a process that should be rushed. As already stated, recognizing the different types of personality styles enables the office manager to see beyond first impressions and understand how each employee operates. Every staff has "dead wood," that is, employees who, for whatever reason, are burned out, complain, and generally fail to meet the standards of the office. It is sometimes possible to motivate an underachiever of this type; however, if 3 to 6 months have gone by and the employee is still not performing adequately, the manager may have to consider letting this employee go. One of the keys to motivating employees is to allow them to make some of their own decisions. This is discussed further in the section entitled "How To Remotivate the Staff."

MANAGER'S ALERT

Keep in mind that it is costly to the practice to fire employees. It is in everyone's best interests to remotivate and communicate openly with existing employees rather than to hire new ones.

THE DEVIOUS REBEL

The office manager knows that the devious rebel is talented. She or he may even be described as a good worker with special talents. This may be why this employee has been able to get away with rebellious behaviors such as constantly coming to work late, dressing inappropriately, and sometimes bucking authority. This individual does not usually benefit by being given more flexibility in scheduling, because her or his reasons for being late are not always related to the hour. The office manager does not want to keep this employee from achieving but knows that the office would run more smoothly if this employee would abide by the standards set for the office. The best way to deal with the renegade employee is to be direct. In being direct, the manager tells the employee how much her or his work is valued but also explains what it is that is troubling about her or his behavior. Because the reprimand is preceded by positive feedback, the blow is dealt with easier and the renegade employee generally is found to straighten up.

HOUDINI

One of the problems that some medical office managers complain about is what they call the "disappearing act." When employees leave their work area without mentioning to anyone where they are going, problems can occur. It should be a common practice in the office that employees tell each other, or the office manager, when they are leaving, where they are going, and when they expect to return. All employees should be held responsible for this, even if they are leaving their area for only a minute. One minute sometimes stretches to fifteen, and important telephone calls should not be put on hold while someone frantically searches for the missing employee. It is a good idea for the office manager to adopt this practice also. The employees should always be able to locate the manager in case of a problem. If the manager is not going to be readily available, she or he should specify to the employees certain times when she or he will call to check on the office and receive messages. By adopting this call-in plan, the office manager will keep up to date on the pertinent events of the day.

JEKYLL AND HYDE

Employees will almost always be polite and well mannered in front of the boss. They will treat the office manager just as Emily Post would, with the most impeccable manners you could imagine. Now, imagine an employee who treats the office manager so sweetly treating co-workers and patients rudely. This type of employee might see her- or himself as more of an equal with the office manager than with the rest of the staff and convey an air of superiority to other employees.

The manager should watch carefully to identify signs of rudeness in staff. Do patients shy away from dealing with a particular employee? Are the employees planning an outing and leaving someone out? Maybe the position that was filled five times in the past 2 years is not a problem with that particular position, but a problem with a rude employee. Listed below are three common ways to discourage rudeness in employees:

- Stress courtesy.
- Set the right example.
- Act immediately to compliment courteous behavior.

Stressing Courtesy in the Medical Office

The importance of being courteous to all the patients should be stressed to each employee at the time of hire. A new employee should be instructed that courtesy is a major part of her or his position and that the lack of it will not be tolerated. Long-time personnel may also need to be reminded with gentle pep talks on an occasional basis. They should be reminded that it is the patients who pay their salary; without patients, they have no work. Patients today are consumers. They will choose their physician on the basis of the service that is given. They will always choose a medical office that has a friendly, polite, and caring staff.

Setting the Right Example

Many office managers do not realize how important their function as a role model is on an everyday basis. Everyone has a bad day now and again; however, the office manager should put on her or his best face for patients, the physicians, and the employees. Inconsistent behavior by the office manager is not advised.

Temper tantrums should be kept out of the office. This type of behavior should not be permitted in an office setting and should be discouraged immediately. If an employee decides to have a temper tantrum, remove her or him from the office and settle the matter away from other employees.

Acting Immediately to Compliment Courteous Behavior

Performance reviews should include evaluation of employees' courtesy. Employees who go out of their way to be courteous to patients, physicians, and co-workers should be commended. Compliment them on their grace under pressure. Positive reinforcement strengthens employees' recognition of the importance of good manners. It boosts office morale and productivity.

Making Teamwork Work for You

DEALING WITH CLIQUES

It is almost inevitable that some employees will group together to make a clique. A clique is a narrow, exclusive social grouping of people with the same interests, objectives, or goals. The exclusionary nature of a clique hampers effective teamwork in the office. However, human nature being what it is, cliques do exist and can be powerful and difficult to deal with. A skilled office manager can sometimes use a clique to her or his advantage by telling the clique about any major changes or decisions slightly ahead of others. If the office manager has usually met with resistance from certain members of the clique, this should help get them on her or his side. Their positive attitude will help sway the others and set the tone for the whole office.

EMPLOYEES' UNDERSTANDING OF WHAT IS EXPECTED OF THEM AS THE FOUNDATION FOR TEAMWORK: THE EXAMPLE OF LUNCH SCHEDULES

The foundation for teamwork is employees' having a clear understanding of what is expected of them. From this, solid working relationships are built. The staff and office manager are able to work together to reach common goals. In clarifying what she or he expects from employees, the office manager may find that the subject of lunch hours is a good place to start. In every practice, large or small, the telephone must be monitored at all times, a factor that influences whether and when employees can take lunch breaks. The office manager must make sure that all staff members understand the office's policy regarding lunch hours. The office manager who is managing a large staff may find it necessary to initiate set lunch periods, whereby each employee is assigned a regular lunch time in which to do whatever she or he wishes. To ensure that the phones are managed at all times, the manager of the smaller office has two options. Lunch breaks can be staggered, which allows for someone to be available at all times to answer the telephone. Alternatively, the office manager can request that employees work through their lunch, merely grabbing a bite of sandwich here and there between calls. If the flexibility is not there to allow each employee to have a set lunch period, the best solution is to stagger the lunch periods so that the employees get a break and the telephones are still answered. It is important that the office manager decide how flexible she or he is going to be about the length and time of lunch breaks. Employees should be made aware of the office policy regarding lunch hour at the time of hire, and this should also be addressed in the *Office Procedure and Policy Manual*.

The Personal Telephone Call Plague

"Alexander Graham Bell did not invent the telephone, he invented a source of entertainment!"
—Anonymous

Office policy regarding personal telephone calls should also be discussed at the time of hire. Giving employees a lot of leeway regarding personal phone calls will result in problems for almost any office. However, the occasional personal telephone call is certainly permissible. It is good to have a certain amount of flexibility in each office, because it builds a productive office setting. By allowing personal phone calls, the manager contributes to the flexibility within the office. However, care must be taken to make sure the privilege is not abused.

Personal Problems and the Employee

Although we are at the threshold of humanizing the workplace by meeting employees' needs for day care, counseling, fitness, and so on, personal problems are still better left at home. Nasty divorces, disobedient children, family drug abuse, car problems, etc. do not belong in the workplace. One of the most important reasons for requesting that employees keep their personal problems out of the workplace is that employees who reveal personal issues in the office may find that they come back to haunt them at a later date. There is something about a personal crisis that lingers in an individual's mind. It has been found that long after the crisis is over, the employee is still perceived as impaired.

When one employee confides in another, she or he is placing a burden on the other not to mention the situation to the rest of the staff. However, co-workers have been found to use this information against each other for personal gain. This can easily happen in a competitive environment, be it a small, single-physician practice, or a large, multispecialty practice.

There may come a time when an employee finds it necessary to mention a personal problem to the office manager—because it may affect the employee's productivity or because the employee might be receiving more personal telephone calls than usual. Even in this case, the less said the better. If the personal problem becomes invasive, the manager might suggest a leave of absence to the employee in order to get matters resolved. The office manager should ask for the minimal amount of information, and that only of a factual nature. The manager should not get into how she or he feels about the situation; it can only lead to problems. The only crisis that warrants more detail is a true personal tragedy, such as a death in the family or a family member with a severe illness, such as cancer. In this instance, sympathy tends to outweigh stigma.

Recognizing the Power of the Grapevine

The effective medical office manager never underestimates the power of the grapevine. Gossip networks exist at every level of every office and company. Yes, even the physicians are sometimes guilty of gossiping. Attempts to quell the flow of information through the grapevine are usually a waste of time; however, the effective office manager tries to ensure that at least some of the information being passed around is on the positive aspects of the practice. There are five ways the office manager can influence the nature of the grapevine:

- informed communication
- give-and-take policies
- performance reviews
- trusted employees
- formal responses

Informed communication starts with better informed employees. Employees who are kept well informed are less likely to turn to the grapevine for information. Whenever possible, the office manager should discuss issues with the employees so that they will not have the need to gossip. If there are no office secrets, there are generally no office problems. Informed employees also make better employees. Regularly sharing information and sending around memos will create less need for an office grapevine and will positively convey the office's version of events.

Give-and-take policies are much more effective than policies set in stone. It is good practice to be known as an office manager who is fair and flexible and open to negotiations. The office manager is often the person to whom the employees turn for confirmation or denial of information traveling through the grapevine. It is good to establish an open and truthful relationship with the employees.

Performance reviews are done on either a quarterly, a semiannual or annual basis and are good sounding boards for employees. When an employee hears through the grapevine that she or he may be in hot water, the office manager should be truthful with the employee during the performance review. Sensitive issues should be confronted head on and not avoided. The manager should simply state the information available to her or him and suggest that any further information will be passed on to the employee as it becomes available. If the office manager does not know the information or is not aware of the problem, she or he should tell the employee she or he will check the appropriate source and get back to the employee as soon as possible.

It is helpful for the office manager to have a trusted employee to whom she or he can turn when in need of an intermediary. This employee can act as the eyes and ears of the office manager and should be someone in the practice who is highly regarded and can be trusted.

Formal responses should be considered only as a last resort, but they may sometimes be necessary to quiet some of the more beastly rumors. A response does give a degree of credence to the rumors; however, it also allows for a clearing of the air and a fresh start.

Staff Supervision

"Leadership is the ability to get men to do what they don't want to do and like it!"

—Harry S. Truman

Some office managers have a difficult time understanding the difference between managing and policing. Good office managers realize that the people in their office come first. This means they know that employees do their best work when they are not afraid to make decisions and feel free to express their opinions. It is not necessary to become the Simon Legree of the medical profession to supervise staff. Supervisors should not act as spies or dictators. More can be accomplished by creating an environment of enthusiasm, commitment, respect, and trust. The slightest lean toward spying and bullying will sabotage this environment every time. Down-to-earth leadership will show that well-supervised employees are more productive and responsible than scared employees. Well-trained office staff will produce more than office staff who are unsure of their job descriptions and office expectations will produce. Good training is designed to build confidence in employees, confidence that is reflected in the way they do their jobs and treat patients. Training is not about standing near employees and pointing out what they are doing wrong. It is about showing them how to do it right. As mentioned previously, teamwork is the answer to a well-run office. Studies have shown that medical offices that use teamwork approaches to their tasks are more organized, efficient, and flexible than are offices ruled by the heavy-handed practices of the past.

HOW TO REMOTIVATE THE STAFF IN TIMES OF LOW MORALE

Motivation is a constant concern of the good office manager. Dealing with sick patients and cranky doctors can quickly wear down even the best employees. When this happens, it is time to re-energize the staff. Offering good salaries is an important factor in obtaining and keeping good employees, but that alone will not necessarily motivate them. It is important for employees to feel in control of and secure in their jobs, respected by their co-workers and superiors; and hopeful about their professional futures. Building trust and morale in a medical office is an art and can be accomplished by encouragement, enthusiasm, and loyalty. There are several tried and true ways of motivating the staff:

- Don't issue commands.
- Delegate, don't dump.
- Set goals with staff.
- Listen.
- Let staff make decisions.
- Offer constructive criticism.
- Provide continuity and consistency.
- Avoid hasty judgments.
- Furnish rewards and incentives.
- Be a friend.

- Follow through with promises.
- Monitor without smothering.

Instead of issuing commands, effective office managers sell a course of action to their employees. They know that persuading and rewarding will get them further than shouting orders like an army sergeant will. Many managers feel that it is necessary to be in control and to be firm, but when they give quick, harsh orders, they can easily start to lose the support of their employees.

Delegating is essential to successful medical office management, yet many office managers do not understand what it means or how it works. By delegating certain tasks, the office manager is free to do other tasks that cannot be delegated. The office manager who delegates only unpleasant tasks is "dumping," and employees view it as an abuse. Delegating means giving an employee a task to accomplish that can further the employee's own expertise and give her or him more responsibility and authority.

Setting goals with the staff improves motivation more than any other technique mentioned here. By sitting down with employees and defining their work in terms of goals and objectives, the manager shows employees that she or he has confidence in them and is counting on them.

In times of low morale, listening to what the employees are saying is a valuable tool. If necessary, the manager should schedule a 15-minute one-to-one talk with each employee. The manager should listen to what the employees have to say and let them know it is important. The manager does not have to agree with everything employees say or suggest, but at least it shows that she or he respects their opinions.

Having the staff make some of their own decisions gives the staff a sense of authority over their own jobs. It is better if they are allowed to make some decisions on their own than if they have to ask the office manager about every single decision. This creates a feeling of ownership. Allowing employees to participate in decision making that relates to their jobs allows them to develop their decision-making ability. As Woodrow Wilson said, "I use not only all the brains I have, but all I can borrow."

Constructive criticism is much better than public ridicule. The office manager should never, ever, criticize any employee in front of others. Neither should the manager get into the habit of telling employees to come into her or his office only when the intent is to criticize them. It is necessary to be fair to everyone, even those in trouble. Yelling, public criticism, gossip, and personal feuds are self-indulgent. Set clear rules and stick to them.

FROM THE AUTHOR'S NOTEBOOK

Always try to couple a criticism with a compliment on a job well done. It takes away the bitter taste of the criticism.

Employees need continuity. They expect the office manager to remember what they told her or him yesterday and the day before. They expect consistency in what they are told, and they expect that if a change in policy occurs, they will be notified as soon as possible. The manager tries to insulate the employees from inconsistencies in the physician's actions and policies. If the manager passes them on, the staff feels as though nobody is in control. The manager weeds out any inconsistencies in information from the physician before passing the information on to the staff.

Avoid hasty judgments about employees' work styles. The office manager who expects employees to work exactly as he or she does is many times disappointed. It is crucial that the manager recognize that employees have different ways of handling different tasks and that her or his way is not always the *only* way. The office manager's disapproval of any decisions that are not identical to her or his own could erode any free flow of ideas that could be coming from the employee. In a productive medical office, the manager is flexible, recognizes different work styles, and avoids hasty judgments.

Rewards and incentives should be provided. The office manager's praise for a job well done immediately after an employee did something well is just as important as a paycheck the following week. People respond to praise; when it is used as often as possible, it will provide the office manager with positive results. The ratio of praise to punishment should be four to one. Some offices also choose to issue bonuses to employees who have performed beyond what is expected of them.

The manager should be a friend and encourage office friendship and camaraderie. Employees who are allowed to talk and socialize at work generally stay on their jobs because they like the people they work with. Teamwork is easier among co-workers who have developed friendships. If employees are allowed to be sociable, they become more energized and creative. This

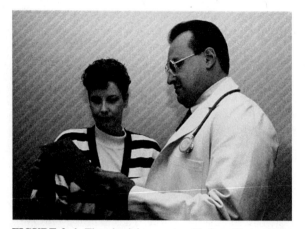

FIGURE 2–1. The physician meets with the office manager to discuss employee projects.

positive atmosphere will be felt by the patients and create a much nicer office environment.

Promises of action must be kept. Employees need to know that matters are being attended to. When the office manager tells employees that she or he will check on something for them, it is imperative that the office manager follow through. The manager's credibility will go down each time employees' expectations are not met. If a decision from the physician is being awaited, the manager should let the employees know that she or he is still working on the problem and hasn't forgotten it.

Monitoring the staff on a daily basis without smothering them is a good way for the office manager to keep problems from becoming major. The manager should talk with each employee regularly and ask for a summary of her or his projects and what her or his work entails. The office manager should create a list of employee projects and provide the physician with updates of this list on a regular basis (Figure 2–1). If the office manager has a regular monitoring system in place, employees will expect the manager to check up on them and will not see this as being smothered. The manager should make sure that all employees are monitored on a regular basis so that no one feels singled out.

THE ART OF INSTRUCTION

As mentioned earlier, the delegation of responsibility is essential to effective medical management. However, delegated projects often come back to the office manager below the standard that the office manager was expecting. Many office managers find themselves saying, "I should have done it myself." In a frustrated state, they point the finger at an employee, saying that

she or he is incompetent. However, the problem may very well lie in the instructions that were given by the office manager, not the incompetencies of the employee. Clear and thorough instructions must be given for each delegated responsibility. In delegating work, the office manager needs to

- Be specific.
- Avoid jargon.
- Explain to the employee why she or he is being asked to handle this task.
- Offer feedback.
- Understand when to give instructions and when to give orders.

The manager needs to be specific and explain exactly what is to be done and when it is to be completed. If the employee is given the latitude to make some decisions, the manager needs to specify which areas of the project should not be changed. The instructions should be presented in easy-to-understand steps. Everyone has a different learning style. Some people like to read directions, whereas others like to be shown. (It is a good idea to assess the learning style of the new employee, so that the training period is easier on both parties.) Regardless of whether they give instructions in writing or verbally, office managers must never assume that employees will know what they mean and therefore leave out steps in the directions. Office managers should check their directive skills by writing down the steps of a certain task from start to finish and then asking someone to perform the task by following only the written directions. This is a proven way of determining whether the manager's directions are vague or clear.

One key to giving clear directions is avoiding jargon. Employees may not understand some terminology and may be afraid to ask for explanations.

When employees are asked to handle a specific project, they need to be told why they must complete it in a certain manner, so that they understand and comply with the directions.

Feedback is important to employees. They need to know when the office manager is pleased with their work. If an employee did not follow the instructions given, the manager should find out why. Communication problems should be identified so that the employee will be able to correct the problem in the future. The office manager needs to know when to give instructions and when to give written orders. The manager may want to use a written order for a task when an employee has successfully handled similar projects in the past or when the office manager is confident that the employee understands her or his expectations. In addition, as already mentioned, some people perform better when given written instructions than when given verbal instructions.

Personnel Credibility

Individuals with good reputations are sought out and listened to. The medical office staff should be concerned about how people, particularly patients and their families, perceive them and the role they play in the health care setting. If patients were asked to describe their physician's office personnel, would they describe them as problem solvers, advice givers, counselors, bookkeepers, physician helpers, teachers, form filers, or obstacles in getting to the doctor? The image of the medical office staff is critical to the patient–physician relationship. If the patient has doubts about the professionalism of the office staff, these concerns are generally transferred to the physician.

The image that medical office personnel display should be professional and compatible with a medical office environment. A good reputation must be earned, and the need to maintain this good reputation must be continuously reinforced by the medical office manager. Each interaction between the medical office staff and patients and their families should be looked upon as an opportunity to enhance the positive professional image of the office.

People are generally influenced more by negative experiences than by positive ones. It has been found that 11 positive experiences are required to neutralize 1 negative experience. One mistake, one incident of inaccurate information, or one instance of rude treatment may negate all of the positive experiences that a patient had with the physician's office. The patient could start looking for a new physician. Many patients in a physician's office are friends, relatives, or co-workers of other patients, which can cause a mass exodus from the medical practice. A bad reputation can be difficult to overcome, and thus mistakes that may give rise to one are to be avoided at all costs. The physician's staff can be a detriment if they are not expressing a solid professional image of the physician and her or his practice.

The Valuable Employee

"Loyalty is like love. You have to give some in order to get some."

—Anonymous

Most physicians don't understand the value of a good employee until that employee has left. A good office manager should recognize the value of each employee and do everything possible to make the employee feel appreciated and valued. The departure of an employee immediately throws the office into a state of confusion, which usually results in less productivity from everyone. Studies have shown that during a transition period, a medical office can lose $5,000 or more. This figure includes the hidden costs involved from a typical "downtime" period, such as the cost of temporary employees; the cost of work delays, which, depending on the position vacated, can be high; the cost of obtaining a new employee (the cost of a classified ad or a fee to an employment agency); and the loss of the office manager's time during the interview process. To prevent the loss of a good employee, the office manager should address the concerns of all employees. These concerns may be conflicts between co-workers, conflicts between the manager and an employee, unclear understandings of job descriptions, and personal crises. It should be the number one objective of each office manager to attempt to know each employee, to interact with her or him, and to communicate with the employee on a daily basis. This will minimize problems down the road.

FROM THE AUTHOR'S NOTEBOOK

Cross-training employees in positions other than their own helps alleviate some of the stress created by the loss of an employee.

The Employee Life Cycle

The employee life cycle has various stages. The first stage is the search for candidates for a position. The second stage is selection of the perfect employee after interviews with several people. The third stage is the training stage. If employees are not properly trained, their productivity will be low. The office manager will ultimately be blamed for this, so it is imperative that the manager take the time to train an employee well or appoint an appropriate person to implement the training.

The fourth stage is the directional stage. At this point, the employee is given direction as to her or his performance and the expectations of the medical practice. Proper direction opens many doors into a solid employee–employer relationship. A person cannot be

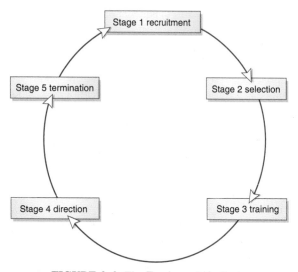

FIGURE 2–2. The Employee Life Cycle.

expected to start a position without being informed of the goals of the practice. Orienting a new employee to the philosophies of the medical practice by way of a mission statement is just as important as informing her or him of the technical aspects of the job. The mission statement is printed in the *Office Procedure and Policy Manual,* but it also needs to be discussed with the new employee. How well this mission statement is explained to the employee affects the overall character and assertiveness with which the employee will approach the position. Simply handing a new employee a *Procedure and Policy Manual* with no explanation is like giving someone a car full of gas and telling them to drive, without ever telling them their destination. The priorities of the office, the benefits of productivity, and the reason for the practice of medicine in that particular area must be explained. This stage can prevent the loss of good employees and should not be skipped.

The fifth and final stage of the employee life cycle is termination. By properly using the first four stages, most office managers can prevent this unpleasant stage. The employee life cycle is illustrated in Figure 2–2.

Mission Statement for the Medical Office

The philosophy of the medical office is an integral part of its success. This philosophy, or mission statement, should be brought to all employees' attention so that they have a clear understanding of the conscience of the practice. The mission statement is generally written by the physician(s) and office manager and simply spells out the philosophies of the practice and the rules and regulations by which the office means to uphold this philosophy. This is very important when an office is attempting to maintain employees and avoid a high turnover rate. The anxiety and time involved every time the office manager must replace an employee are not to be taken lightly; having a clear mission statement about the office philosophies may help make the office objectives easier to obtain. A sample mission statement that can be personalized to fit any medical practice is shown in Box 2–1.

The Three Basics of a Successful Employer

All managers want to be successful and have the support of quality staff. There are three basic rules to remember to become a successful employer. Follow these rules, and success will follow:

1 Hire the best person for the job.
2 Pay the person what she or he is worth—have a pay raise table.
3 Explain the expectations of the position.

BOX 2–1. **SAMPLE MISSION STATEMENT OF A MEDICAL OFFICE**

---

*Our office is pleased to welcome you as a member of our health care team. We want you to have an understanding of the objectives of our practice and why we have many established patients and referrals. The primary objective of our office is **to respond to all our patients' needs in a caring and personal manner.** We focus our complete attention on each and every patient, because without them, we have no practice. With our primary focus on patient care, we are able to think less of our own personal problems and tensions and by this, we eliminate many interpersonal conflicts. We strive to ensure that our personal problems are not brought into the office, and this allows us to promote an atmosphere that maximizes the morale of the entire staff. We have carefully developed a list of policies and procedures that reinforce our thoughts on our objectives. We respect our co-workers, managers, doctors, patients, and, most of all, ourselves.*

BOX 2–2. **JOB DESCRIPTION SHEET**

Job Title: _____

Supervisor: _____

Date of Original Description: _____ By: _____

Date of Updated Description: _____ By: _____

1 Transcribes from cassette to patient's chart by using word processor or typewriter.
2 Maintains a correspondence file of all letters dictated.
3 Maintains a list of temporary agencies in event of illness or vacation of any member of the secretarial pool.
4 Sorts and opens mail and distributes it to the appropriate persons.

5 Answers the telephone when others are busy.
6 Posts checks from mail in absence of secretary, who usually does this job.
7 Prepares all physicians' C.O.D. and manuscripts.
8 Performs special duties when asked.
9 Is in charge of lunch room clean-up.

Job Descriptions

It is essential to keep a list of up-to-date job descriptions in a file that is easily accessible. A job description is nothing more than a list of the duties and expectations of each position in the medical office. A job description should contain the following elements:

- title of the position
- responsibilities of the position
- duties of the position
- educational requirements
- job requirements
- accountability statement

The list of duties should be prioritized so that new employees are not found tidying up the lunch room when they should be confirming patients for the next day. Most employees will welcome the direction that a job description gives them because it clarifies their roles and provides specific guidelines.

FROM THE AUTHOR'S NOTEBOOK

It is always a good idea to ask a leaving employee to provide a list of her or his duties. This will give a good overview of how the job is actually being done.

Job descriptions can be used when hiring a new employee, when interviewing and selecting a new employee, for training purposes, for employee evaluations, for salary evaluations, and for termination. Box 2–2 shows a sample job description that can be used as a model.

Hiring That "Right" Employee

It is important to hire an employee with the exact mix of characteristics that a position requires. In the medical office, employees' performance in their job is directly related to patient satisfaction. The right person for the job is the one who smiles; is polite to co-workers, patients, and supervisors; and is responsive to the needs of the office.

When looking to fill a position in a medical office, the office manager should be aware that a person who is interactive in a certain environment may become unglued in a hectic medical office environment. Picture the telephones ringing off the hook, a patient waiting to make an appointment, and a patient contesting her or his bill and Medicare coverage . . . this scenario can turn a calm, cool, and collected person into a frazzled, quick-tempered individual. Most patients are not happy to be at the physician's office and therefore are not in good moods. They feel anxiety, pain, apprehension, and a variety of other emotions. These are the people who need empathy from the medical staff. When patients walk into the office, they should first encounter a friendly and caring receptionist who is eager to greet them and welcome them to the office. The clinical staff of the office should also consist of warm, empathetic, and concerned individuals who give the patient a sense of security. Knowing that the individuals in the office *care* means a lot to a patient. Caring is not a taught behavior; caring is inborn, and it is a valuable commodity in a health care employee.

When faced with the dilemma of searching for a new employee, the office manager may want to consider the following methods to find applicants:

- Contacting an agency.
- Putting an ad in the newspaper.
- Contacting a technical school or college for work-study students.
- Paying a headhunter.
- Letting people know by word of mouth.
- Posting notices on bulletin boards in a hospital.

EMPLOYMENT AGENCIES

Most medical office managers have hectic daily schedules and do not always have the proper amount of time to allot to the interviewing process. They are not swayed by fancy clothes or pretty faces. They are trained to dig deep into the employment history of the individual and extract the qualities that the individual best exudes. When they do not have the time to do this, the employment section of the telephone book presents a long list of employment offices that are ready and willing to help them. These offices hire trained employment counselors who know just the right questions to ask of the individual seeking employment. They are experienced in what to look for and are familiar with certain behaviors that send "red flags." Some agencies specialize in finding temporary personnel, and others specialize in finding permanent staff.

Such agencies greatly benefit a medical practice. A prospective employee can be hired as a temp for a set amount of time and then be brought on board as a permanent employee. If the temp is not exactly what the office is looking for, she or he can be exchanged for a different one. There is a lot of flexibility in this type of system. This type of system can also be costly. For many agencies, the buyout figure for a temp is less at 2 weeks of employment than at 1 to 3 months of employment.

There is a fee for this service that can be paid by the person seeking employment. It is best paid by the employer, because this shows the employer's commitment to an employee. An employee whose fee has been paid by the employer tends to start the job with a reservoir of good will toward the new job. Many times, a medical office will reimburse a new employee

two-thirds of the fee after a reasonable probationary period has been met and satisfactory work has been completed. If the physician is willing to allow the office manager to use an employment agency, it can be a definite plus to the office manager!

THE EMPLOYMENT APPLICATION

"The closest to perfection a person ever comes is when he fills out an employment application!"
—Stanley Randall

There are several different formats that can be used for an employment application. A preprinted employment application form may be used, but some offices prefer to design their own form, integrating important subjects that uniquely apply to their office. Once the office manager has designed an employment application that suits the particular needs of the practice, it can be either typeset and printed at a local print shop or formatted on the practice's computer and copied onto a better grade of paper. Formatting the form on the office computer and printing it out and making photocopies is much less expensive than having it typeset and printed by the local printer and is done by many offices today in an effort to contain costs. Important issues that should be addressed in the employment application are

- Education history
- Employment history
- Salary from last employment
- Special qualifications
- Reason for leaving previous position
- Current salary requested
- Long-range professional goals
- Flexibility of applicant
- Date of availability

A sample employment application is shown in Box 2–3. If an interviewee arrives with a resume, she or he should be instructed to skip the areas on the application that are covered by the resume.

THE ART OF THE INTERVIEW

The office manager who interviews and then hires only on the basis of a gut reaction may be headed for big problems down the road. As Figure 2–3 shows, the two main areas to examine during the interview are technical skills and people skills. Managers should listen to their gut feelings; only they know their own needs. However, coupled with this should be a systematic approach to the decision to hire.

BOX 2–3. EMPLOYMENT APPLICATION FORM

Name: _____

_____

Address: _____

_____

_____

Phone: _____ Answering machine _____ Y _____ N

Social security number: _____

Education:

1] _____

_____

2] _____

_____

3] _____

_____

Experience: Name, address, telephone number, supervisor

1] _____

_____

_____

Hourly rate: _____ Reason for leaving: _____

2] _____

_____

_____

Hourly rate: _____ Reason for leaving: _____

3] _____

_____

_____

Hourly rate: _____ Reason for leaving: _____

4] _____

_____

_____

Hourly rate: _____ Reason for leaving: _____

Continued

BOX 2–3. **EMPLOYMENT APPLICATION FORM** *Continued*

Do you speak any languages other than English? _____ Y _____ N

If so, what? _____

Are there any physical problems that could keep you from performing the duties of this position? _____ Y _____ N

If so, what? _____

Have you ever been convicted of a crime? _____ Y _____ N

Are there any areas in which you think you need improvement? _____ Y _____ N

If so, what are they? _____

Like most doctor's offices, occasionally there are days that employees have to work later than their usual quitting times. Is this a problem? _____ Y _____ N

What qualities do you possess, if any, that make you more qualified than others? _____

_____

_____

Are you willing to be bonded? _____ Y _____ N

Do you have any previous commitments that might interfere with this position? _____ Y _____ N

If so, how will you handle them? _____

What are your long-range plans? _____

_____

List 3 Professional References: Name, address, telephone

1] _____

_____

_____

_____

2] _____

_____

_____

_____

3] _____

_____

_____

_____

What hourly rate are you looking for in this position?

$ _____

Date of availability _____

Date of interview: _____

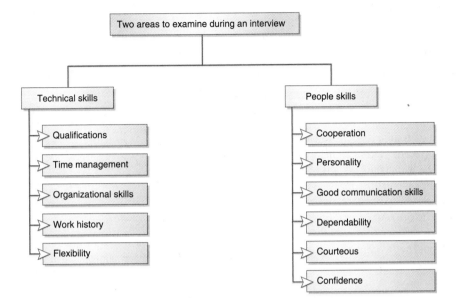

FIGURE 2–3. Two areas to examine during a job interview.

The first thing the office manager should do before beginning an interview is obtain a piece of paper on which to jot down notes during the interview or a form that has been designed to be completed during an interview. Later, these notes will be invaluable to the process of remembering and comparing the applicants.

The manager should remember to let the prospective employee talk and should listen intently to everything that is said. Some applicants will offer much more information than is asked for and should be listened to, because this information can be very helpful later. Applicants' answers to the questions will help to pull the whole picture together. Their body language can also be helpful.

First impressions are not always the right ones. *Never, ever* hire an applicant on the first interview. Many times, the second interview provides a completely different picture of the applicant than the first. During the first interview, all aspects of the job should be covered, along with the nuts and bolts of office policy, such as vacation time, benefits, salary, etc. The applicant should always be allowed time to ask questions.

Second interviews should be scheduled for applicants who possess the qualities that are necessary for the position. In the second interview, the manager talks with the applicants about a trial period of employment and why the applicant wants this particular position.

It is then time to check the references on the final applicants. More information will be obtained by calling the person given as a reference than by sending her or him a letter. When speaking with an applicant's past employers or professional references, the manager should always ask the million-dollar question: "Would you hire this person again?" In addition, information should be obtained on the applicant's health history, dependability, general personality traits, and compatibility. It is a good idea to give applicants only salary ranges until an applicant has been chosen. At that point, a starting salary may be offered. All details of office policy should be explained to the individual at that time, such as the lunch policy, whether there is a lunch room (microwave, refrigerator, etc.), when the applicant should start, and who will be training the applicant.

The office manager should be well versed in the job requirements of the position available. The manager should thoroughly evaluate the demands of the position before beginning to conduct interviews for the position. At this time, the office manager might want to make some long overdue changes in the job description. The position should be carefully analyzed as to the specific personality traits it demands, the physical capabilities it requires, and the mental and emotional demands associated with it.

Most physicians do not want to be involved in the interviewing process and give their office manager a "green light" in the hiring department. Some physicians want the office manager to do all the preliminary interviewing and choose the best applicants to interview with the doctor. In a group practice, one physician may handle personnel matters, and it may not be necessary for all of the physicians to interview the applicants.

ISSUES TO CONSIDER DURING THE INTERVIEW

There are several issues that the medical office manager needs to consider when interviewing an applicant:

Where does the applicant live in relation to the location of the office? This is an important concern. In conjunction with this, it needs to be determined whether the applicant has her or his own transportation or will be using public transportation.

Does the applicant's job history indicate job stability?

In what type of practices has the applicant worked? Are they close to the type of practice that contains the available position?

What is the applicant's educational background? Does the applicant have a teaching degree along with a medical receptionist's certificate? Experience has shown that this type of applicant will generally not stay, and is probably just using this position as a stepping stone. However, to deny someone a position for this reason might be considered discriminatory, so care must be taken when interviewing this type of individual.

FAIR AND SENSITIVE QUESTIONING OF APPLICANTS

Beware of questions that could promote a lawsuit down the road. Federal and state laws protect individuals from job discrimination, and what an office manager might think is an innocent question can result in a discrimination suit! Hiring employees used to be an easy task; find the person you like and hire her or him. Not any more! There are many laws in place to protect individuals against discriminatory questioning. The manager must be careful not to ask any questions that might relate to the applicant's credit history. Care must be taken to avoid any questions that might constitute an invasion of privacy or discrimination. The following are some questions to avoid. These questions may seem harmless enough, but they are not. A medical office may be slapped with a lawsuit before it knows what hit it.

Instead of
"Will you have any difficulty obtaining child care?"
Ask
"If you have to work late some day, will that be a problem?"
Instead of
"Will you be using public transportation, or do you have a car?"

Ask
"Will you have any difficulty in getting to work?"
Instead of
"Do you have any plans for a family in the next few years?"
Ask
"Where do you see yourself in the next five years?"

Before asking a question, office managers should always ask themselves, "How does this relate to the job?" They must stick to asking questions regarding the job; after all, that is what the applicant is there for. Education, work history, and technical skills should be important areas of discussion. They should not try to slip any trick question to the applicant in an effort to obtain information. They should always check with the state laws, because each state has different guidelines to be followed.

Even after a person has been hired, care must be used. For example, An office manager should never say, "Keep up the good work, you have a future here!" This simple phrase can come back to haunt you. If down the road it becomes necessary to fire that employee, those simple words spoken a year ago can make it difficult for the manager to prove she or he has a legitimate reason for letting that individual go. Words can be a dangerous thing and can create situations that may not have been intended.

"At Will Employment"

In the past, the concept of "at will" employment made it possible for an office manager or physician to fire an employee at any time for any reason, or without a given reason. In more recent years, however, individuals and the court systems have become more sophisticated, and employers must be very careful of what they do and how they do it. Congress has expanded employees' rights and with that, taken away employers' rights. In today's litigious society, employers must follow the guidelines of each state and make sure that everything is in order. During performance reviews, employees should always be asked if there is a comment they want to make regarding their poor performance, or whatever it is that is the problem. Sometimes, an office manager will find extenuating circumstances that may warrant another look at the situation. When firing an employee, the manager must make sure that there are documented memos to the employee giving warnings about the problem. The firing should not come as a surprise. Experience tells us that one of the easiest ways to avoid a possible discrimination suit may be offering a week's severance pay.

Giving Employee References

The threat of a lawsuit also makes it tricky to give a reference for a former employee with a negative work history. The medical office manager must know the state laws regarding conditional privilege (that is, some degree of protection against a claim of defamation of character) in giving employment references. Each state handles this differently. If an office manager gives an employee whom she or he fired a very good reference, that employee may decide to file a wrongful-discharge suit against the office, and the employer does not have a leg to stand on, since the office manager gave such a glowing reference. If the office manager gives a detailed, derogatory reference about an employee who was fired, the office could be hit with a suit for slander (that is, defamation of character). If the office manager discloses little to no information about a former employee, the office could be sued for defamation under the self-publication act. For example, if a receptionist was fired for stealing from the daily receipts and the office manager does not tell a prospective employer calling for a reference the reason for dismissal, the prospective employer could sue the office if she or he hired the individual and the individual did not disclose this to the new employer. It is best to consult the office attorney when dealing with a reference on a former employee with an unfavorable work history. Many medical offices and hospitals have adopted the policy of providing only the dates of the individual's employment and verification of the position held. This protects the office and the office manager from any problems down the road.

The Frazzled Employee

No matter how much a patient complains to a health care giver, the patient must be treated with respect and understanding at all times. There are various levels of stress found in medical offices, and the office manager must be able to identify them in employees and deal with them. An employee who argues with a demanding patient not only upsets the patient more, but becomes just as tense and out of control. An employee must be able to adapt to various situations that might arise in a medical office. The employee must show this adapt-

ability when relating to patients, physicians, co-workers, and any ancillary services that the employee might be using.

FROM THE AUTHOR'S NOTEBOOK

When choosing between an individual with excellent technical abilities and an individual with a genuine caring ability, ALWAYS choose the individual with the genuine concern for others. Skills can be taught, but caring and concern can't!

The Enthusiastic Employee

One very important lesson for the office manager to learn is the power of positive reinforcement. There is an old saying that goes, "You can catch more flies with honey than you can with vinegar!" It has been proved that employees will go the extra mile for the office manager if they are receiving some positive reinforcement. For example, by simply stopping by an employee's workstation and thanking her or him for doing such a good job on a report, the office manager increases the confidence of that employee. Confidence, coupled with genuine appreciation, gives a benefit to the employee, which in turn means more productivity for the office. Everyone benefits from a compliment from time to time, and medical office personnel are no exception. They possess a certain amount of pride in their work, and for many a word of appreciation is just as important as a weekly paycheck.

Employee Performance Evaluation

The size of a medical office does not dictate whether there should be a performance review system in place—*every* medical office needs a review system. It is of vital importance to evaluate staff performance on a scheduled basis (Figure 2–4). If there is not some type of systematic review system in place, unproductive employees can go unrecognized for years, and prized employees can look for new positions where they will be recognized. There are three basic steps to employee evaluation:

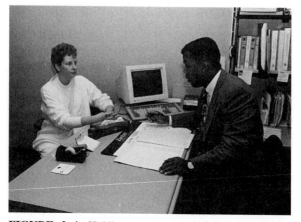

FIGURE 2–4. Holding regularly scheduled performance evaluations with employees is an important responsibility of most office managers.

1 For each employee, maintain a file that contains the employee's performance evaluations; an employee data sheet (Box 2–4); a copy of the employee's resume; and records of vacation days, sick days, raises, and promotions).

2 On a quarterly basis, review and assess the information that has been inserted into the file.

3 Meet with the employee at an appointed time to discuss her or his performance (a note with details of this meeting should be inserted into the file). Recognize that taking care of the employee is just as important as taking care of the patients!

Most physicians do not want to be involved in employee performance reviews and leave their office managers in charge of this task. If there is an impending problem with an employee, the office manager may want to ask the physician to sit in on the review session. Some offices use an evaluation sheet to evaluate each employee. This sheet may be completed by only the office manager, or it may be a collective effort between the office manager and the physician or physicians in the group. Regardless of who completes the evaluation sheet, it is important that it be completed as objectively and affirmatively as possible. New hires should receive a review at 1 month and then again at 90 days; thereafter, reviews should be conducted on a yearly basis. Yearly reviews should be scheduled by seniority so that no one will think there is a specific pattern in the way in which the reviews are scheduled. The most logical time to schedule a review is on the anniversary date of the employee. Offices that do not raise salaries on anniversary dates may conduct reviews at the time of year at which the salaries are raised. It is generally best to start off the evaluation with any problems that may have arisen and need to be addressed. The end of the interview should address the strong points of the employee and can end with a statement of whether the employee will receive a raise and how much. When reviews are conducted in this way, employees leave the evaluation session feeling confident and good about themselves.

BOX 2–4. EMPLOYEE DATA SHEET

Name: _____

Address: _____

_____

Phone: _____

Social Security Number: _____

Number of Exemptions: _____

Spouse Name: _____

Spouse Number at Work: _____

Person to Notify in Case of Emergency: _____

Relationship to Employee: _____

Daytime Phone Number: _____

BOX 2–5. **EMPLOYEE EVALUATION SHEET**

Employee name: _____

Position: _____

Date of review: _____

Date of last review: _____

_____

Reviewer: _____

CONFIDENTIAL
[1] excellent, [2] good, [3] adequate, [4] needs work, [5] poor
Enter the evaluation figure that best rates the area being rated.

Attendance _____	Job perception _____
Cooperation _____	Quality of work _____
Dedication _____	Quantity of work _____
Dependability _____	Versatility _____
Disposition _____	Total _____
Flexibility _____	Total from last review _____
Initiative _____	Raise _____ Y _____ N Percent _____

Comments: _____

If there is a problem that needs to be addressed with an employee, the office manager explains the problem or deficiency that exists and sets a certain period of time in which the matter must be corrected. The time period granted must be fair—30 to 60 days is more than fair for an employee to correct the situation. If it is not resolved by the end of 60 days, this can be used as a step toward the employee's dismissal. The manager must be sure to document the conversation held at the end of 60 days and insert the documentation into the employee's file, especially if she or he gave the employee a warning that if the situation is not rectified, termination will occur. The manager always allows the employee to participate in the evaluation and to express any concerns or ideas on how to improve a specific situation or task. The office manager listens intently and remains objective. In fact, the office manager might learn something about the managerial aspects of the office that might not be apparent but may need reworking. Medical offices that use the performance evaluation system find that it improves productivity and morale. Employees feel that someone cares about their work and recognizes their accomplishments. A sample evaluation sheet is shown in Box 2–5.

THE SIPS WAY TO AVOID ERRORS IN EMPLOYEE EVALUATION

Many office managers make mistakes during an employee evaluation that can be costly to both them and the practices for which they work. The SIPS acronym helps the office manager identify and avoid these common errors and prevents turmoil in the office. As shown in Box 2–6, SIPS identifies the errors of Softness, Influence, Particularity, and Strictness.

Softness refers to an office manager's tendency to overrate every aspect of the employee. Such a manager wants to be nice and therefore gives all employees higher ratings than perhaps they deserve. This might win them a popularity contest, but it often hinders the practice. Employees do not get an accurate accounting

---

BOX 2–6. **COMMON ERRORS IN
EMPLOYEE EVALUATION: SIPS**

Softness
Influence
Particularity
Strictness

---

of their work and therefore do not know to correct certain aspects of their job.

Influence refers to an office manager's becoming friends with one or more of the employees. When this situation arises, the office manager cannot help but show favoritism toward these employees. All office managers have favorites among their employees; however, this favoritism should never be shown.

Particularity is probably the most common error in employee evaluation. The office manager tends to focus on one particular task that was done well and rate the employee's entire performance according to that single task. The manager can avoid this by, first, being aware of the potential problem and, second, carefully evaluating each area on the employee evaluation slowly and accurately.

Strictness refers to using the position of office manager to exhibit power. Strict managers are managers who boast that no employee deserves the highest rating on the evaluation.

THE EMPLOYEE SELF-EVALUATION

"Only the mediocre are always at their best."
—Anonymous

The office manager might want to use employee self-evaluation as a tool for reviewing employees' productivity and work habits. One way to obtain employee self-evaluations is to provide employees with the Employee Task Sheet (Box 2–7) 2 weeks before their scheduled evaluation. They should be instructed to take their time and fill out the form carefully. It must be returned to the office manager 1 week before the evaluation appointment. It is often interesting to find out how employees view their jobs.

A tool that can be used in conjunction with the Employee Task Sheet is the Employee Self-Evaluation Form (Box 2–8). Again, employees should take the time to judge themselves carefully. Many managers will find that the employees are harder on themselves than they are.

The Employee Task Sheet and Employee Self-Evaluation form can be altered to suit a particular office's needs, or they can be copied and used as is straight from this book. All office managers will find these tools to be invaluable in evaluating the employees. The Employee Task Sheet can be given to each employee midyear so that the office manager can gain an understanding of the tasks the individual performs and her or his goals. This has been found to be a valuable tool in increasing productivity and job satisfaction.

BOX 2–7. **EMPLOYEE TASK SHEET**

Name: _____

Date: _____

The tasks that I perform now are:

Other tasks that I feel I could do are:

BOX 2–8. EMPLOYEE SELF-EVALUATION FORM

Name: _____

Date: _____

I feel my deficiencies are:

I feel my accomplishments are:

Individual Rating Factors: (5 = superior, 4 = good, 3 = adequate, 2 = needs work, 1 = poor)

_____ Quantity of work done

_____ Quality of work done

_____ Understanding of job

_____ Cooperation

_____ Dependability

_____ Productivity

_____ Neatness

Areas in which I feel I need improvement:

Raises

Medical offices handle raises in many different ways. The three most common ways of handling pay increases are merit, fixed, and variable raises. One thing is certain: If good employees are to be kept, they must be paid a median salary or better. If they do not get the salary they deserve, they will begin to look elsewhere for employment.

MERIT RAISES

Merit raises are usually a direct result of employee evaluations. Merit raises, generally awarded in addition to cost-of-living raises, can be an invaluable tool in boosting morale and increasing performance. When the merit raise approach is used, the employee who performs beyond the call of duty is rewarded. It also provides incentives for others to increase work performance so that they might increase their salaries as well. For example, if Jill is doing commendable work and is staying late on occasion to finish projects, the office manager might want to increase her pay, say, an additional 4% on top of her cost-of-living raise. At the same time, if Julie has slacked off on collecting overdue accounts and the accounts receivable figures are beginning to soar, she might receive only the cost-of-living increase. Ned, who is working at an adequate work level and doing only the amount of work that is expected, might receive a 2% merit raise in an effort to boost his work performance by renewing his morale.

FIXED PAY RAISES

Fixed pay raises are generally given in smaller offices. These raises are generally a cost-of-living increase or the cost-of-living increase plus a small percentage. The difference between the fixed pay raise and the merit pay raise is that in the fixed pay raise, everyone in the office receives the same percentage of increase. For example, the cost-of-living increase may be 3% for the year, and because the physician feels that all the employees are doing a good job, he adds an additional 2% to that figure to give everyone a 5% raise for the year. Because one percentage is the same for everyone, employees who draw a larger salary, of course, will receive more of an increase. For instance, Mary makes $8.00 per hour and Ann makes $12.00 per hour. With the 5% raise, Mary's new hourly rate would be $8.40 per hour, whereas Ann's new rate would be $12.60 per hour.

FLEXIBLE PAY RAISES

Flexible pay raises are generally not a good idea in any office. This type of raise has been used in small, one-physician offices, but it is not without its problems. If a physician has two employees, a medical assistant and a receptionist, she or he might choose to increase their salaries by different amounts. For example, the medical assistant's salary might be increased 7%, whereas the receptionist's salary might be increased only 4%. A word to the wise: people talk! They always want to talk about their salaries, and in a close-knit office such as this the medical assistant and receptionist probably know what one another had for breakfast in the morning! The issue of favorites comes into play in a situation like this, and there are enough problems that can occur in a medical office without creating new ones! To save a lot of headaches and gnashing of teeth, the office manager should advise the physician to avoid a flexible pay raise system in favor of a fixed pay raise system.

Discipline

The wise office manager makes all employees aware of the various infractions that can result in disciplinary actions. When a list of disciplinary actions is made available to each and every employee, it may be presumed that all employees understand the seriousness of certain types of behavior (Box 2–9). It is far better to have typed a Levels of Disciplinary Actions list than to discipline an employee and hear "I didn't know that!" In addition to making all employees aware of behaviors that may result in disciplinary action, the list provides the office manager with a paper trail that can be referred to should termination be necessary. Some offices include this list in every employee's personnel manual. Other offices post it in a common area, such as a lunchroom or lounge.

Wherever this sheet is placed, it will be most helpful during employee warning sessions, where it can be referred to for a policy backup. The list shown in Box 2–9 can be customized to suit a particular office, but it

---

BOX 2–9. LEVELS OF DISCIPLINARY ACTIONS LIST

Secondary Offenses That Require Disciplinary Action:

- Excessive tardiness
- Inappropriate dress
- Conducting personal business during work hours
- Smoking
- Minor damage to office property
- Uncontrolled emotional outburst

Primary Offenses That Require Disciplinary Action:

- Excessive absenteeism
- Conduct unbecoming a professional
- Obscene language or behavior
- Insubordination

Severe Offenses That Require Disciplinary Action:

- Use of obscene/abusive language to patients
- Lying and/or stealing
- Loss of temper with patients
- Fighting with co-workers
- Drugs and/or alcohol use
- Falsifying records
- Violation of confidentiality
- Any other behavior deemed objectional by the office manager

should include every type of scenario that might arise in a medical office.

Managers who use this technique for discipline must realize that it is most important that a follow-through occurs. An office manager who merely threatens and does not follow up is not an effective manager. She or he will not be respected by any of the employees, making future managing very difficult. The purpose of this Employee Warning Notice is to create a paper trail, in other words, a record of infractions by the employee that were severe enough to warrant written confirmation. The office manager should use common sense when choosing between verbally reprimanding and completing an Employee Warning Notice that would become part of the employee's permanent record. When the office manager chooses to use an Employee Warning Notice, she or he has made the decision that the problem was highly serious. A sample warning notice is shown in Box 2–10. It may be altered to suit a particular practice's needs.

As a general rule, the first warning becomes a "W," or warning. The second becomes a "P," or probation, and the third becomes a "T," for termination. This form is for use only with employees who appear to need discipline on a regular basis and when the office manager feels that an employee has the potential to become a problem employee. It is not intended for use as a daily tool, for every reprimand or incident. This form should be placed in the employee's file and kept confidential in a locked drawer in the office manager's office.

✓ Termination

Poor job performance, violation of an office policy, or illegal activities may make it necessary to terminate an employee. It is important for the office manager to document all conversations and dealings with the employee. She or he should keep in mind that this documentation might end up in a court of law. Therefore all notations must be clear, concise, objective, and properly dated. The number of times the employee's work habits were discussed must be documented.

In confronting the employee, the manager reviews the job description and compares the employee's strengths and weaknesses to this description. It is important that strengths not be forgotten. During the conversation with the employee, the manager points out dates and times of incidents and information that was reviewed for improvement or change. At the end of the conversation, the office manager may suggest ways in which the employee could improve in her or his next position. Ideally, the employee will be able to learn from this experience. It is usually best to have this conversation at the end of a workday, preferably on the last day of a workweek. The manager must make sure that the employee understands that the termination is a fact and must explain clearly, with no emotional involvement, the basis for this decision.

As mentioned, the use of employee warning notices is a good way for the office manager to create a paper trail for a termination. The employee warning notice is signed by the employee; therefore, there can be no accusations of miscommunication about the problems. The warning notice is recognized by the signature.

Orienting the New Employee

INTRODUCTIONS

New employees have a certain level of skill; however, they need to be taught the system of the new office and to be oriented in a manner that makes the transition from the old employer to the new employer as smooth as possible. Well-oriented employees are more likely to stay; since there is a certain amount of cost associated with rapid turnover of employees, it is advisable to orient all new employees as effectively as possible.

BOX 2–10. **EMPLOYEE WARNING NOTICE**

Employee name: _____

Type of incident: _____

_____ Attendance

_____ Tardiness

_____ Rudeness

_____ Unsatisfactory work

_____ Disregard of policies or procedures

_____ Insubordination

_____ Working on personal matters

_____ Other

_____ Other

	Date	Code
1st Occurrence:		
2nd Occurrence:		
3rd Occurrence:		

W = Warning   P = Probation   T = Termination
O = Other

Employer Statement: _____

_____

_____

_____

_____

_____

Signature of Office Manager

_____

Signature of Employee

_____

Date

The best approach to orienting a new employee is the team approach. The transition period is faster and smoother when everyone on the staff helps in the training process. Just as important as training the employee in the aspects of the new job is explaining the rules and regulations of the practice. Explaining the mission statement of the practice and its goals and philosophies is essential in establishing a solid relationship with the new employee. The bonding that must take place between the existing staff and the new staff member is an important part of the orienting process. Co-workers should be introduced to the new staff member and should make a special effort to ensure that she or he feels comfortable. One way to do this is to have each member of the staff spend a few minutes chatting with the new employee.

The office manager should give the new hire some information about her or his manager's role in the medical office and how the new hire will interact with her or him. Volunteering a little personal information may help ease the situation and will help the new employee to better understand the office manager. Training should also include explanation of how the new employee's position interacts with all others on staff.

The office manager should also introduce the new employee to the building security guards, maintenance workers, parking lot attendants, and housekeepers. This will be valuable if the new employee needs any of their services. If the bookkeeping is not done by the office manager, the new employee should be introduced to the bookkeeper and accountant when they come to the office. Depending on the new employee's job responsibilities, the office manager might want to take her or him to the bank or hospital to introduce her or him to staff there.

SHOWING THE NEW EMPLOYEE THE ROPES

The new employee needs to be given a thorough tour of the office so that she or he doesn't have to waste time looking for certain areas. It is helpful to show the new employee where coats are hung and where personal belongings can be kept during working hours. Because of security problems, some offices have a designated area for such items.

Explaining lunch procedures is also very helpful. Many offices have lunchrooms equipped with refrigerators, microwaves, and coffee pots. Some offices send out for lunch, and some take a lunch hour in which they can leave the office to get lunch or do errands.

All of these regulations must be explained to a new employee either at the time of hire or on the first day of work. The *Office Procedure and Policy Manual* will help to explain these procedures and should be given to the new employee on the day of hire. Although their contents vary from office to office, procedure manuals can be helpful in explaining telephone and scheduling techniques, billing procedures, physicians' schedules, etc.

Both clinical and logistical procedures vary from office to office, so it is imperative that the new employee be oriented properly to how the office works: The closest person to the phone when it rings answers it, only the receptionist can call the answering service at the beginning and end of each day, only the data entry employee is allowed to turn on the computer in the morning, etc.

It will take time for the new employee to feel at home in this new environment, and anything that the office manager or staff can do to help is always appreciated. The manager should remind all employees and physicians to be patient with the new employee during this transition period and that a kind word or gentle suggestion is better than impatience and snarling.

If the new employee is new to the area, the office manager should have the local Chamber of Commerce send materials on churches, community services, and other activities to the office for her or him. Many of the other employees may want to suggest entertainment possibilities, reputable car repair shops, good bakeries, dry cleaners, etc. This will help to make the new employee feel at ease in unfamiliar territory. If parking at the office is not possible, the office manager should acquaint the new employee with the closest, cheapest, and safest off-site parking lot available. If there is a parking garage, the new employee should receive a parking card on her or his first day at work and be reimbursed for any parking expense she or he had that day.

A final word about orienting the new employee: Care should be taken not to overload her or him with too much information about all the quirks of the practice or the employees.

JOB AWARENESS AND FEEDBACK

The office manager should encourage the new employee to express any ideas she or he might have for improving current procedures. Many times, employees will bring ideas with them from other practices that can be useful to the new practice. Feedback from the new employee after the first week on the job is very important. It is important to learn of any concerns the new employee might have; however, she or he may feel reluctant to speak out. The manager can make the new hire feel invited to express her or his concerns by asking some very nonthreatening questions, such as "How do you like it here?" or "Is there anything you need help with?" The manager may want to ease into the conversation by saying, "The first month in a large practice like this can be very stressful. It took me a few months to. . . " This becomes a sharing situation between the office manager and the new employee, the basis for a bond. Remember, the office is looking for loyal and dependable individuals, and a little bit of kindness and caring will go a long way toward this end.

The Appearance of the Medical Professional

The image that an employee presents to patients and their families is another important factor that will influence others. Appearance, posture, vocabulary, tone of voice, and manners are all part of the medical office employee's image and have been found to influence patients and their families. There have been several texts written on the health care worker's appearance, but there is no right or wrong way to dress in the medical office environment. Some physicians require office staff to wear crisp, white uniforms that will inspire trust and suggest credibility. Others prefer a low-key, relaxed atmosphere and allow colored scrubs and uniforms in the office. More and more offices today allow the staff individuality in their attire as long as it is appropriate. Depending on the type of medical office, some office managers allow clinical personnel to wear street clothes under white lab coats to show an air of warmth and confidence. Dressing for a professional role in a medical office has become increasingly important and must always be neat and clean. Each individual physician's office will establish a dress code which should be part of its *Office Procedure and Policy Manual.* An office manager should always convey a sense of authority in her or his attire, whether it is a uniform or street clothes. With image playing such a big role in the medical office, the staff should be guided by the patients', the patients' families', sales representatives', and physicians' reactions to their appearance. First impressions of a medical office are important and are generally long-lasting. As in other professions, such as the military and law enforcement, appearance that commands respect and authority has a very positive effect on individuals.

Employee-to-Physician Ratio

Four factors affect the number of employees a medical office has on staff (Fig. 2–5):

1 The type of medical practice
2 The type of physician practice
3 The location of the practice
4 The style of the practice

The most widely used method of determining the number of staff that a medical office needs is allowing three employees per physician. As the number of physicians increases, so should the ancillary staff. For instance, because of the variety of treatments involved in family practice, a family practitioner may require slightly more staff than a general surgeon. A recent study by *Medical Economics* magazine showed that, on average,

Family practices employed two assistants per doctor.
Specialty surgeons employed one assistant per doctor.
Ophthalmologists employed four assistants per doctor.
Neurologists employed one assistant per doctor.
Obstetricians/gynecologists employed three assistants per doctor.
Anesthesiologists employed zero to one assistants per doctor.
Internists employed two assistants per doctor.

Many physicians make the mistake of thinking that if profits are down, they must decrease their expenses, with payroll being the most likely place to start. This could be a big error in judgment on the physician's part. It has been proven that medical offices that employ three people see 50% more patients in a typical week than the medical office that employs only one person. The

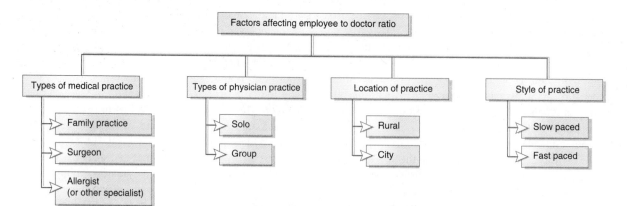

FIGURE 2–5. Factors that affect the employee-to-doctor ratio.

problem is getting the physician to believe in this statistic! If hiring another employee allows the physician to see just two more patients a day, the system is working. This figure can only grow, constantly increasing the patient volume of the office.

Some physicians will become overzealous and add too many employees as the practice grows. A surplus of employees can also result when two medical practices merge, because neither physician wants to let employees go. What should be done if the office finds itself overstaffed? The solution to this problem is easy. The situation should be viewed as an opportunity to get rid of dead wood and trim the staff down to the employees who are necessary for the office to run efficiently. Those employees who have just been along for the ride for the past year will be let go and in the case of a merger of two practices, replaced with employees from the other practice who are doing top-notch work. This might sound harsh, but many consultants asked to evaluate the size of a practice's staff will take this approach and decisively make changes in personnel as they see fit, without consideration of the employees. This is a business decision and is not based on the employees personally.

An effective way for the office manager to establish whether the office is overstaffed is to have each employee list in order of importance, the 10 most important things she or he does. The manager then collects all the lists and compares to see if any of the tasks are repeated on any lists. If a task appears on two or more lists, the office manager might want to take this time to revise the job description and responsibilities of each employee. The addition of new office equipment might also have an effect on the productivity of the office. Reorganization can be very helpful in making the staff more efficient and in determining the amount of staff necessary for a particular medical office. This practice is commonly called "right-sizing."

Office Romances

Romances between physician-bosses and employees or between office managers and employees can turn into living nightmares for everyone involved. In the first place, the people involved may think that no one knows what's going on when, in fact, everyone knows and the couple have become the topic of conversation in the lunchroom. Romances can also lead to embezzlement in the blink of an eye. For example, an office nurse was having an affair with a physician-boss and, during this fling, decided to help herself to monies from bank deposits every day. Because the physician had become partial to the nurse, he gave her more responsibility, which included making all the bank deposits from the office. Because the nurse was always working late, she was the last employee to leave the office, and it became increasingly easy for her to change bank deposit slips. This office did not have an acting office manager, and when the receptionist spoke with the doctor about the suspected problem, the receptionist was immediately labeled a troublemaker and asked to leave. The doctor finally saw the error of his ways $35,000 later, when the nurse moved out of state unexpectedly.

An office manager should always be aware of personal relationships that might be brewing and attempt to put a stop to them. Of course, if one of the players is the physician, the office manager might have a difficult time. There is no way an office romance can go on without its hurting the practice. It is not uncommon to hear from job applicants that their reason for leaving their last position was that "the doctor was having an affair with the receptionist and I just didn't want to deal with it any more!" Office romances give rise to irreversible morale problems and complaints about favoritism. Office romances have been the start of divorces, dissolutions of partnerships, and embezzlement proceedings. The smart office manager stays away from them!

Sexual Harassment

Sexual harassment can be as open as a physician's or supervisor's offering an increase in salary in return for sexual favors or as elusive as making a comment about an employee's dress. Every office should have a policy in place regarding sexual harassment issues. The Equal Employment Opportunity Commission (EEOC) defines sexual harassment in a very loose manner that can, however, be translated into TROUBLE for the medical office. Some feel that sexual harassment is merely an issue between the two people that it involves. This is incorrect! The office manager should recognize that sexual harassment not only affects those involved, but also creates tension, low morale, and reduced productivity in the office.

Fewer than 10% of harassed individuals file formal complaints. Those in the medical profession tend to feel we are immune to such nasty issues as sexual harassment, when, in fact, sadly, there is much of it going on. A survey conducted by *Nation's Business* magazine showed that 9 out of 10 medical profes-

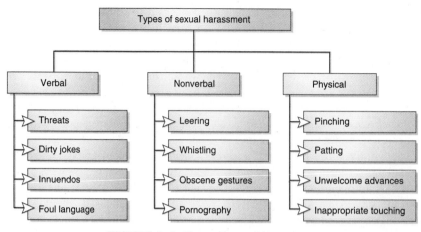

FIGURE 2–6. Types of sexual harassment.

sionals had either witnessed or been involved in sexual harassment on the job.

THE EQUAL EMPLOYMENT OPPORTUNITY COMMISSION'S DEFINITION OF SEXUAL HARASSMENT

Since 1963, Congress has passed a series of laws protecting the rights of each individual with respect to employment. These laws place responsibilities on employers by specifying certain job requirements. For example, when an employer or manager is interviewing an applicant for a job or considering whether to continue to employ a particular person, she or he can consider only job-related criteria. For instance, an employer or manager cannot ask questions during an interview that are not job related. A person's sex and race are not job related. Whether the person is married or has children is not job related.

The EEOC defines sexual harassment as follows: unwelcome sexual advances, request for sexual favors, and other verbal or physical conduct of a sexual nature. These constitute sexual harassment when the following exist:

An individual surrenders to a conduct that was made either explicitly or implicitly a term or condition of the individual's employment.

An individual surrenders to or rejects a conduct that is used as a basis of employment decisions affecting the individual's employment.

Such conduct has the purpose or effect of unreasonably interfering with an individual's work performance or creating an intimidating, hostile, or offensive working environment.

BOX 2–11. SEXUAL HARASSMENT POLICY STATEMENT

Jones Medical Clinic is committed to providing a working environment in which its employees are treated with courtesy, respect, and dignity. Jones Medical Clinic will not tolerate or condone any actions by any persons that constitute sexual harassment of any employee.

Sexual Harassment is defined as unwelcome sexual advances; requests for sexual favors; and other verbal, written, or physical conduct of a sexual nature by employees or supervisors where such conduct is either made an explicit or implicit term or condition of employment, is used as the basis for employment decisions affecting employees, or has the purpose or effect of unreasonably interfering with an employee's work by creating an intimidating, hostile, or offensive working environment.

Deliberate and repeated comments with sexual overtones, sexual jokes or ridicule, physical gestures or actions of a sexual nature, and solicitations for sexual favors are examples of violations of this policy and will subject the offender to discipline, including discharge. A sexual harassment complaint should be directed to the medical office manager or practice administrator, who will promptly and fully investigate. Confidentiality will be maintained to the maximum extent possible, consistent with the need to investigate the complaint fairly and thoroughly.

BOX 2–12. SEXUAL HARASSMENT COMPLAINT FORM

Date and time of incident: _____

Allegation: _____

_____

_____

_____

_____

_____

_____

Victim's name and position: _____

Alleged harasser's statement: _____

_____

_____

_____

_____

Action victim wants: _____

_____

_____

Action taken: _____

_____

_____

Witnesses: Name   Position

1) _____

2) _____

3) _____

To understand how sexual harassment cases are defined, it is necessary to understand that the standard used to determine the validity of sexual harassment acts is that of a "reasonable person." The law judges cases from the victim's perspective. There is a lot of latitude in the interpretation of what constitutes sexual harassment. This means that everyone must be very careful of how they act in their place of employment.

TYPES OF SEXUAL HARASSMENT

The three types of sexual harassment as shown in Figure 2–6 are physical, verbal, and nonverbal.

Physical sexual harassment is just as it seems: being touched, rubbed against, pinched, or assaulted or receiving *any* unwanted physical contact. *Verbal sexual harassment* consists of innuendoes, sexual jokes, foul and unacceptable language, sexual comments, and threats. *Nonverbal sexual harassment* consists of obscene gestures, leering, whistling, and suggestive objects or pictures. The legal system recognizes sexual harassment by "quid pro quo" (demanding sexual favors for economic compensation, such as a promotion or money) and "hostile work environment." Each medical office should compose a policy statement regarding sexual harassment. A sample statement provided by the Medical Group Management Association is shown in Box 2–11.

THE SEXUAL HARASSMENT COMPLAINT

The costs of a sexual harassment suit can be substantial, whether the medical office wins or loses. Sexual harassment suits increase absenteeism, tardiness, and employee turnover; result in low productivity; and ruin the image of the office in general. If the suit is lost, the physician could be responsible for paying back wages, punitive damages, and reimbursement for pain and suffering of the victim.

Every complaint should be handled with dignity and proper documentation, whether it is a small incident or a large one. Any other employee who might have witnessed the act should be interviewed. The person committing the act should also be interviewed and advised of the allegations against him or her. Disciplinary actions can be oral; however, it has been found that written disciplinary actions are much more effective. A copy of this action should be made a part of the employee's personnel file. It is important to obtain correct and accurate information before taking any action against the employee. Failure to do so can result in a wrongful-termination suit against the office. A sexual harassment form can be implemented to resolve sexual harassment

---

BOX 2–13. EMPLOYEE COUNSELING REPORT

Date: _____

Employee name: _____

Problem: _____

_____

_____

_____

_____

Employee response: _____

_____

_____

Corrective steps taken: _____

_____

_____

_____

Office manager's signature: _____

Employee's signature: _____

complaints; the one shown in Box 2–12 can be revised to fit the personal needs of each office.

Liability and the Medical Office

The physician is responsible for any acts of her or his managers or administrators. If a co-worker is responsible for the act of sexual harassment, the employer can still be held liable, especially if the employer knew about the act and did nothing to prevent it. Physicians can also be held responsible for the actions of individuals not in their employ, for instance, pharmaceutical representatives, patients, and delivery people. The best way to avoid all this is to create an atmosphere of loyalty and positive employee relations.

Employee Counseling

Office managers may occasionally find themselves in the position of confidant or counselor. Employees may look to them for advice on various matters from personal to professional. A good office manager always has time for the staff and good listening skills. If the employee is experiencing a problem involving the office, the personnel, or the employee's role in the practice, it is important to use an employee counseling report (Box 2–13). This should be filled out and placed in the employee's permanent file.

References

Caplan, C. "A Guide To Hiring and Keeping Good People." *Physician's Management,* March 1993, pp. 122-138.

Coleman, D. "What You Must Know Before You Hire or Fire an Employee." *Physician's Management,* May 1992, pp. 60-70.

Curry, G. "Temporary Help Market Continues To Grow." *The Office,* July 1993, pp. 8-10.

Davis, M. "Hiring the Overqualified." *Management Review,* August 1993, pp. 35-38.

Farber, L. *Encyclopedia of Practice and Financial Management.* Oradell, NJ: Medical Economics Company, 1988.

Gray, R. "How To Deal with Sexual Harassment." *Nation's Business,* December 1991, pp. 28-32.

Hirsh, R. "Office Romance: A Sure Way To Shatter a Practice." *Medical Economics,* February 1991, pp. 118-120.

Regel, R., & Hollmann, R. "Gauging Performance Objectively." *Personnel Administrator,* June 1987, pp. 74-78.

Schneier, C., Beatty, R. & Baird, L. "Creating a Performance Management System." *Training and Development Journal,* May 1986, pp. 74-80.

Sevel, F. "The Most Effective Ways To Train A New Employee." *Physician's Management,* November 1992, pp. 97-115.

3

The Front Office: The Telephone, Communication with Patients, Scheduling, and Correspondence

Why Bad Things Happen to Good Offices

The patient who walks into a medical office today is quite different from the patient of the past. In today's hectic society, many physicians find themselves so busy that they do not have the luxury of developing a rapport with the patient, as the physicians in the past did. Decades ago, physicians knew all the family members by name and often had delivered them. In our busy urgent care facilities today, the physician generally deals with demanding, hectic schedules that preclude the opportunity for closeness. In our changing world, the physician is no longer seen as almighty, as a god on a pedestal. Many of the older physicians feel relief that this change is taking place. They feel it is a more desirable position to be in, to be perceived as a human, not a god. When patients walk into the medical office today, they walk in as consumers, knowing what they need, looking for the right price, and knowing how they plan on getting it. There are some potential danger zones into which a medical office can fall. The following is a list of potential problems that the medical office manager should be aware of and possibly correct before they occur:

1 Patients rarely understand that some problems do not have easy answers.
2 Patients seldom understand that delays in scheduling occur despite the best efforts of the office staff.
3 Some patients are "doctor hoppers" and arrive at your office with quite a history of conflicts with other physicians. They're in your office simply to put you to the test.
4 Patients never understand fully their insurance coverage and think they have much more coverage than they do.
5 Patients are consumers. They believe they know what they need and are there to get it.
6 Newspapers and television programs instruct patients incorrectly and tend to be biased about how the physician *really* feels about the patients. Patients are exposed to book titles like *Drugs That Don't Work,* magazine articles like "How to Demand the Most From Your Doctor," and local news broadcasts such as "Mammograms: Are They Really Necessary?"
7 Patients believe that they require intensive treatment when, in fact, they do not.

Many patients are more interested in whether they are entitled to a particular service under their insurance plan than in whether they really need that service. Managed care seems to be bringing a lot of this type of patient to the surface. One important factor to remember is if the office excuses itself to patients who are angry with it, some patients will see this as a weakness and walk all over the office. Patients have a right to sound off about their grievances; however, if the medical office overreacts, it only makes the situation worse. Many patients feel better if they make an issue out of a delay, a bill, or whatever might be bothering them on that particular day. The office staff should be trained to remain unruffled and to let these difficult patients clamor on and on. Often, when patients see that they are not receiving the response they expected, they will quiet right down.

The Telephone System

There are more than 40 manufacturers of telephone systems today. According to the North American Telecommunications Association, more than four million desk telephone systems are sold each year. With this kind of competition, the office manager should call a number of telephone system companies in the area and ask them to send information on their products and services to the office. After reviewing the information the manager should invite four or five of the top companies to come in and present their products and service. Before contacting these companies, the office manager should try to determine just how many phone lines and phone sets are going to be needed.

> ### MANAGER'S ALERT
>
> Don't forget to forecast the amount of growth expected in the practice in the next 5 years. You don't want to purchase a system that doesn't have expansion capabilities.

It is not easy to predict the growth of a practice, but a basic rule in purchasing a telephone system should be that the system purchased today should be large enough to allow for double the amount of lines and units over the next 5 years. Many systems have growth modules that can be purchased to expand the system as the time draws near.

The office manager can determine how many telephone lines the office needs by asking the telephone company to conduct a traffic study or what they call a "busy study" on the lines. This study shows how many times a patient got a busy signal instead of the office staff. If the last line regularly rings busy, the general rule is to add two additional lines. The sales representative will need the following information from the office:

- About how many calls the office receives
- About how many local calls the office makes
- About how many long-distance calls the office makes
- Whether the office wants customized calling, whereby certain lines are designated to certain individuals (for instance, the office manager might want a certain number to ring directly at the billing department or at the appointment secretary's desk)
- Whether there is a need for any of the special features offered

SPECIAL FEATURES

A variety of special features offered by telephone companies may be useful to the medical office. The office manager needs to think about the needs of the office ahead of time so that they can be discussed with the sales representative. An office's needs may require certain telephone equipment or may require certain services that the company provides. The following are some of the special features available:

Call forwarding—The office can forward calls that come in on the main line to another designated line (used in conjunction with many answering services).

Conference calling—Three-way phone calls can take place.

Toll restrictions—Any attempts to call toll numbers are rejected.

Direct inward station dialing—Direct access to a particular extension is provided.

Call cost display—A running total of the cost of a call is displayed as the call goes on.

Privacy buttons—With the press of a button, the physician can ensure that the conversation she or he is having on one of the phones on a line cannot be overheard by someone picking up the receiver of another phone on that line.

Intercom—One employee can summon another through a buzz; they can then talk on the intercom.

Display messaging—Some phones have a screen on which a message can be left, such as "I'm at lunch until 2:00."

Secure off-hook voice announcement—Co-workers can interrupt phone conversations with important messages and without the other party's hearing.

Battery backup—This ensures the availability of telephones that are plugged into outlets.

Repeat call—The last number dialed is redialed for up to 30 minutes.

Return call—The person who called can be called back, regardless of whether the phone was answered or not.

Call waiting—A beep indicates that someone else is trying to call on the line.

Speed calling—Regularly used numbers can be preprogrammed for faster dialing.

Call trace—This mechanism traces the number of the last call and sends it to the telephone company's annoyance department.

Select forward—Up to six calls can be transferred to another location.

The office manager must be careful not to buy features that the office really doesn't need. An array of features and fluff should not sell the product. The wise office manager buys the system that allows for growth, provides the necessary features, and demonstrates the most telephone for the money.

WHY NOT USED EQUIPMENT?

With technology changing as rapidly as it does, there is a lot of used equipment available for purchase. This equipment can be purchased anywhere from 30% to 70% of the original price. There are a couple of things to keep in mind about buying used equipment. First, the company selling the used equipment must be a reputable one. It's a good idea to ask for a list of references and call them. Second, what is the warranty on the used equipment, and who will provide repairs if needed? Just remember, you get what you pay for!

Telephone Savvy

THE IMPORTANCE OF THE TELEPHONE

The government's creation of diagnosis-related groups in the 1980s (see Chapter 5) has resulted in competition among physicians and decreased the censuses of many hospitals. This increased competition has required that both hospitals and physicians market their services more effectively. In Chapter 15, we will discuss the medical marketing necessary in today's economic environment. The medical field has been able to step back and view patients as consumers. These new-wave patients shop around for their physician, just as they shop around for a new car.

The upshot of this is that patients today expect to be treated in a courteous, friendly, and professional manner by both their physician and their physician's staff, and if they are not treated in this way, they'll go elsewhere. Often, it is the staff member on the phone who gives the patient her or his first impression of a physician's office. When a business depends a lot on the person answering the phone, it is most important to have staff who are trained in the courteous and productive use of the phone. No one gets a second chance to make a good first impression.

The professional treatment should not stop when a patient is no longer new to the practice. The physician works hard to establish a relationship of mutual trust and confidence, and this must not be destroyed by staff blunders or unprofessional treatment of patients. The overall tone of the office is set by the office staff, and the personal interactions patients have with the staff will color their view of the physician.

A MAJOR SOURCE OF DISCONTENTMENT

The telephone has the potential to be a major source of discontentment for patients. The telephone is a very important part of the medical office and should have skilled personnel answering it. Receptionists and secretaries spend more than 50% of their day dealing with patients on the telephone. Thus they are the key individuals in creating the initial bond between the prospective patient and the physician's office. Once the patient is in the office, the receptionist or secretary can communicate the office's environment by nonverbal means, such as projecting a welcoming personality and a friendly, caring, professional appearance. Over the phone, however, the responsibility is all in the way the office staff talks to the patient. The telephone should always be answered after no more than three rings. The office that is too busy to be able to adhere to this rule on a regular basis might have a need for additional personnel. If a delay occurs, it is appropriate to answer the telephone and say, "Hello, Dr. Miller's office, Jan speaking. Sorry for the delay. Can I help you?" If a delay of 2 minutes or less is anticipated, it's okay to ask the caller for permission to put her or him on hold. The conversation should always resume with a thank-you to the caller for waiting. "Thank you" should also end

every conversation, regardless of the nature or reason for the call.

Staff should be instructed to follow the **PHEE** principle:

Positive
Helpful
Empathetic
Efficient

If patients complain that they can never get through to the office because of busy signals, it is time to call the local telephone company and have it do a study to evaluate what the practice needs. This study generally takes 2 weeks. Anxious patients only become more anxious as the telephone rings repeatedly. Even if the patient simply wants to set up an appointment, the constant ringing of the telephone can convey an impression of a disorganized, chaotic practice. This could cause the patient to hang up and call another physician. Prompt answering of the telephone builds a reputation of efficiency.

In some form or other, Bell Telephone is found in every state. They continually hold Improving Telephone Skills workshops. They usually offer group discounts and on-site training for larger office staffs. The Education Services department of your local Bell Telephone company will provide information regarding these workshops. It will also send newsletters such as *Business Communications Update* on a regular basis which helps the office manager keep abreast of new services and seminars and offers helpful hints.

What one patient feels is an emergency may not be an emergency to another patient. However, no matter what the problem is, if the patient feels it's an emergency, it is the office staff's responsibility to take the time to listen and advise the patient according to the guidelines established by the office manager or the physician. The patient on the other end of the telephone neither knows nor cares that you had an emergency patient walk into the office first thing this morning, that the physician was an hour late for office hours, that the first five patients of the day were staring holes through you from the waiting room, and that it looks like you will not get lunch again today! All the patient cares about is her or his problem and when the physician's office will solve it.

THE VOICE OF A FRIENDLY, COMPETENT MEDICAL OFFICE

Tone of voice is the key factor in handling the patient on the telephone. Office staff should practice the technique of smiling with their voices. If they are thinking with a friendly smile on their face, they will present a caring, pleasant image. Niceness is almost always contagious. Killing with kindness works in many cases and diffuses the most difficult of situations. When attempting to solve a patient's problem, be it medical or clerical, office staff will find that their chances greatly increase if the patient perceives them as competent and caring (Figure 3–1). It is important to portray an impression of interest in the patient's problem and efficiency in attempting to solve it. Staff must guard against representing themselves through their voices as having had a busy day and being tired. Since moods are contagious, an employee's negative tone of voice can easily be adopted by the patient, resulting in the patient's becoming unpleasant and uncooperative. Situations like this have no happy ending.

The voices of the office staff reflect their thinking. Canned enthusiasm doesn't fool anyone. Staff's voices should be natural and well modulated and should contain the appropriate inflections. One way to answer the telephone that is a very effective icebreaker is to say, "Hello, Dr. Smith's office, Ann speaking. How may I help you?" Having personnel automatically give their name projects a familiarity that allows the patient to become better acquainted with her or his physician's office. It forms a bond between the patient and the staff and adds a personal flavor to the staff's professionalism. Saying the patient's name several times during the conversation implies that the office recognizes the patient and is familiar with her or his problems. This personalizing puts the patient at ease and sends the message that she or he is special. Each patient wants to be thought of as the only patient the office has, and

saying the patient's name is a very effective way of depicting this.

Staff should *never* be allowed to answer the telephone and, before asking who is calling, say, "Can you hold please?" This technique is guaranteed to provoke a negative response from the caller when the employee returns to the line—either angry words or, worse yet, a dial tone. Many patients feel they are an emergency, or at the very least the most important case of the day, no matter what their ailment is. The liability involved with putting a caller on hold before asking her or his name is great. Suppose the patient *was* an emergency! In a busy office setting, it is possible to have more than one telephone line ringing at the same time. Staff should be instructed that in this situation, they should answer the telephone by saying, "Hello, Dr. Smith's office, Rob speaking. May I ask who is calling? Mrs. Johnson, I'm on a call on the other line. May I ask you to hold the line for a minute?" This courtesy allows the patient to understand the situation and to voice any emergency that might be taking place. This ensures cooperation from the patient and is another way of saying that the office cares about the patient.

Office managers need to decide whether they will take all calls that come in for them or would like to have their calls screened and inform the receptionist or secretary of their preference. Even if the office manager answers the telephone as a matter of course, the secretary can still be asked to pick up calls when the office manager is in meetings or interviews.

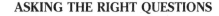

FROM THE AUTHOR'S NOTEBOOK

Constant interruptions to take phone calls can disrupt the work of any office manager or physician and should be kept to a minimum.

ASKING THE RIGHT QUESTIONS

When patients call the office to request an appointment, the staff can better assist the physician by asking the patient the right questions. The patient should first be asked, "Have you seen Dr. _____ before, either in the hospital or in one of our offices?" This is asked first so that as the patient is talking, her or his medical record can be looked up on the computer. If staff do not ask about the hospital, they could spend hours looking for an office chart that doesn't exist. This also helps in determining how much time to allot for this

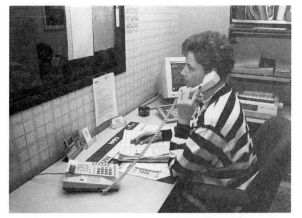

FIGURE 3–1. The medical office receptionist should be a friendly voice on the phone.

patient's appointment. A list of questions that should be asked of each patient who calls to schedule an appointment should be mounted by the front-desk telephone. The following are some of the questions that should be on the list:

"Have you ever been seen by any of our doctors before, either in the hospital or in the office?"

"Who referred you to our office?"

"What will you be seeing the doctor for?"

"Have you had any blood work or x-ray exams done regarding this condition? If so, please bring copies with you."

"Can we please have your daytime and evening phone numbers?"

"What type of insurance do you have? Please bring your cards with you to the office. If your insurance requires a referral from a primary doctor, please make sure you have a referral with you. We will not be able to see you if you do not come to the office with a referral." (Insurance questions are asked if the physician requires payment for services at the time of the visit.)

"Our charge for an initial office visit is xxxx dollars, and this must be paid at the time of the visit."

THE CHOSEN FEW

Every office has some patients who have special privileges and require special treatment. The office manager needs to give the receptionist or secretary the names of the people who are important to her or him and the names of the people who are important to the physician, so that the receptionist can make the appropriate decisions when these people call:

- Whether to interrupt the office manager or physician.
- What questions to ask the patient.
- Where to route the call in the event the party with whom the patient wished to speak is absent.

Employees should not be expected to know which patients get special privileges. The manager should provide them with a list of such patients and should update the list periodically.

THE CORRECT HANDLING OF TELEPHONE MESSAGES AND RESPONSES

If a telephone call requires an answer from the physician, it can be handled in two ways. If it is not an emergency situation, it is best for staff to advise the

patient that they will check with the physician and get back to her or him. This way, staff do not hinder the patient care that is currently being handled in the office. The physician can be asked the question at a more convenient time, and then the return call to the patient can be placed by the staff.

Staff should be instructed that if the patient feels that it is necessary to talk directly with the physician, they should say, "May I take the message and have the doctor return your call later today?" They should always ask the patient how long she or he will be at that particular number, and that information should be noted with the message. It is always a good idea to assign a staff member to be responsible for checking the physician's messages intermittently, so that if there is a message that needs urgent attention, the staff member can direct it to the physician sooner.

FROM THE AUTHOR'S NOTEBOOK

One medical office put together a "New Patient Packet" and sent it to all new patients who scheduled an appointment on the telephone. This packet specified the routine lab tests that the physician ordered on all new patients and asked the patients to have them done before the initial visit. At the time of the visit, the physician already had the lab results in the new patient's chart. It saved a lot of time, and the patients and physicians were grateful!

THE MESSAGE BOOK

Messages taken for the physician should be kept in either a spiral notebook or a telephone logbook. This way, there is a record of all calls. This is helpful for many reasons—when the physician wants to talk to a family member from out of town who called last week and when a medical–legal issue arises—as well as preventing the loss of little pieces of paper with messages written on them. All messages for the physician should contain the following information:

- The patient's name
- The caller's name and relationship to the patient, if the caller was not the patient
- The patient's/caller's phone number and how long she or he will be at that number
- The reason for the call

- The result of a lab test, if the patient is looking for a result (if the result has not yet come in, call for it)
- The pharmacy's phone number, if the call is for prescription renewal

Telephone message books can also be used by the office staff. These books allow the staff member taking the call to fill in the blanks of the message form, pull off the physician's copy, and leave a hard copy in the book for reference at a later date. Many physicians prefer this system and like the messages put on a spindle on their desk for them. The patient's chart should be pulled and handed to the physician along with the patient's phone message. The patient, like the consumer, is important to the business. Patients who are happy with their physician's practice are an excellent source of referrals for new patients.

FROM THE AUTHOR'S NOTEBOOK

To make sure that telephone messages are complete, make a list of questions that should be asked when each patient calls. This list will provide the information needed to determine the urgency of the call and is helpful to all staff members, clinical and nonclinical.

Communication That Connects

ACTIVE LISTENING: A NEW APPROACH TO PATIENT–STAFF RELATIONSHIPS

Good communication is a fundamental tool in practicing good medicine. Listening is essential to good communication. Today, however, many people have a difficult time listening, and health care professionals are no exception. We find ourselves finishing sentences for people, misinterpreting what they are saying, and allowing our mind to wander as patients ramble on about their problem. Communication is a very important aspect of dealing with people. If the office communicates effectively with the patients, patient compliance will be better. Physicians and health care workers find it difficult many times to bridge the gap between scientific, logical thinking and effective communication with people. One person's perception of what was said can be quite different from another's.

One of the most important factors that make up effective communication is *active listening*. When talking with Mrs. Porter, staff should not be thinking that Mr. Rimer's thermometer is probably ready to be read or that Mrs. Benning is undressed and waiting for her cardiogram. They should be concentrating on what Mrs. Porter is expressing to them at that time. The act of active listening involves asking the right questions and then analyzing the facts before making a decision. Staff should be trained to rely not only on their ears, but also on nonverbal communication. In a face-to-face situation, staff can often learn more from their eyes than from their ears. Active listening consists of a series of dialogues with the patient that involve listening and reacting. There are five steps to active listening.

Avoid Distractions. The first step in active listening is to *avoid distractions*. Distractions hamper the ability to listen and to process the information received.

Jot Down Notes. The staff member should jot down *notes* as the patient is speaking. This enables her or him to review certain aspects of what the patient said, making it easier to recreate the story for the physician.

Gain Clarification. It is a good idea, as the third step, to question the patient to *gain clarification* of some of the details. The staff member should try to ask questions that cannot be answered by a simple yes or no. As an example, it is better to say, "Tell me about the arm pain you've been having" than to ask a series of questions such as "Does it hurt around your elbow? Does it hurt if you lift it above your head? Is it a sharp pain?" Once the patient has told her or his story about the pain in the arm, the staff member can ask the appropriate questions to gather any information the patient might have left out of her or his story. Staff should be cautioned against interpreting and reacting to what they thought the patient said. It is important for them to be correct in all aspects of the patient's history. It is sometimes helpful for the staff member to interject phrases so that the patient is aware that the staff member is still listening and is interested in what she or he is saying. A simple "Um-hum" or "Go on" may do the trick.

Use Reflective Technique. As a fourth step, the staff member may need to get the patient to explain a certain complaint. This step is called *reflective technique.* When patients say they have had arm pain for a week, do they mean 7 days? If staff respond, "So, you've had arm pain for a week?", patients may then say, "It actually started four days ago." The details of the patient's condition have been made much more accurate.

Restate the Patient's Comments. The fifth and final step in active listening is to think like a patient. This requires *restating the patient's comments.* Staff will be better qualified to deal with patients' concerns if they comprehend what patients are saying and are able to understand patients' points of view. Staff should be warned against responding to a patient's needs before they have clarified all the details of the patient's situation. Once they have done this, staff should be able to provide an intellectual and caring response to the matter. The purpose of restating the patient's comments is to think and feel like the patient, and thus it isn't quite the same as using reflective technique, the purpose of which is to verify a particular complaint the patient made.

TELEPHONE ADVICE

When staff have been instructed by the physician to give advice to a patient over the phone, they should have a thorough knowledge of the subject about which they're talking. They should not attempt to answer questions they are not sure of. If they are uncertain how to answer a question, they should defer to the physician, explaining to the patient that they would like to clarify the physician's instructions. This response will command respect from patients, who will feel that any information staff members relay to them is accurate and complete. *Never* allow staff to use such phrases as "I guess" and "I think so." This type of response creates havoc and may cause a loss of confidence in both the office staff and the physician. It is always important to remember that the physician is liable for everything that staff members say.

COMMUNICATION THAT REFLECTS PATIENT AWARENESS

The outcome of a patient's medical treatment depends on effective communication. Effective communication takes place when the health care provider "connects" with patients, that is, enables patients to understand something by speaking to them on a level that they can understand or doing whatever else it takes. To be effective, communication must acknowledge the cultural and religious beliefs that patients bring with them to the office. For example, Jehovah's Witnesses cannot receive blood or blood products from another person.

It is important for the medical office manager to help the staff develop strong communication skills. Patients are concerned with a few basics when entering the

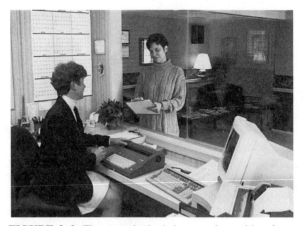

FIGURE 3–2. The receptionist helps a patient with a form.

medical office: what is wrong with them, will they be all right, and did they cause this problem to occur? All medical office staff should be carefully trained in patient awareness and patient instruction so that they can provide clear and concise explanations (Figure 3–2). It is important to remember that patients are generally upset when they are at the physician's office, which causes confusion and lack of understanding. Patient fallibility is an important recognition of the health care worker and should not be played down.

FROM THE AUTHOR'S NOTEBOOK

Many offices provide written information to patients, so that when they return home and are no longer anxious, they can read the information provided. They will often understand much more if information is given to them in this way.

COMMUNICATION TIPS FOR MEDICAL PERSONNEL

There are certain behaviors that are exhibited during communication. An office manager should provide an in-service training session on communication behaviors in order to ensure the best possible lines of communication between staff and patients. The following are some common behaviors that are necessary for open communication.

- Let patients speak. If staff are speaking more than 40% of the time, they are talking too much.

- Don't rush patients. Give them the time necessary to explain their thoughts.
- Explain everything in easy-to-understand words and phrases.
- Be aware of nonverbal language, such as shrugging or avoidance of eye contact. Body language often speaks louder than words.

WHETHER TO INVOLVE THE FAMILY

When considering whether to involve family members in the care of the patient, staff must assess the wishes of the patient. This can be done by observing the patient's age, sex, and culture. The patient's family plays a major role in her or his welfare. Some patients do not want their family members involved in their care or, for that matter, in any of their business! One must be careful of patient confidentiality in certain cases, and the health care worker should be careful to "read" the patient in order to determine whether to involve the family. Some patients are hesitant to inform the staff that they want patient confidentiality. The physician can be most helpful in many of these cases, and the health care workers can take their cues from her or him.

Other patients want and need the support of their family, and the office staff must be cognizant of involving the family in their care.

PATIENTS, PATIENCE!

Mr. Angry

Now that medical professionals must view patients as consumers, the old adage, "the customer is always right," applies in the medical office just as it does in any other place of business. Even the rude and angry patient should be handled with a certain degree of respect and friendliness. Office personnel can accomplish more at a faster rate by disarming the angry patient than by feeding the patient's anger with their own. Patients should be allowed to vent their problems, and staff should refrain from interrupting them. Some patients need to talk out their problems and feelings. Letting patients verbalize their problems gives staff time to assess the situation and come to the appropriate perception of exactly what the problem is and what the patient wants the office to do about it. Empathy works very well in situations like this: an example of an empathic response is, "I'm sorry that you are so upset, Mr. Brown." Agreeing with the patient can also be

helpful. For example, a good response to a patient who is angry about a delay in getting x-ray exam results is, "I would be upset too if I had to wait a week for the result of my x-ray." The staff member then asks the patient where the test was done, what was done, and when. She or he then calls the appropriate hospital or laboratory to obtain these results. The *Office Procedure and Policy Manual* should be referred to for guidelines for looking for test results. Generally, these results are reviewed by the physician, and then the staff is directed as to how to handle each specific case. Patients requiring prescription renewals should also be handled according to the guidelines in the manual. Staff must *never* renew a prescription without first checking with the physician, no matter how much they know about the patient.

The Noncompliant Patient

The office staff can be invaluable in interactions with the physician's noncompliant patients. They can coax them into compliance when the physician has exhausted all efforts. Patients who will not cooperate with the physician will cooperate with office staff for several reasons. One of the most common reasons is very simple. The office nurse or medical assistant might favor the patient's grandchild, whom the patient loves dearly. When an office assistant shows caring, the patient feels secure and trusts that person. Don't forget: staff build relationships with patients just as much as or more than the physician does. The office manager should recognize this and attempt to use it in a positive fashion. Much can be accomplished!

Scheduling

"There cannot be a crisis next, my schedule is already full!!"

—Henry Kissinger

TAMING THE APPOINTMENT BOOK

The medical office appointment book is the lifeblood of the office. The duties of all members of the staff revolve around it. Physicians find themselves slaves to it. It commands the respect of everyone and is the most difficult part of the practice. It changes like the weather and therefore enforces change around it. It is a powerful tool and should not be taken lightly. Making patients wait for their appointments is bad for any practice. Surveys on patient satisfaction have shown that the main complaint is excessive waiting. The appointment schedule that handles all situations has not been designed yet. A seasoned medical office manager knows that the number of patients scheduled for one day is not necessarily the number of patients seen on that day. It is important to remember that the appointment book is the key factor in the office manager's day. It should be used as efficiently as possible to maximize the physician's time.

FROM THE AUTHOR'S NOTEBOOK

To avoid having patients "stack up" in the waiting room, use the signal on the telephone and buzz once each time a patient is ready and waiting. Three buzzes over a period of 5 to 10 minutes tells the physician to pick up speed. If there are no buzzes, the physician knows she or he can chat with the patient and not get behind.

THE GENTLE NUDGE

Not all patients are willing to adjust to policies regarding office scheduling. Most of them do not care about the events of the day—they just want to see the doctor! Once a medical office establishes an appointment scheduling policy, it is important to attempt to stick to it. Patients must be dealt with in a firm, yet tactful manner. If they are late for an appointment, they can be told gently as they leave that the office is sorry about their wait, but they were a little late for their appointment and the schedule began to run behind. Positive reinforcement is just as important. Patients who arrive on time should always be told how much their promptness is appreciated. Gentle nudges such as these can do a world of good in getting the office policy on promptness across without offending patients.

Some patients want appointments on certain days and at certain times. They must be told gently that the office hours are such and such and that the physician has the following appointments available. It is unfair to the staff, the physician, and other patients to attempt to accommodate some patients' personal schedules. Box 3–1 gives a true story about an attempt to schedule an appointment for a patient.

Every receptionist's motto should be "Firm, but Tactful." As the story in Box 3–1 shows, the receptionist can bend over backwards in an attempt to schedule an appointment for a patient, and yet it will not be enough. These situations can be very difficult when dealing directly with a referring physician. The internist in the example in Box 3–1 began to show a bit of exasperation as the conversation progressed, but he never actually verbalized it. The same scenario

---

BOX 3–1. **A RECEPTIONIST'S SCHEDULING DILEMMA**

Dr. Bush was a busy internist in a small metropolitan area. He had a patient, Jeffrey Schwarz, who needed an appointment with a cardiologist. Dr. Bush called the cardiologist to whom he referred all of his cardiology patients and asked to set up an appointment for a patient of his. The receptionist very efficiently looked at the cardiologist's schedule and offered an appointment the following day, Wednesday, at 11:30 AM. The internist checked with Jeffrey and found that Jeffrey could not make it at that time. The receptionist then offered the next available appointment, which was 2 days later, on Friday, at 1:30 PM. Dr. Bush soon confirmed that his patient could not make that appointment either. The receptionist again checked the schedule and offered

Monday, at 3:00 PM. Again, Dr. Bush checked with Jeffrey and found that he could not make the appointment. Dr. Bush then added that his patient had stated that he worked at those times, but Tuesdays were his free day and he would like to come into the office on Tuesday. The receptionist politely told Dr. Bush that the cardiologist was not in that particular office on Tuesdays; however, he did take appointments at his other office across town. Jeffrey decided that he could not travel to the other office on Tuesday, because it was too far. At this point, the receptionist held firm to the previous dates that had been offered and was told by Dr. Bush that he would have to discuss this further with Jeffrey and call back.

happens when some patients call and try to schedule an appointment around their busy personal schedules. When this situation happens with a patient, and the patient ends the conversation with a promise to call back, it is extremely important for the receptionist to call the referring doctor (if there is one) and explain the course of the conversation with the mutual patient. This is good public relations. After all, it is important for the office to protect its relationships with its referring physicians.

THE BASICS OF MEDICAL OFFICE SCHEDULING

Because patients cannot be seen when *they* decide to be seen, the office should follow these simple, basic scheduling criteria in an attempt to prevent chaos.

- Maintain quality of care at all times.
- Schedule patients with emergency or urgent problems immediately.
- Maintain an on-time schedule as best as possible.
- Realize that patient satisfaction is important to the success of a medical practice.
- Realize that although the office aims to please, it must maintain a schedule by being firm, yet tactful.
- Be fair to the physician—don't schedule patients during her or his lunch break, etc.
- Use foresight and knowledge of the office operations to keep the schedule running smoothly.

SCHEDULING BY SPECIALTY

The appointment book should be clear and uncomplicated to prevent chaos in the front office. How patient appointments are scheduled greatly depends on the type of practice. Plastic surgeons and psychiatrists find it better to schedule their patients every hour. This means that each patient scheduled has an hour slot blocked off for her or him. Many surgeons prefer half-hour sessions. The normal scheduling for a physician's office is one patient every 15 minutes (Box 3–2).

AFFINITY SCHEDULING

Affinity scheduling is frequently used in dentists' offices, and it works well in some medical offices. In affinity scheduling, for Monday morning, the dentist schedules appointments only for patients who need fillings, for Monday afternoon, the dentist schedules

---

> **BOX 3–2. SAMPLE PHYSICIAN'S OFFICE SCHEDULE**
>
> OFFICE SCHEDULE FOR DR. QUINN
> AUGUST 1, 1995
>
> | | | |
> |---|---|---|
> | 9:00 | Debbie Bilardo | 221-9045 |
> | 9:15 | Charles Harmon | 321-6775 |
> | 9:30 | Laurie Bass | 221-0234 NP |
> | 9:45 | Ref: Dr. Babinetz | (MC & 65 Spec.) |
> | 10:00 | Christopher Stridiron | 221-6656 |
> | 10:15 | Shirley Beckton | 321-4556 |
> | 10:30 | ************* | |
> | 10:45 | Joseph Michaels | 221-1243 |
> | 11:00 | Hilary Smits | 321-0300 |
> | 11:15 | Rob Reinhardt | 221-2387 |
> | 11:30 | Jean Goralski | 532-7312 |
> | 11:45 | Linda Conklin | 722-9754 |
> | 12:00 | LUNCH | |
> | 1:00 | Charles Whalen | 221-0765 |
> | 1:15 | Samuel Weller | 445-7769 |
> | 1:30 | Michael Guidice | 321-4655 |
> | 1:45 | Jean Safin | 455-8231 |
> | 2:00 | Albert Roye | 321-7809 |
> | 2:15 | Ed Worthington | 633-7741 (US Healthcare) |
> | 3:00 | Consult | Ref: Dr. Doe |
> | 3:15 | Dolores Keifer | 633-2550 |

only patients who require fittings for dentures, etc. This type of scheduling is found in many other professions and can be a time-saving tool. Bunching patients by the type of service they require can increase efficiency and patient flow. For instance, in the medical office, all physicals may be bunched, all hospital follow-up visits may be bunched, all well-baby visits may be bunched, and so on.

APPOINTMENT BOOK STYLES

Many companies sell appointment books preprinted with blocks of 15 minutes, half hours, or hours. There are also appointment books that allow staff to customize a schedule according to the needs of individual physicians. There are appointment books designed for solo practices and appointment books designed for group practices. It is best to sit down with the physician and ascertain her or his needs before setting up an appointment book.

It is important to take as much information as possible from the patient at the time she or he calls to schedule an appointment and enter it into the computer. The phone number of the patient is most helpful, especially when the staff is calling to confirm the appointments for the next day.

WORKING EMERGENCY PATIENTS INTO THE SCHEDULE

Many offices consider the appointment book their worst nightmare. To be a scheduler in a medical office, a person must possess a great deal of flexibility and composure. Physicians will often go to the front desk and tell the staff that they have just instructed a patient to come right into the office. The best laid plans of the day go down the drain at that point. The scheduler may have already fit an emergency patient into the afternoon because there was no available appointment time. The office also has to contend with the patient who came to the office with one complaint and ended up spending double the time she or he was allotted, throwing a monkey wrench into even the best of schedules. This is all in a day's work for the medical office appointment scheduler.

TIME STUDY

If the office is constantly behind schedule, the office manager should sit down and evaluate the reasons for this. There may be too many patients booked in the course of a day, or there may not be enough time allotted for each patient, or there may not be enough staff to make patient flow efficient. Whatever the reason, the office manager should assess the situation and resolve it. One tool that is helpful is the *time study*. To conduct a time study, the office manager has the staff keep track of each patient as she or he progresses through the office. An example is as follows:

Patient Name: Colleen Murphy
Arrival time: 3:12PM
Appt. time: 3:30PM
Dr. time: 3:50PM
Discharge time: 4:16PM

Studying these times can help the manager determine where the trouble spots are located within the office.

TIPS FOR KEEPING THE SCHEDULE UNDER CONTROL

FROM THE AUTHOR'S NOTEBOOK

A way to keep the physician on time is to post a list of patients for the day either on the physician's desk or in any central location. This way, the physician can monitor her or his own time and will be able to work more efficiently. It keeps patients waiting less and the physician from missing dinner!

There are a few ways the scheduler can keep the appointment book under control. If the physician is using a 15 minute interval for patients, the staff might want to leave open one 15-minute slot every 2 hours. This allows some time for the physician to get caught up. This also helps the schedule accommodate the "Oh, by the way . . ." patient. This is the patient who is scheduled in the office for one problem and while there, discusses three other problems.

The office can also leave a half-hour slot open every day for the emergency patient. The half hour is left open until that day. The biggest problem with using this system is that other office staff will want to steal that slot beforehand. For the system to work, the slot must be left open until that day.

Some physicians like to leave a 15-minute slot open in the morning and one in the afternoon to make a few telephone calls, especially to patients who cannot wait until the end of the day for a call.

MANAGER'S ALERT

Never bind the practice to a schedule that the physician cannot possibly keep. Unrealistic scheduling will come back and bite you.

Many computer systems are equipped for appointment scheduling. This type of scheduling works well for some practices but is too inflexible for others. If the computer system that is already in place does not have appointment scheduling, there is an excellent chance that the company has it available as an option and it can be easily installed.

BOX 3–3. OFFICE STAMP FOR NO-SHOWS

Date: _____

_____ No show   _____ Cancelled

Follow-up _____

_____

_____

Initials: _____

FROM THE AUTHOR'S NOTEBOOK

Do whatever it takes to ensure that the physician is on time to begin office hours. It will keep the gray hairs from growing rapidly on your head!

NO-SHOWS

How to deal with those nasty no-shows!!! These patients are a constant challenge to the front-desk personnel. The patient who repeatedly doesn't keep appointments should be denied appointments in the future unless it is an emergency. What the office may find is that the patient who did not show for the appointment on Monday may call on Wednesday with an emergency. If there seems to be a pattern to this type of behavior, it should be brought to the physician's attention. The physician and office manager should then create a policy for the office to follow in dealing with no-shows.

No-shows should have documentation on their charts explaining what took place each time they missed an appointment. An office stamp can be made to contain the information shown in Box 3–3. The patient's chart is stamped each time the patient either did not show up for appointment or called at the last minute to cancel. If the patient did not show up, the staff should be trained to call the patient to follow up on why she or he did not keep the appointment. At this time, a new appointment can be scheduled. Two attempts to call the patient regarding a missed appointment are sufficient. The staff member who speaks with the patient initials the note stamped in the chart. Patients should always be called the day before their appointment to remind them of their appointment. A code or checkmark should be placed in the appointment book by the receptionist so that the office is aware that the reminder call was made. The codes shown in Box 3–4 can easily be used.

NEW-PATIENT BLOCKS

Some offices prefer to block off hour slots for new patients. This works well if the staff looks through the appointment book and blocks off hour slots in red pencil. The growth of the practice dictates the number of hour slots needed. If a new-patient slot is not completely used up, the remaining time can be used for emergency patients, phone calls, or catch-up. This slot, if unused, can also be helpful in dealing with office personnel or business-related problems that require the attention of the physician on that particular day.

THE LATENIK

When patients are late for appointments, it is best to explain to them that they are late and should expect to wait to be squeezed in to see the physician. The receptionist can also ask if the patient would like to

---

BOX 3–4. APPOINTMENT SCHEDULING CODES

N/A—no answer
L/M–left message with person
L/MM—left message on machine
Check mark—a confirmed appointment

reschedule. This generally works better for the office and the patient. Some patients will become indignant, and some will stomp out of the office; however, this is the only fair way to handle this situation. This office policy should be explained to all office staff and should be included in the patient information booklet (see Chapter 11). It is unfair to let the late patient go in to see the physician ahead of other patients who are on time for their appointments and are quietly waiting to see the physician.

FROM THE AUTHOR'S NOTEBOOK

To help patients to make appointments for specialists, keep business cards from specialists' offices at the receptionist's desk. Patients can simply call the specialist at their convenience by looking at the phone number on the card.

THAT PESKY PHARMACEUTICAL REPRESENTATIVE

Your day is already going bad and it's only 10:00 in the morning. In walks a pharmaceutical representative who wants to tell the physician about all the wonderful drugs her or his company has on the market! To save your sanity and your day, it is imperative to have a policy for dealing with pharmaceutical reps. Some offices see them by appointment only. Other offices have them buy lunch and sit and talk about their products while the doctor and staff are busy eating. An office that allows reps to walk in at any time and be seen is asking for trouble. Such a policy will take even the best of schedules and throw it out the window. Of course, each rep feels that her or his product is far superior to the others on the market and would like to spend an hour or so telling you why. This is where a firm, but tactful receptionist will come in handy. She or he must be instructed to stick to the policy that the office has set up and not let them past!!

Most reps understand the hectic schedule of the physician and simply leave the appropriate samples, requiring only a signature from the physician (Figure 3–3). This is very helpful in a busy practice, and because the office staff and physician appreciate this understanding, they may make time at a later date for the physician to listen to the rep talk about new products. Some reps are pushy and get agitated when told they cannot see the physician. The receptionist is in the driver's seat, and the

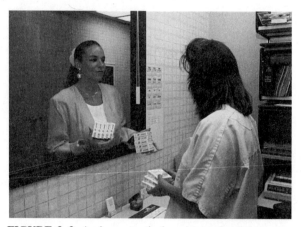

FIGURE 3–3. A pharmaceutical representative brings samples to the office.

policy will work only if she or he stands firm. The physician's schedule can be set up to allow the rep to see her or him at certain times on certain days. It is important that this time be closely monitored so that it is not exceeded. Pharmaceutical reps usually come into the office loaded with "toys." This is a good way for the office to restock with pens, pencils, scratchpads, and Post-It Notes advertising a company's favorite drug. It saves the office from having to buy pens and papers, too!

Beating the Waiting Room Blues

Waiting rooms should be warm, friendly places. However, most patients get irritable when made to wait for any period of time. Even patients who come a half hour early for their appointment will complain that they have waited for 35 minutes before being seen. These are sometimes impossible situations to try to dispute with angry patients.

WAYS TO MAKE THE WAITING ROOM A MORE CHEERFUL PLACE

Although there are no tried and true cures for the waiting room blues, there are some tricks that have worked for some offices. One trick is to put a television in the waiting room. Even though the physician is late in seeing the patient, the patient becomes engrossed in a television program and does not realize that time has marched on. The office might even want to invest in a VCR and keep a large supply of general-audience movies on hand for patients to watch.

For patients who like to become better acquainted with their illnesses, or even read about what their friends have, it is a good idea to keep various educational brochures available in the waiting room. For instance, a pamphlet on toilet training can be of great interest to a new mother. Another on hypertension can be of interest to many. Older patients might be interested in pamphlets on strokes. Many pharmaceutical companies provide these pamphlets at no charge to the physician. Some companies print specialized pamphlets that they sell for a nominal price per copy. Pamphlets can also be designated as waiting room reading only: simply use a marker and write across the pamphlet "Waiting Room Copy. Do Not Remove." Many of these pamphlets still grow legs and walk away, but writing this on the front cover lengthens the period of time they remain in the waiting room.

There are also pamphlets available from various organizations explaining what they are all about and the people to contact should patients wish to become active in them. Examples of these organizations are the American Liver Foundation; the American Diabetes Association; the Ostomy Club; and other organizations, such as day care centers, transportation services, and senior centers.

If the physician is a general practitioner, family practitioner, pediatrician, or obstetrician, it is a good idea to have children's books and toys easily accessible in the waiting room. Children need to be occupied, whether they are there with an ailing adult or they are the patients. Many pediatricians' offices have little tables and chairs for children to use while waiting. Some pediatricians physically split their waiting room into one room for sick children and one room for well children

(Figure 3–4). Parents find this concept appealing. If their child is scheduled for a "well visit," that is, for a routine checkup and immunization, the child is not exposed to the child who is in the waiting room with measles. Puzzles and quiet toys are also helpful and will be appreciated by the parents, other patients, and office staff. Don't buy coloring books and crayons . . . you will find yourself or other office staff constantly cleaning up messes!

MANAGER'S ALERT

Use caution when choosing toys for the waiting room. You do not want to increase liability by buying toys with small pieces that can easily be swallowed.

There have been instances of an office manager's buying what she thought were innocent toys for the waiting room and later finding that Mr. Potato Head had many small pieces that children could easily swallow, put in their ear, or shove up their nose. Office managers who do not have experience with children's toys should consult the mothers they have working for them; they will be experts on dangerous toys.

FROM THE AUTHOR'S NOTEBOOK

Don't let the doctor tell you that she or he has a lot of magazines at home and will bring them in to the office for the waiting room. This is fine as an addition to the subscriptions, but the office managers with happy waiting rooms are those with a few good magazine subscriptions of their own!

The office manager should take the time to address the magazine issue with sincerity. It is an old joke that if you're looking for an older issue of a particular magazine, go to a doctor's office—that's all they have. Because patients can spend some serious time in a waiting room, it is a good idea to keep current with various magazines to accommodate various tastes. Along with the general magazines like *Time, Newsweek, People, Ladies Home Journal,* and *Sports Illustrated,* more specialized magazines that parallel the specialty of the office might be provided. *Arthritis Today* and *Parents' Magazine* are good examples of specialty

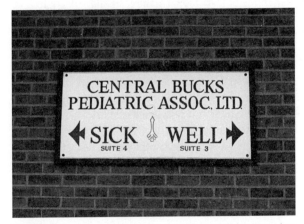

FIGURE 3–4. One pediatrician divides his waiting room into sick children and well children.

magazines that might be found in a medical office. The goal is to try to keep the patients happy. This makes everyone's day a little easier.

Patients love to read about health problems, whether their own or their Aunt Myrtle's. Having educational materials available in the waiting room has been found to be very helpful and also keeps the patients busy while waiting. Installing a bookcase and filling it with hardbound books and pamphlets is a great way to start. By stocking books (acquired through discount bookstores or from drug reps), the office introduces patients to a variety of issues that they might find they are interested in learning about further. Topics can range from Alzheimer's disease, to parenting tricks, to how to deal with rheumatoid arthritis. All books should be stamped with the office's name and address and should be allowed to be taken home by patients. Index cards can be used to track the location of borrowed books. The office can set a deadline as to when they want the books returned. A library generally allows 2 weeks for lending of books, but the office staff can set up any deadline they think is appropriate. The office can also accept books donated by area businesses and individuals. This idea can also be expanded to educational videos. For instance, patients with Crohn's disease might appreciate a video on how they can adapt their lifestyle to their disease. The lending library is a great public relations tool!

PATIENT FLOW

In a group practice, it is sometimes difficult to find a system to direct each doctor to her or his next patient. When there is more than one physician in an office at a time, "traffic jams" are common. One way in which to handle this problem is to use a color-coded flag system. In this system, a set of different-colored flags is mounted on the wall outside the examination room. Each doctor is assigned a different flag. When a patient is taken to an examination room, the appropriate flag is manually raised to indicate which physician has a patient in that

room. These flags can be purchased from Medical Arts Press or Tab Office Environment or many other office supply stores.

A very simple method is to position the chart in such a manner that it becomes a code for the physician. This type of system works well only for a small group office, but it does the job effectively and inexpensively.

A more sophisticated system from Veratronics can also be used. Veratronics designed a system of lights that enables the physician to ascertain which room her or his patient is in. The system is programmed to represent each physician as a different color. When a staff member takes a patient into the examination room, she or he pushes the color button representing the physician whose patient is in the room. Outside the room, that physician's light will flash, showing which patient is ready for the physician. (A light that is not blinking indicates that there is a patient in the room but the patient is not ready for the physician at this time.) When the physician finishes with the patient, she or he pushes the blinking light out. This is also helpful in aiding the staff when they are looking for a physician and might not be sure which room she or he is in.

Correspondence

DEALING WITH WHEELBARROWS OF OFFICE MAIL

The average weight of a physician's yearly mail is just under one ton. The most efficient way for the physician to manage this mountain of mail is to receive it secondhand. The office personnel should be able to open any mail that comes to the office (Figure 3–5). (Anything of a personal nature should, of course, be mailed to the physician's home.) However, all mail should pass over the desk of the physician at some point, unless it clearly states that it is a payment or insurance form for billing.

About half of a physician's mail is made up of pharmaceutical advertising. Some offices have set policies on how to handle advertisements. Many offices instruct their staff to automatically discard all junk mail that comes in. It is important that the person designated to do this job has a complete understanding of what is important and what is not. The office manager may choose to sort the mail in an effort to obtain useful information, such as advertisements for a new copier, a less expensive long-distance service, etc. Some offices set advertisements aside and go through them at a later date.

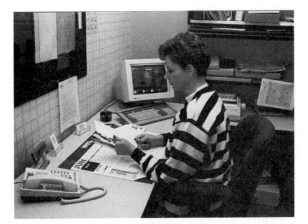

FIGURE 3–5. Some medical offices keep the receptionist busy just opening the day's mail.

The staff member who will be doing the mail should be instructed to check all return addresses on envelopes to see if there is a change from the information that is currently in the office. This will save time when bills go out to the wrong address and return 2 weeks later stamped "Forwarding Address Expired" or "No Such Address."

FROM THE AUTHOR'S NOTEBOOK

Always have stationery printed with "Address Correction Requested" on the lefthand side of the envelope. This way, when the mail is returned, it will have a yellow sticker on it with the correct address.

A properly trained office staff will save the physician a lot of time and will be appreciated by hospitals, referring doctors, insurance companies, etc. The office manager should provide adequate training in front-office policies, and perhaps even conduct workshops on streamlining the efficiency of the office. A brainstorming session involving all staff members can be helpful. Brainstorming sessions are appreciated by the staff, because they give them the opportunity to provide input into the daily workings of the office. The office manager can make a game out of front-office problems, asking for staff members to come up with workable solutions. The individual with the winning idea may be treated to lunch that day by the office.

TYPES OF MAIL

Many types of mail are handled in a medical office. They are:

- First-class/regular mail
- Second-class mail
- Third-class mail
- Fourth-class, or book-rate, mail
- Registered mail
- Certified mail
- Two-day economy mail
- Express/overnight mail

First-class/regular mail is the most common method of mailing and is used to mail most business envelopes, postcards, notecards, and business reply mail.

Second-class mail consists of "flats" (those 9 × 12 inch or 10 × 15 inch tan envelopes) and packages. This is the type of mail that delivers the medical journals to the office. This mode of mail transportation is slower and less expensive than first class.

Third-class mail includes circulars and advertisements that weigh less than 16 ounces. Third-class mail is slower and less expensive than second class.

Fourth-class mail consists of catalogs and books. This is the mode of mail transportation that may deliver office and medical supplies catalogs and books. The office manager should be aware that if the office needs to send books, they can be sent quite inexpensively with the fourth-class or book rate.

Registered mail is first-class mail that is usually insured. Any item of value that needs to be mailed should be sent via registered mail. This mail route is more expensive, but it is sometimes necessary. This type of mail can also provide the sender with a receipt.

Certified mail should be used when the office requires confirmation of a letter's or package's arrival at the specified address and acknowledgment of receipt at that address. This is more expensive than regular mail, but it is commonly used in a medical office. Certified or registered mail should be used for mailings of important documents such as

- Hospital and insurance company recertifications
- Letters of termination to a patient
- Documentation required by peer review organizations
- Application for staff privileges
- Requests for information from the Physician National Data Bank

For important and urgent mailings, the U.S. Post Office offers *second-day mail* and *overnight express* mail. If you use second-day mail, the package you send on Monday should arrive on Wednesday. Overnight express mail is hand delivered and guaranteed to arrive by noon or 3:00 PM (depending on the destination) the day after it's mailed.

Other companies also offer express mail services such as second-day delivery, standard overnight delivery, and priority overnight delivery. Standard overnight delivery is the most commonly used. It guarantees delivery by 3:00 PM the next business day and is slightly less expensive than priority overnight delivery, which guarantees delivery by 10:30 AM the next business day. The well known and commonly used express delivery companies are the following:

- United Parcel Service (UPS)
- Federal Express (FedEx)
- Airborne Express
- DHL
- TNT
- RPS

METERED MAIL

Some offices with heavy mailings choose to use metered mail. Metered mail is simply mail that has been entered into a machine for the imprinting of postage, as opposed to using the regular stamps that are purchased in the post office. Mail that is metered is delivered faster than regular postage mail and is faster than using postage stamps. To use metered mail, the office leases a postage meter, a piece of equipment that stamps the envelopes, and buys the postage from the U.S. Post Office. It costs more to use metered mail than regular mail; however, the time saved by not having to affix stamps on envelopes or wait in line at the post office for accurate postage on flats and large envelopes saves the office money in the long run. Whether to use metered mail is a decision that must be weighed carefully.

OUTGOING MAIL

On any staff member's desk, at any given time, there can be found a fair number of items that are quietly waiting to be processed and mailed—lab work to be copied and mailed to referring doctors or patients, letters to physicians, RSVPs to various social events and workshops, membership applications to insurance companies, recertification forms for hospital privileges, etc. The office manager might want to call Pitney Bowes to see if they can save the office money on postage and employees' time in processing.

The Postmaster General prefers businesses to use abbreviations whenever appropriate. Box 3–5 lists common addressing abbreviations.

Other outgoing mail items may be notices to patients. They may take the form of recall notices or notices of missed appointments. In any event, they need to be processed. An example of a recall notice is provided in Box 3–6.

The office might send a letter to a patient who did not show up for her or his last treatment and has not been heard from since. An example of such a letter is given in Box 3–7.

When the office has been asked to obtain copies of records from another physician, a note like the one shown in Box 3–8 may be used. The other side of the coin is when a patient wants to see another physician, and the other physician's office requests a copy of the patient's chart. If the patient has not signed a release form, it is necessary for the office to write or call the patient to request a signature permitting release of the records. This is discussed in depth in Chapter 7. Once permission from the patient is obtained, the records can be copied and mailed. If the office chooses to write for the patient's permission, it may send the letter shown in Box 3–9.

The office might find itself in a situation in which the insurance company pays a patient's bill and so does the patient. No, both monies cannot be kept! A simple note explaining the situation to the patient along with a refund of the monies will create goodwill. After all, how many patients receive checks from their doctors?! Not even considering the fact that it is illegal to keep both, the patients perceive this as an honest gesture on the part of the physician's office. With everyone always talking about Medicare fraud, it is good to hear a patient saying the doctor sent a refund. A letter to accompany the refund can be found in Box 3–10.

BE POLITE . . . ALWAYS SAY THANK YOU!

One way an office manager can make patients feel special is to institute a thank-you note system. When the office treats a patient who has been referred by another patient, the office should send a thank-you note to the first patient. This can take the form of a simple handwritten message on a plain card, or the office can have preprinted thank-you cards made that the physician can simply sign. It is also appropriate for the office manager to send the note, if the physician prefers not to. Sometimes, patients will refer more than one patient to the office, so it is important to write the name of the referral

BOX 3–5. COMMON ADDRESSING ABBREVIATIONS

Miscellaneous Abbreviations

APT	Apartment	DR	Drive/Doctor
ASSOC	Associates	EXPY	Expressway
ASSN	Association	FL	Floor
AVE	Avenue	FWY	Freeway
BLVD	Boulevard	GRP	Group
BLDG	Building	LN	Lane
CO	Company/County	PKWY	Parkway
CIR	Circle	RD	Road
CORP	Corporation	RFD	Rural Free Delivery
CT	Court	ST	Street
DEPT	Department	STE	Suite
DIR	Director	TER	Terrace
DIV	Division		

Abbreviations for States, Territories, Commonwealths, and Districts

AL	ALABAMA	NE	NEBRASKA
AK	ALASKA	NV	NEVADA
AZ	ARIZONA	NH	NEW HAMPSHIRE
AR	ARKANSAS	NJ	NEW JERSEY
CA	CALIFORNIA	NM	NEW MEXICO
CO	COLORADO	NY	NEW YORK
CT	CONNECTICUT	NC	NORTH CAROLINA
DE	DELAWARE	ND	NORTH DAKOTA
DC	DISTRICT OF COLUMBIA	OH	OHIO
FL	FLORIDA	OK	OKLAHOMA
GA	GEORGIA	OR	OREGON
HI	HAWAII	PA	PENNSYLVANIA
ID	IDAHO	PR	PUERTO RICO
IL	ILLINOIS	RI	RHODE ISLAND
IN	INDIANA	SC	SOUTH CAROLINA
IA	IOWA	SD	SOUTH DAKOTA
KS	KANSAS	TN	TENNESSEE
KY	KENTUCKY	TX	TEXAS
LA	LOUISIANA	UT	UTAH
ME	MAINE	VT	VERMONT
MD	MARYLAND	VI	VIRGIN ISLANDS
MA	MASSACHUSETTS	VA	VIRGINIA
MI	MICHIGAN	WA	WASHINGTON
MN	MINNESOTA	WV	WEST VIRGINIA
MS	MISSISSIPPI	WI	WISCONSIN
MO	MISSOURI	WY	WYOMING
MT	MONTANA		

on the note. This note is a great patient satisfaction tool and can generate much goodwill and future referrals to the office.

PATIENT CORRESPONDENCE

When a patient writes to the physician regarding her or his medical condition, the staff should be instructed to pull the patient's chart and attach the letter to the front of it. The physician will be grateful for the time-saving effort. This is especially helpful in a group practice, where the physician may not be familiar with the patient. Even if the physician knows the patient, being human, she or he cannot possibly remember all the details of all patients' treatments. The physician will probably never admit this to the staff, but she or he will

---

BOX 3–6. SAMPLE RECALL NOTICE

Dear Mrs. Smith:

I would like to take this opportunity to suggest that you call our office at your earliest convenience and schedule an appointment for a checkup. Our patients with chronic illnesses require periodic checkups and reevaluations of their medications and treatment.

Sincerely,

Dr. Matthew Wells

BOX 3–7. SAMPLE NO-SHOW LETTER

Dear Mrs. Vail:

It has been six (6) months since your last visit to our office. Your condition requires continuous medical treatments, and we are concerned about your health. We would be relieved if we knew you were obtaining medical care elsewhere, and we would be happy to send copies of your medical records to your new physician. Please call our office to set up an appointment as soon as possible, or if you would like your records sent elsewhere, please call our office and the staff will be happy to assist you.
    Thank you.

Sincerely,

Dr. Carolyn Babinetz

BOX 3–8. SAMPLE REQUEST FOR PATIENT RECORDS

Dear Dr. Babinetz:

Mrs. Nancy Vail, a patient of yours, has placed herself in the care of our office. She tells me that she has been a patient of yours for the last ten years. I would appreciate your sending me copies of all her medical records up to her last visit with you. A signed release from Mrs. Vail is enclosed.
    Thank you.

Sincerely,

Dr. Margaret Brennen

BOX 3–9. **SAMPLE REQUEST FOR RELEASE OF PATIENT RECORDS**

Dear Mr. Jones:

   We received a request in the mail today from Dr. McDonald for a copy of your medical records. Before our office can send your records to him, we request a signed release from you that will authorize us to do so. Please sign and date the attached form and mail it back to our office.

   Upon receipt of your release, we will copy and forward your medical records to this physician. Thank you for your cooperation in this matter.

Sincerely,

Dr. Simon Simms

BOX 3–10. **SAMPLE LETTER REGARDING DUPLICATE PAYMENT**

Dear Mr. Smith:

   A check arrived in the mail today from Patient Health Insurance for $400.00, payable to our practice. The check should have been sent to you, since you have already paid for these services.

   Since insurance companies have a difficult time dealing with refund checks, we have taken the liberty of depositing this check into our account and sending you our check in the same amount.

   This will avoid any lengthy delays in waiting for the insurance company to correct their records and send a reimbursement check to you. If you have any questions, please do not hesitate to call my office. My staff will be happy to explain this further.

Sincerely,

Dr. Nathanial Hall

---

greatly appreciate the effort and thought put into the gesture.

   Some patients will write short notes requesting prescription renewals. These can be handled in the same manner—by pulling the patient's chart and attaching the note to it. However, this can be delegated to the office nurse or medical assistant. The staff member can then follow previous instructions on how to handle this type of request. Any correspondence that requires a reply should be handled as soon as possible. If staff are instructed to take care of these items on a daily basis, it will not be difficult to keep up with the mail that floods the office. Many staff members can handle a large majority of this tedious mail if properly instructed to do so. It is important to keep in mind that everything is done to streamline the workings of the medical office and the physician.

FROM THE AUTHOR'S NOTEBOOK

When sending important correspondence, always take the time to send it certified mail and request a return receipt. This way, there is a record of the day it was received and who received it.

4

The Medical Record

The Medical Record

The medical record, or patient's chart, can be the medical office manager's best friend or worst nightmare. Records are an indispensible part of modern health care, yet they are not usually given the respect they deserve. They are often taken for granted and can be found to be in deplorable shape. Ragged edges and tears with enough repair tape on them to last a lifetime are only a few of the indignities to which these important files are subjected.

All physicians and office managers know the importance of the medical chart. Accurate medical records are an indication that good care was delivered, whether it was a routine blood pressure check or the transfer of a patient to another doctor. Because of the medical-legal environment today, the physician's office must be extremely careful about what is written in the chart, how it is written, and by whom it is written. Documentation of the entire visit is extremely important, not only for insurance auditing, but for defensive medicine. Under the resource-based relative value scale system of reimbursement (discussed in Chapter 5), the documentation must be in the patient's chart to justify the level of visit billed. If a procedure is billed with a modifier, simply stating "The procedure was unusually complicated" is not enough. It is necessary to document the reasons for this billing, or the procedure could be downcoded by the insurance company.

Putting aside for a moment the mere legal functions of the medical record, accurate and neat medical records symbolize quality care and a well-informed physician. The office manager should realize the importance of the medical record and should stress to the office staff the value of neatness and clarity of each and every patient's chart (Figure 4–1). This will result in an efficient office, and the physician will appreciate the staff's attention to detail when she or he is looking at a chart for a specific test or note.

It is important to remember that the medical record is the physician's professional lifeline.

INDIVIDUALS WHO USE THE MEDICAL RECORD

According to the American Medical Association, the patient's chart is used by several people. It is helpful for the office manager to understand who might have a need

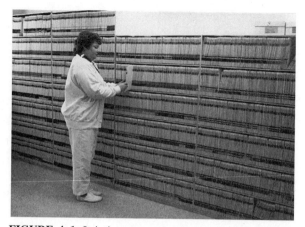

FIGURE 4–1. It is important to maintain neat and orderly medical records.

for the medical record. The following people are likely to consult the chart:

- The medical personnel involved in the patient's care
- The patient
- Clinical researchers
- Peer reviewers
- Reimbursement technicians
- Professional licensing and accreditation

> **MANAGER'S ALERT**
>
> If a practice has several patients with the same name, have a label printed that says: "Warning— there is more than one patient with this name." This label should be placed on the cover of the chart to prevent mix-ups.

Each patient's chart should include a Patient Registration Form that specifies the patient's demographics: name, address, telephone number, workplace and phone number there, social security number, date of birth, referring physician, allergies to medications, insurance information, etc. The Patient Registration Form is discussed in more detail later in this chapter. Having clear and neat medical records not only helps the physician, but also aids the office staff when they have to locate certain information in the chart.

The physician will discuss in detail the allergies of each patient, however, it is prudent to have a foolproof method of informing the office staff and reminding the physician of patients' allergies. Some offices have rubber stamps custom-made to say "ALLERGIC TO _____." They stamp the front of the patient chart and then fill in with red pen the name of the medication to which the patient is allergic.

FROM THE AUTHOR'S NOTEBOOK

Preprinted labels can be purchased in bright colors advising of allergies to certain medications. Due to the importance of this information, it is good practice to place these labels both on the front and inside of the patient's chart to call attention to this allergy.

RECOGNIZING PROPER RECORDS RELEASING

A *subpoena* is a document issued by the court system that requires an individual to appear in court on a specified date. A *subpoena duces tecum* is a subpoena for documents to be produced at a specific time at a specific place. This subpoena is usually addressed to the **Custodian of Records.** When a medical office is issued a subpoena for a patient's medical records, the custodian of records is expected either to arrive at the designated date with the original chart or to photocopy the records and mail to the record copy service. A record copy service is in business to obtain records for various different law offices. If the medical office does not have time to photocopy the medical records and mail them to the record copy service, the copy service will come to the office at a designated time and photocopy them themselves.

MANAGER'S ALERT

NEVER allow the original medical chart to leave the office through the mail. If the court will not accept a photocopy, someone from the office staff must go in person with the chart.

Records subpoenas are sometimes served by a local constable or sheriff's office and sometimes are simply mailed. Subpoenas can be sent through regular mail, or they can be sent certified mail, with a return receipt requested.

When the office receives a request for records from another physician's office, the staff should be instructed to obtain a signed records release form from the patient before copying and mailing the records. (See Chapter 3 for a sample letter requesting a patient's signature on a records release form.) Once the records release form has been signed, records should be copied and mailed to the designated physician within 2 weeks. It is a good idea to send records certified mail with a return receipt requested, so that there is no question as to whether they were received. The office should *never* refuse to send copies of a patient's medical record! The patient might sue the office on the grounds of neglect. Some states have laws that apply to this situation that carry criminal penalties, so the bottom line is *once the patient has signed the records release form, send the copies of the records within 2 weeks.* Records release forms can be purchased from many different vendors and generally come in tablets of 50. They look like the one shown in Box 4–1.

HANDLING INSURANCE COMPANIES' REQUESTS FOR RECORDS

Insurance companies often request the medical records of patients applying for insurance. They generally request a recent and past medical history, along with blood pressures, weights, and copies of lab tests, x-ray exams, and electrocardiograms. To expedite matters, the office manager should write a policy statement as to how the office handles these requests. With each request, the insurance company must send a release from the patient that is current. If the release is missing, the records cannot be released. Insurance companies will pay the medical office a fee to fill out the form and make copies of the test results and send them with the form. The office manager should have a set fee for the preparation of such requests, so that when insurance companies call the office, they can be told that a clerical fee of $____ must accompany the request. The average charge for copies of medical records is $0.25 per page. It is always a good idea to check with the practice's lawyer to see if there is a state law that limits copying fees to a certain price. These requests should be done in a timely fashion, so that the patient's insurance coverage is not held up.

BOX 4–1. **MEDICAL RECORDS RELEASE FORM**

Name: _____

Address: _____

_____

Please release any and all records on the above patient
for the dates

_____ to _____

to the office of
Dr. Carolyn Dibler
111 Main Street
Nicetown, USA

Patient's signature: _____

Witness: _____

Date: _____

> **MANAGER'S ALERT**
>
> Never, under any circumstances, give to insurance companies patient information over the telephone. It must all be done in writing after the patient has signed the release form.

- The office manager should contact references to check on the transcription service's dependability.
- The office manager should discuss with the service the turnaround time of the correspondence.

> **FROM THE AUTHOR'S NOTEBOOK**
>
> It is helpful if a list of commonly used diagnoses, procedures, and medications are given to the transcription service at the start. The office also might want to provide the service with a list of frequently used referring physicians and their addresses, so the physician won't have to repeat this information every time.

DICTATION . . . SINCE THE BEGINNING OF TIME

Dictation Systems

Dictation started with the Babylonians, was improved by the Egyptians, was perfected by the Romans, and is still going strong today. Dictation, whether by manual method or more modern technology, has long been a timesaver. Dictation can be handled through the physician's office or by an outside transcription service. If the office chooses to use an outside service, several things should be kept in mind:

- The physician must give all information as to where the letter is to be mailed, because the chart is in the office and is not available for reference.
- The physician should spell the patient's name and any other diagnostic or procedural terms that might be foreign to the transcriptionist.

Today's modern technology affords much flexibility, both for the physician and for the medical transcriptionist. It is no longer necessary for the physician and the transcriber to be in the same country, let alone the same room! Everyone involved can work at her or his convenience and from any location. If many users are tied to one system, the work is completed with more accuracy and efficiency. The units available today can be used by almost anyone, since they are user friendly. With a minimal investment in equipment and personnel, today's medical office can increase its productivity dramatically.

It has been proven that a nondictated general business-type letter will take a person 10 to 30 minutes to write. The varying segments of time depending on the technical aspect of the letter and the speed of the individual writing it. Dictation takes us away from those cumbersome constraints and brings us into the world of advanced technology. Most individuals talk five times faster than they write, which is one reason that dictation is so successful (Figure 4–2). Dictation is definitely a great time management tool and should be considered by any medical practice operating today.

With available equipment ranging from portable units to whole systems serving a large medical office, the needs of any physician and her or his staff can be met. The physician can use either a handheld microcassette tape recorder or a desktop unit. A small medical practice's needs are best addressed by simple dictation units that rely on cassette tapes for information storage and retrieval. The sizes of the tapes range from micro, to mini, to full size, the most popular being the microcassette. The sizes of the portable dictating units vary considerably, with the smallest weighing only a few ounces.

The Olympus Model L400 is the smallest fully featured microcassette tape recorder available and is about the size of a cigarette lighter. It is designed to provide 3 hours of continuous recording. The desktop unit is used by simply picking up the microphone and beginning to dictate. The handheld microcassette recorder is the most popular, because of its versatility. This unit usually weighs a few ounces and can easily be used

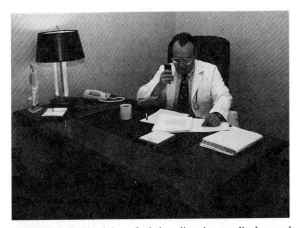

FIGURE 4–2. Physicians find that dictating medical record notes saves time.

in a hospital setting, at home, or even in the car. This portability increases the popularity of this method. The office manager should assess the needs of the physician so that the appropriate equipment is purchased.

Digital and analog dictation systems are available for large-volume practices. An analog system is a tape-based system in which an "endless" loop tape or cassette tape can be used. The physician either goes to a specific dictating location and dictates into a tank or dictates into a handheld dictating unit. A transcriptionist then plays the tapes on a transcribing unit and converts them into hard copy.

Digital dictation systems are electronic systems that are not tape based. These systems use a chip or speech board to accept the physician's voice. The voice, or sine wave, is then broken down into 1s and 0s (hence the name "digital") and stored in a computer's hard drive. Information can be called in from any location. This system also allows information to be inserted into the body of a letter without destroying the rest of the letter. If a physician needs to make an addition, she or he simply inserts the material and new space is created on the disc for it without the already-dictated work's being deleted. (In contrast, the portable tape units erase the previous material, and the new material is dictated over it.) In addition to this insertion feature, digital dictating technology eliminates the need to label and erase tapes on a continual basis. Digital dictation equipment is basically designed for multiple users, which in the health care profession would be large medical groups, clinics, or hospitals.

Telephone interfacing provides similar advantages, except that there is no delay in getting the tapes from the physician to the medical transcriptionist. The physician may be in another town or may be driving home from the hospital and can simply pick up the telephone to dictate progress notes reflecting work just completed. The dictated material is entered into the system at the office, where it will wait for the transcriptionist. Dictaphone Corporation has developed a product called "Straight Talk Plus" that is a voice-processing system that allows for dictation and voice mail.

Dictation of Chart Entries

Dictation is the tool that keeps doctors out of trouble when others cannot read their writing. It is imperative that medical records can be read and understood. Typing the progress notes is not vital to all practices, but it is a good habit. The office manager for a group practice will find it necessary at times to pull patient records to provide information over the phone to a member of the group who is covering for a colleague who is out of town. This task becomes stressful when the physician is requiring specific information, but the manager and office staff cannot read the entries in the chart. In a solo practice, there may be times that the physician is away and a colleague is covering for her or him. The colleague may call the office and ask for names of medications or progress note information, but the transfer of information may be stymied by sloppy writing.

Dictated and transcribed case histories, initial examinations, progress notes, and medications can be helpful to everyone whose job brings her or him in contact with patient records. Even if the physician chooses to handwrite the progress notes, dictated and transcribed case histories and initial examinations can be helpful. It has been found that physicians who dictate their charts generally provide more information than do physicians who write their charts. If the physician is dictating medical records, the office manager should assign a staff member to proofread the dictation before giving it to the physician to sign. *Remember, all chart entries must be signed by the person entering the note.*

In an office that uses dictated records, it is important for the physician to state the date every time she or he dictates. If the transcriptionist is given the record several days after the dictating was completed and no date is mentioned, she or he will be confused as to when the patient was in the office. The correct date is an important part of the medical record. All precautions to prevent error should be taken. It is better not to use nonmedical abbreviations when typing a medical record, because this can cause confusion at a later date. There are acceptable medical abbreviations that can be used as timesavers and also as spacesavers in the medical record. A partial list of approved medical abbreviations is presented in Appendix C.

The physician should be reminded to spell out the patient's name and any procedures or terms that might be unfamiliar to the transcriptionist. If the physician does not do this, the result will be many questions for the office manager from the transcriptionist throughout the day. It is also necessary for the physician to provide the name and address of any physician to whom she or he is dictating a letter. Routine referring physicians' names and addresses should be kept in a Rolodex at the transcriptionist's desk. It is a good idea for the office manager to check the transcription before it is placed in the chart for accuracy. It is always better to find an error in the office than in the courtroom.

BOX 4–2. DICTATION TECHNIQUES

Identification

Doctor's name
Date
Patient's name
Text to be typed
Sequence of material

Verbalization

Speak clearly
Speak slowly
Enunciate properly
Spell difficult names, diseases, and diagnoses
Do not mumble
Do not have loud background noise at time of dictation

Grammar

Indicate paragraphs
Indicate numbering
Indicate any special punctuation
Indicate capitals
Indicate indentations

FROM THE AUTHOR'S NOTEBOOK

If the physician does not have the time to dictate after each patient, she or he can place a Post-It Note on the front of the patient's chart with any pertinent information regarding the patient's visit. This will assist dictation at the end of the day.

A smart office manager trains not only the transcriptionist, but also the physician. If the physician follows simple dictation techniques, the transcriptionist can be saved hours of time per week. By simply sitting down with the physician and explaining the techniques that she or he can use while dictating to increase productivity and efficiency, the office manager can put an end to many of the complaints that typically come from transcriptionists. Some offices have physicians who talk fast, mumble, or dictate diagnoses that they couldn't spell even on a good day! This is the type of dictation that the office manager wants to eliminate! Box 4–2 presents a simple chart on dictation techniques . . . share it with the physician!

DOCUMENTATION

The Importance of Documentation

There isn't a single part of the medical record that isn't subject to the eyes of insurance auditors, peer reviewers, quality assurance investigators, or the law. In today's medical environment, the medical chart not only must include the diagnosis, prognosis, and plan of treatment, but also must justify the necessity of the treatment. In some cases, after insurance review, the office gets paid according to the documentation present. There is no such thing as over-documentation. Lack of documentation has always been a legal issue. Now, it is a reimbursement issue, too!

SOAP Method of Documentation

SOAP is the acronym for a method of organized and comprehensive documentation. Documentation performed according to this method includes

Subjective view of the case
Objective data
Assessment
Plan for treatment

By faithfully following this method of documentation, the physician imposes organization on the information she or he compiles about a patient and reduces the chances of forgetting information (Box 4–3). Some physicians are slow to use this method, because they think it is not comprehensive enough. This method does, however, serve as a basic system for preparing a medical record.

BOX 4–3. SOAP METHOD FOR DOCUMENTING PATIENT CASES

Patient Name: _____

Date: _____   Patient Account #: _____

Subjective Review _____

_____

_____

_____

Objective Review _____

_____

_____

_____

Assessment _____

_____

_____

Plan for Treatment _____

_____

_____

Liability and Documentation

Negligence is legally defined as the "failure to do what a reasonably prudent person would do under the same circumstances." "Reasonable prudence" means that a professional is required by law to act in a manner in which the average professional would act. To establish a claim for professional negligence, a patient must claim that there was duty owed to her or him, that that duty was breached, that damage was incurred, and that there was a relationship between the damages and the breach of duty. Professional negligence is discussed further in Chapter 7. Medical personnel have a duty to practice within the standards set for them by licensing or regulatory agencies. Documentation becomes a key issue in liability when a patient claims malpractice or negligent behavior. Having office personnel who are trained to do extensive documentation will reward the practice should defense in court become necessary. Most claims of this nature are filed years after the event, when most individuals would not remember the details of the event. Proper documentation will help the physician and office staff recall specific details and the series of events that took place.

Until lately, the importance of documentation of care in the physician's office was not clearly defined, although it has always been a standard of practice in the hospital setting. Medical office personnel should be trained so that they are governed by the same principles that underlie documentation in other professional contact situations. Any information that may change treatment and any patient response to medications or treatment should be recorded in the medical chart in a timely manner.

Documentation must be a concern for not only the medical staff, but also the physician. Under the doctrine of "respondeat superior," the employer is responsible for the actions of her or his employees. Because of this doctrine, the physician can be held accountable legally for the actions of any and all personnel working in the office. A properly trained office staff will eliminate worry. There are no guidelines for the documentation of the specific content of a patient's chart; however, the office manager should implement a policy wherein certain basic information is recorded in the patient's record at the time of each service. All entries into the patient chart should be made in ink or should be typed.

THE LIFE OF THE MEDICAL RECORD

From a legal viewpoint, the length of time that a physician's office should keep a medical record varies from state to state. Each office manager should check with the practice's legal counsel or with the local medical society to find out the state's statute of limitations for medical malpractice. This has a direct impact on the length of time the office must retain its patient records. From a strictly medical viewpoint, a medical office should retain medical records as long as the patient is an active patient in the practice or if the patient has undergone a procedure that could have an impact on her or him later in life.

In most cases, medical records should be maintained for 7 to 15 years for patients who are no longer seeing the physician. For deceased patients, records should be maintained for 5 years from the date of their last service. Pediatrics practices and family practices that treat children must maintain medical records for 7–10 years past majority (that is, the age at which full civil rights are accorded, or age 21). In other words, if you treat an infant and the infant's family moves out of town, the infant's medical record may be in your office for as long as 30 years! The x-ray films of inactive patients should be maintained for 5–10 years after the patient is no longer active. Many consulting agencies will advise a medical office to condense the patient's chart if the patient has been inactive for 3 years. This means that not every piece of paper has to be kept in the chart, just pertinent information containing medications, certain procedures, specific treatments and tests, etc. If a copy of the patient's chart was sent to another physician

---

FROM THE AUTHOR'S NOTEBOOK

Inactive patient charts are an excellent source of future revenue. Inactive patients can be contacted and reminded that they have not been in the office for quite some time. Give them an update on your practice—for instance, that you have a new associate. Potential revenue is waiting in these old charts!

FROM THE AUTHOR'S NOTEBOOK

A purged chart can be recycled by inverting the chart, covering the name and number, and using the chart as a manila folder for papers in the office. This saves on overhead and the environment.

during the physician's care of that patient, a copy of the record release should remain in the chart also.

COLOR ELIMINATES CHAOS: THE USE OF COLOR IN OFFICE TASKS

Filing Systems

Everyone has heard the old saying "Time is money!" The time spent looking for a lost chart or filing and pulling charts for the next day costs the practice hundreds of dollars a month. It has been estimated that the cost of looking for and replacing one patient's chart can reach $100 and that the time spent looking for it can take as much as 25% of a working day. More than half of that time is spent looking for lost or misfiled information.

Color-coded filing systems have taken the worry out of filing and pulling charts. With the help of colorful tabs located on patients' charts, the office manager can create a filing system that works for the medical office. Color coding can shorten the length of time spent on training new employees. It can also shorten the amount of time spent looking for charts that seem to have sprouted legs and walked away! Manila folders can be bought with the color coding already on the edges, but many offices purchase plain folders and the color coding stickers to apply in the fashion that they prefer. This last method allows for greater flexibility in the filing system.

Color coding schemes are based on either alphabetical or numerical systems. In alphabetical systems, 13 colors represent the first half of the alphabet, and the same colors are repeated to represent the last half, but with variations of stripes to delineate the differences. Some medical offices use the first three digits of the patient's last name, and some use the first two digits of the patient's last name along with the first digit of the patient's first name. For example, in an office that uses the first method, the chart for the patient William Snyder would be labeled **SNY**. In an office that uses the second approach, William Snyder's chart would be labeled **SNW** (Figure 4–3). In either method, each letter is in a certain color.

Numeric filing allows for the addition of new files without the hassle of moving all existing files and can be a straight or consecutive filing system. Numeric systems use 10 colors to represent the digits 0 through 9. Each patient is assigned a number and charts are filed according to that number. The following is a list of patients and their file or patient numbers. They may not look in order to you now, but in a minute you will see that they are.

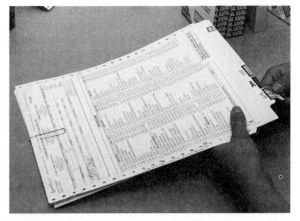

FIGURE 4–3. Coding systems help offices locate medical records.

Linda Conklin **02 78 00**
Joanne Waldron **00 12 01**
Tyler Keiper **00 99 01**
Christine Stern **02 34 02**
Julie Miller **20 10 10**
Angelina Anders **13 64 31**
Jessie Anders **13 65 31**
Anne Harris **00 00 65**
Gail Rinehart **01 00 65**

All files that end in the same last numbers are grouped together. Then the files are grouped together using the middle digits. Lastly, the files are grouped together using the first two digits. For example, Joanne Waldron **00 12 01** comes before Tyler Keiper **00 99 01,** because both have the same last number but the second digit 12 comes before the second digit 99. In the case of Anne Harris **00 00 65** and Gail Rinehart **01 00 65,** the second and third sets of digits are the same, so the filing is done with the first set. Anne's 00 comes before Gail's 01. Each number is in a specific color.

If the office wants to do alphabetic color coding by using colored file folders, it is generally done by assigning colors to certain letters of the alphabet. Red folders are used for last names beginning with the letters A, B, C, D, or E. Green folders are used for last names beginning with F, G, H, I, and J. Blue folders are used for last names beginning with K, L, M, N, and O. Yellow folders are used for last names beginning with P, Q, R, S, and T. Purple folders are used for last names beginning with U, V, W, X, Y, and Z.

For example, patients with red folders would be

Marge Brennen
Amy Carr
Karl Erickson

Patients with green folders would be

Anne Hale
Steve Gant
Jim Jones

Patients with blue folders would be

Kayla Keiper
Marilyn Miller
Betty O'Brien

Patients with yellow folders would be

Missy Presti
Gail Rinehart
Florence Tarantino

Patients with purple folders would be

Philip Waldron
Carol Vail
Sophie Zither

The office manager can customize a system to meet the office's individual needs. Many companies make color-coding systems; some of the more popular companies are Tab Products and Smead. There are many vendors in this business, but you will find that all of them use the same colors for each system and use them in the same way. This way, it allows for changing of vendors with little to no effort.

Other Ways Color Can Help Office Tasks

Many other tasks can be made more efficient by the use of color. Index cards in different colors can be used to designate different types of tickler files, while keeping the information well organized. Color used in the appointment book helps to draw attention to the most important meetings. For instance, using a red pencil to write hospital meetings in the book and a blue pencil to write personal appointments of the physician helps keep schedules straight and clear. The use of highlighters in the practice is becoming more fashionable these days. They can be used for a variety of different tasks and can be very helpful in pointing out important information.

If the office manager uses overheads for office meetings or meetings with the physicians, the overheads should always be in dark colors, such as purple or blue. It has been established that people remember more of the material from a meeting if it is presented in color as opposed to black and white.

WHO GETS THE RECORDS?

When a physician retires, there is the question of who gets the records. Many physicians send their patients a letter advising them that they are retiring or leaving the practice. This letter contains instructions for the patients as to what will happen to their charts. Some physicians will have already made arrangements with other physicians to accept these new patients. The patients are given the opportunity to come to the office between certain dates and at certain times to pick up a copy of their records to take to their new physician. Some local medical societies will act as records custodians. If the practice is being sold, arrangements should be made between the physicians that the sale includes maintaining the old records. If there is an employee who wishes to take on such a task, the records can be left in her or his custody for future copying when needed. This last method should be used only as a last resort, however. Microfilming the records is another avenue that the office can pursue, but it is a costly one. Whichever method is preferred by the physician or office manager, patients must be notified and given ample time to pick up their charts.

SIGNATURE STAMPS

Signature stamps can be the office manager's best friend or worst enemy. These stamps can save a lot of time in a medical office; however, if their use is not closely monitored, they can cause big problems (Figure 4–4). The areas in which the medical office could use signature stamps are

- Insurance forms
- Membership applications to insurance companies
- Notes for patients to return to work or school
- Order forms for patient testing
- Letters

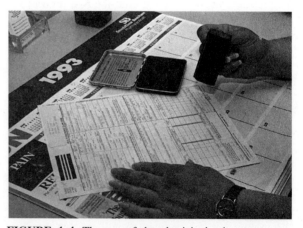

FIGURE 4–4. The use of the physician's signature stamp must be monitored closely.

The dark side of the signature stamp is its potential for abuse. There a couple of ways to protect the use of signature stamps:

- Assign the stamp to one employee, who would be accountable for its use.
- Have different stamps made and issue them to different employees. For example, the stamp "R. H. Hale, M.D." would be issued to one employee, the stamp "Robert H. Hale, M.D." would be assigned to another, and the stamp "Dr. Robert H. Hale" would be assigned to yet another. This way, you can track how each stamp is being used.

COMPUTERIZED PATIENT CHARTS

Many medical offices use computers for billing, accounting, and word processing. Few offices, however, allow the computer to aid them in maintaining their patient medical records. This is the most tedious and cumbersome task in the medical office today, so it only makes sense that it should be done with the help of a computer.

Not all medical offices are candidates for computerized medical records. Each office should weigh the costs against the benefits to see if their practice would benefit from using a computerized system of maintaining medical records. With the growth of managed care companies, computerized records are becoming more desirable. Managed care insurance companies require not only the financial records on a patient, but also increasing amounts of information on the patient's care. The Institute of Medicine of the National Academy of Sciences has identified a computerized medical chart as a crucial element for improving patient care in the twenty-first century.

Advantages and Disadvantages

There are several advantages to a computerized patient chart system. The following is a short list of advantages as seen by one physician's office:

1 The system flags patients for recall.
2 Files can be retrieved faster.
3 Records take up less storage space.
4 Analysis reporting is easier.
5 Charts are misplaced less often.

The disadvantages of a computerized medical chart system are that it is expensive and the time needed to file information into a patient chart is increased.

For a computerized medical chart system to work in a medical office, the physician must be in favor of automation. The staff must be enthusiastic and approach the system as a valuable friend, not a monster about to bite!

Entering Data

Generally, a preprinted patient encounter slip is used for each visit. The physician checks off items and adds notations where necessary, and then a data entry clerk enters the information into the computer. If the physician dictates her or his record, the medical transcriptionist types the information on the tape directly into the computerized chart. Results of laboratory tests and x-ray exams are typed into the patient's chart by the medical transcriptionist or data entry clerk. Letters of referral and letters from consultants are summarized and then typed into an archival storage area in the computer. Electrocardiogram tracings are interpreted, and the interpretations are then added to the patient's computerized chart. Hard-copy tracings are filed in alphabetical order in a file elsewhere in the office. It is important to keep the hard copy for comparison with other tracings the patient might have.

TROUBLESHOOTING CHART PROBLEMS

Every office should be aware of risk management where the patient's medical chart is concerned. The office manager should instruct the staff to follow these simple guidelines:

1 All laboratory results, x-ray films, and electrocardiogram tracings should be initialed by the physician before they are charted.
2 All telephone calls regarding the patient's care should be noted in the chart.
3 A certain procedure should be followed for missed appointments; for example, staff should write the date and the words "Patient missed appointment" in the patient's chart each time the patient misses an appointment. (Some offices have a stamp made and use red ink pads.)

If the office manager trains the staff to follow-through on these details, the office records will stand a better chance if audited or subpoenaed.

CARE AND HANDLING OF MEDICAL CHARTS

Each chart should be well maintained and handled properly to ensure a long life. Before filing the chart, staff should check to make sure that the proper coding, the year sticker, the label with the patient's name, and any stickers indicating special situations ("HMOs," "ALLERGIES," etc.) are clearly visible on the chart. The staff member filing the chart should always check to make sure the charges for the visit were entered into the computer. In the chart, all items of like nature should be filed together. All laboratory studies should be together, with the most recent on top; all progress notes should be together, with the most recent note on top; and so on. This makes filing a more pleasant task. Next, the chart is placed in its appropriate place in the file.

FROM THE AUTHOR'S NOTEBOOK

OUT guides can be very useful and can be purchased from a variety of vendors. They are plastic, chart-shaped guides that are inserted when a chart is pulled out. OUT guides make it easy to return a chart back to its correct place in the file without hesitation.

THE RIGHT WAY TO HANDLE A WRONG ENTRY

There is a right way and a wrong way to correct an error in a patient record. In an in-service session, the office manager should instruct the entire staff on the correct way to make corrections. To correct an error, a staff member should put a line through the mistake, write in the correction near it, initial it, and date it. For legal purposes, the date is very important. It shows the date the correction was made, providing evidence that it was not made after a subpoena was served or a suit was filed. Any addenda should be acknowledged as such and dated. The appropriate time frame for an addendum is generally 1 week. Most computer software packages even have a correction function that runs a line through an error. WordPerfect is one software package that contains such a feature.

ALTERATION OF MEDICAL RECORDS

Don't even think about altering medical records. According to a recent report by St. Paul Fire and Marine Insurance Company, any change made to a medical record could become a crucial part of a plaintiff's malpractice case. Many times, forgotten copies of records or portions of records will show any changes made to that record. Any missing pages or test results

can easily be noticed and can suggest that the patient did not receive proper treatment.

THE PATIENT REGISTRATION FORM

The Patient Registration Form is one of the most important parts of the medical record. This information allows the office staff to function in its various capacities. *There is no such thing as too much information.* A Patient Registration Form should include patient demographics, insurance and billing information, emergency information, and referring physician. Various companies provide preprinted forms for this purpose. Medical Arts Press, Colwell, and Histacount are a few of the more popular companies. This form should be updated every 6 months by each patient. Patients' address, telephone number, or insurance information often changes, and they tend to assume they have given the office the changes. If the office manager institutes a policy requiring that an updated form be completed every 6 months, there will be few problems with billing and contacting the patient. The office manager should make the secretary/receptionist responsible for carrying out this policy. This can also be done by the medical assistant or nurse, depending on the structure of the office (Figure 4–5). The important thing to remember is that someone must be made accountable for this task. A sample Patient Registration Form is presented in Box 4–4. Patients who receive Medicare must sign a Medicare Lifetime Signature Authorization, shown in Box 4–5. This is then a permanent part of the patient's chart, enabling the office to bill Medicare continually, while having the patient's signature on file. A sample Universal Authorization of Benefits Form is

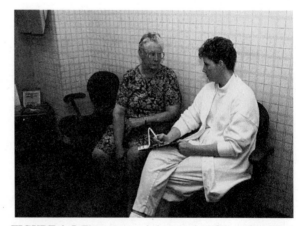

FIGURE 4–5. The secretary helps a patient fill out the patient information form.

BOX 4–4. **PATIENT REGISTRATION FORM**

PATIENT'S NAME: _____

PATIENT'S ADDRESS: _____

_____

_____

SEX: _____ F _____ M DATE OF BIRTH: _____ SS# _____

MARITAL STATUS: _____ S _____ M _____ D _____ W

OCCUPATION: _____

NAME OF EMPLOYER: _____

EMPLOYER'S ADDRESS: _____

_____

_____

EMPLOYER'S PHONE NUMBER: _____

SPOUSE'S EMPLOYER: _____

EMPLOYER'S ADDRESS: _____

_____

_____

SPOUSE'S EMPLOYER'S PHONE NUMBER: _____

REFERRED BY: _____

RELATIONSHIP: _____

PERSON TO NOTIFY IN CASE OF EMERGENCY: _____

_____

RELATIONSHIP: _____

PHONE #: _____

INSURANCE INFORMATION

PRIMARY INSURANCE COMPANY: _____

_____

ADDRESS: _____

_____

_____

Box continued on following page

BOX 4–4. PATIENT REGISTRATION FORM *Continued*

PHONE: _____ GUARANTOR: _____

ID# _____ GROUP# _____

SECONDARY INSURANCE COMPANY: _____

_____

ADDRESS: _____

_____

_____

_____

PHONE: _____ GUARANTOR: _____

ID# _____ GROUP# _____

BOX 4–5. MEDICARE LIFETIME SIGNATURE AUTHORIZATION FORM

_____

Name of Beneficiary

_____

HIC Number

I request that payment of authorized Medicare benefits be made to me or on my behalf to Dr. _____

_____ for any services rendered by that physician. I authorize any holder of medical information about me to release to the Health Care Financing Administration and its agents any information needed to determine these benefits or the benefits payable for related services.

I understand my signature requests that payment be made and authorizes release of medical information necessary to pay the claim. If item 9 of the HCFA 1500 claim form is completed, my signature authorizes releasing of needed information to:

_____

Name of specific Medigap insurance company

In Medicare assigned cases, the physician agrees to accept the charge determination of the Medicare carrier as the full charge, and the patient is responsible only for the deductible, co-insurance, and noncovered services. Co-insurance and the deductible are based upon the charge determination of the Medicare carrier.

_____

Beneficiary's Signature

_____

Date

BOX 4–6. UNIVERSAL AUTHORIZATION OF BENEFITS FORM

I request that payment of authorized Medicare and/or insurer benefits be made to me or on my behalf

to Dr. _____ for services furnished to me by said physician. I authorize

Dr. _____ to release to my insurance company any medical information needed to
determine the benefits payable to related services.

I understand that if, under Medicare program guidelines, a necessary service is determined to be noncovered,
I will personally be responsible for any amount denied or partially paid by the third-party payer.

_____   _____

Signature   Date

_____

I request that payment of authorized Medicare and/or insurance benefits be made either to me or on my behalf

to Dr. _____ for any services furnished me by said physician. I authorize any holder
of medical information about me to release to the Health Care Financing Administration and its agents any
information needed to determine the benefits payable to related services.

_____   _____

Name of Beneficiary   HIC Number

_____

I request that payment of authorized Medigap benefits be made either to me or on my behalf to

Dr. _____. I authorize any holder of medical information about me to release

to: _____
         Name of Medigap Insurer

any information needed to determine these benefits payable for related services.

_____
                        Name of Beneficiary

_____   _____

Medigap Carrier   Medigap Policy Number

_____   _____

Medigap Address   Medigap Policy Number

_____   _____

Medigap Address   Medigap Policy Number shown in Box 4–6 and can be used for all patients in the office.

TRANSFERRING MEDICAL RECORDS

There are three types of medical record: current, inactive, and closed. *Current files* are files of patients who have been seen in the office in the last year. *Inactive files* are files of patients who have not been seen in the office in more than a year. *Inactive files* are of patients who have not been seen in the office in more than a year. *Closed files* are files of patients who no longer come to the office because they have moved, are seeing another physician, or are deceased. Medical charts are generally purged from the mainstream of charts every year and are filed in the Inactive File area of the filing system, which should be easily accessible for retrieval. The type of practice dictates the circumstances under which charts are to be purged. For instance, if a practice recalls patients every 3 years, purging would not be done every 2 years. The charts should have year stickers on them, which can be bought from Tab Products or any other company selling similar products. They can be found with the alphabetical color-coded stickers. These color-coded year stickers help with purging and should be updated yearly as patients return to the office for treatment.

STORAGE OF THE MEDICAL RECORD

Patient charts can be stored in several ways. The vertical two- to four-drawer cabinets are still in use, but in a limited fashion. They are being replaced with larger, open cabinets, which make it easier to use color coding systems. There are four styles of files generally used in the medical office:

- Lateral file
- Shelf file
- Rotary file
- Vertical-drawer file

The style of file cabinet a medical office chooses to use depends on many factors, including cost, number of records, stage of medical practice, and space. The office manager will want to assess the office's present and future needs to determine the type of filing cabinet best for the practice.

The lateral file is generally found in the physician's office or the office manager's office. Lateral files use a fair amount of wall space, but they do not require room in front for extending drawers. They are made of wood, metal, or a composite, and most furniture sets for offices have lateral files that match the desks and other furniture.

Because of their design, shelf files allow for more storage than do lateral files. Drawers do not pull out, shelves can assist in filing, and they can be high to hold a large number of files. More than one person at a time can be filing in a system like this.

Rotary files are expensive filing cabinets and are generally used by offices with very limited space or a high volume of patients and new offices without previously existing files. Or they may be used by an existing office that is moving. The files rotate in a circular motion and can be accessed by more than one person at a time.

Vertical-drawer files should be used when conditions are right. They do not take up wall space; however, they require a great amount of space in front of each drawer so that each drawer can be fully extended to retrieve the files. Only one person at a time can be accessing these files, and, in fact, many filing cabinets will not permit the opening of a second drawer if one is already open.

THE HEALTH HISTORY QUESTIONNAIRE

"To avoid delay, please have all of your symptoms ready."

Anonymous

Some practices like patients to fill out a Health History Questionnaire (Box 4–7) on their first visit to the office. This information can be extremely helpful to the physician and office staff in determining the needs and problems of the patient. The questionnaire can be sent to the new patient before the date of the first appointment, so that the patient can bring the completed form to the office at the time of the visit. Having the patient fill out the form at home avoids slowing down the patient flow in the office. In addition, by completing the form at home, the patient will take more time and the information provided by the patient is much more thorough. The Health History Questionnaire is an integral part of the patient's chart.

THE PATIENT'S FAMILY AND THE MEDICAL RECORD

Any medical receptionist will tell you that the first words the patient hears when she or he returns to the

BOX 4–7. HEALTH HISTORY QUESTIONNAIRE

Please circle the answer which seems best:

Yes	No	Do you need glasses to read or see far away?
Yes	No	Do you see better with one eye than the other?
Yes	No	Do you have any eye pain or blurred vision early in the morning?
Yes	No	Do you see haloes (circles) around lights?
Yes	No	Has your eyesight changed recently?
Yes	No	Are you having trouble with your hearing?
Yes	No	Have you ever had a running ear?
Yes	No	Have you ever had sneezing spells or frequent stuffiness of the nose?
Yes	No	Do you have frequent sore throats or hoarseness?
Yes	No	Do you have frequent nosebleeds?
Yes	No	Have you ever had tuberculosis or any chest condition?
Yes	No	Have you ever had hayfever, asthma, hives, or any other allergic condition?
Yes	No	Have you ever had a close contact with a tuberculosis patient?
Yes	No	Do you have a cough?
Yes	No	If so, do you cough up phlegm?
Yes	No	Has your cough gotten worse in the last six months?
Yes	No	Have you ever had a wheeze?
Yes	No	Have you ever coughed up blood?
Yes	No	Have you ever had rheumatic fever, high blood pressure, or heart disease?
Yes	No	Have you ever had pain, tightness or fullness in your chest?
Yes	No	Does your heart pound or skip or miss beats?
Yes	No	Do you ever have distress, pain, or shortness of breath when walking?
Yes	No	Have your ankles ever swelled?
Yes	No	Do you smoke?
Yes	No	Have you ever smoked?
Yes	No	Do you need pillows or a bolster in order to sleep?
Yes	No	Do you suffer from severe headaches or pressure in the head?
Yes	No	Do you have dizzy spells or feel faint frequently?
Yes	No	Do you have cold hands or cold feet?
Yes	No	Do you have leg cramps when walking or lying in bed?
Yes	No	Is your appetite poor?
Yes	No	Do you have trouble swallowing?
Yes	No	Do you have indigestion, heartburn, belching, or stomach pain?
Yes	No	Have you ever vomited blood?
Yes	No	Have you ever had a stomach ulcer or duodenal ulcer?
Yes	No	Have your bowel movements or habits changed recently?
Yes	No	Do you have loose bowel movements?
Yes	No	Are you constipated?
Yes	No	Have you ever had bloody or tarry (black) bowel movements or blood on the toilet tissue?
Yes	No	Do you have hemorrhoids (piles)?
Yes	No	Have you ever had yellow jaundice, liver trouble, or gallstones?
Yes	No	Were you ever anemic?
Yes	No	Do you bruise or bleed easily?
Yes	No	Do you have any pain, stiffness or swelling in any muscles or joints?
Yes	No	Do you have trouble with your back?
Yes	No	Are you bothered by itching?
Yes	No	Have you had rashes or boils?
Yes	No	Do you have numbness, tingling, or weakness in any part of your body?

Box continued on following page

BOX 4–7. **HEALTH HISTORY QUESTIONNAIRE** *Continued*

Yes	No	Were you ever unconscious or paralyzed?
Yes	No	Have you ever had fits or convulsions?
Yes	No	Are you passing urine more often than usual in the day or night?
Yes	No	Have you had bloody urine?
Yes	No	Have you had cloudy urine?
Yes	No	Have you had any pain or burning on urination?
Yes	No	Do you sometimes lose control of your bladder, especially when coughing or sneezing?
Yes	No	Were you ever treated for syphilis, gonorrhea, or another venereal disease?
Yes	No	Do you prefer warm weather to cold weather?
Yes	No	Do you prefer cold weather to warm weather?
Yes	No	Are you ever unusually hungry or thirsty?
Yes	No	Have you ever had a goiter?
Yes	No	Have you ever had any operations, broken bones, or a serious injury?
Yes	No	Have you gained more than five pounds in the last six months?
Yes	No	Have you lost more than five pounds in the last six months?
Yes	No	Have you noticed any lumps, growths, or sores?
Yes	No	Do you take medicines, laxatives, vitamins, or other pills?
Yes	No	Do you take two or more alcoholic drinks, including beer and wine, a day?
Yes	No	Have you ever had a hernia or rupture?
Yes	No	Have you ever been turned down for life insurance, employment, or the military?
Yes	No	Do you make friends easily?
Yes	No	Are you a nervous person?
Yes	No	Is it hard for you to make up your mind?
Yes	No	Do you often feel tired?
Yes	No	Do you sleep poorly?
Yes	No	Do you often feel unhappy or depressed?
Yes	No	Have you ever had a nervous breakdown?
Yes	No	Have you ever seen a psychiatrist?
Yes	No	Have you taken hard drugs?
Yes	No	Have you ever smoked marijuana?

Men Only:

Yes	No	Has there been any change in the urinary stream in starting, strength of flow, or emptying?
Yes	No	Have you ever had any discharge or bleeding from your penis?

Women Only:

Yes	No	Are you having hot flashes or flushes?
Yes	No	Date of last menstrual period? _____
		Usual number of days of period? _____
		Usual number of days between periods? _____
Yes	No	If your periods have stopped, have you had any vaginal bleeding since then?
Yes	No	Do you have any pain or discomfort with your periods, bleed between periods or too heavily with periods, or have irregular periods?
Yes	No	Have you ever had a vaginal discharge?
Yes	No	Have you ever noticed any lumps in your breasts or discharge from the nipples?
Yes	No	Are you now pregnant?
Yes	No	Have you ever been pregnant?
Yes	No	Have you ever had any trouble with any of your pregnancies?
Yes	No	Are you currently taking birth control pills?

Courtesy of Gastrointestinal Specialists, Inc.

BOX 4–8. **PATIENT FAMILY UPDATE NOTE**

---

a note about my patient . . . .

Jeffrey M. Rienhart, M.D.

patient's diagnosis _____

_____

plan of treatment _____

_____

_____

_____

_____

_____

_____

---

front office from the physician's office are, "Well, what did he say?" These words are spoken by the family members who have been patiently waiting in the outer office for the return of the loved one. The office manager should educate the physician to this situation so that it can be handled to everyone's satisfaction. If family members are not satisfied with the answers they are receiving from the patient, they will want the staff to disrupt the physician's office hours and come out to speak with them. The disruption of office hours is what all good office managers want to prevent! One way to eliminate the need for this is to provide the patient with a note specifying a brief diagnosis and treatment plan for the family to read.

Many patients bring their family members into the physician's inner office so that the physician can speak with them at the same time she or he speaks with the patient. However, if this does not occur, the use of the note can save many hassles in the course of a day. The office manager can design a note and keep a pad of these notes on the physician's desk for easy accessibility. A sample Patient Family Update Note is shown in Box 4–8.

Business Files

All filing and records of a business nature should be kept in their own file in the office manager's office. This file should come equipped with a key so that the manager can lock it every evening before leaving the office. This cabinet should probably be fireproof because of the valuable nature of its contents. Business records that should be included in this file are

- The lease or deed for the office
- The property insurance policy for the office
- The health insurance policy for employees
- Pension and profit-sharing statements and guidelines
- Financial records
- Checkbook and deposit slips
- Petty cash
- Prescription blanks
- Employee records
- The physician's on-call schedule and vacation schedule
- Equipment booklets and warranties
- Tax records
- Files containing the physician's

  Medical license
  Drug Enforcement Administration registration
  Current Continuing Medical Education certificate
  Malpractice policy
  Updated curriculum vitae
  Personal correspondence

- The office manager's personal correspondence

Miscellaneous Files

HOSPITAL RECORDS

Some offices prefer to keep their hospital records separate from the office records. This can be done by using a separate filing cabinet or by using colored folders. In other words, all hospital files would be filed in folders that are red. All hospital patients in these folders would be filed in alphabetical order.

OTHER RECORDS

A separate file can be kept for miscellaneous filing, such as patient records that come into the office before the patient. These records are filed in the miscellaneous file until the patient calls or appears for an appointment. Alternatively, some offices choose to make up a patient chart as soon as records come to the office. This way, the chart is already started when the patient comes in. One problem with this approach is that many patients do not follow their referring doctor's orders and decide to never come to see the physician. The office is then stuck with a chart of records that will not be used. It is difficult to keep track of this type of file, because of the number of patients seen in a physician's office. The office manager should assess the situation in the office and make policy as to how these records should be handled.

Shop Around

Box 4–9 lists several vendors from which the office manager can purchase the necessary supplies for the front office. There are many vendors across the country that sell the same type of product. The wise office manager contacts several to check on pricing, availability, and service before deciding on which company to deal with. Even though it might be easier to use the local office supply store, it is not always the most cost-effective. One of the office manager's main goals is to contain costs while maintaining quality care and

---

BOX 4–9. VENDORS/SUPPLIERS OF OFFICE PRODUCTS

Tab Products
1400 Page Mill Road
Palo Alto, CA 94304
(800) 672-3109

Medical Practice Management Products
United Ad Label Medical Division
650 Columbia Street
P.O. Box 2216
Brea, CA 92622
(800) 423-4643

Colwell
201 Kenyon Road
P.O. Box 9024
Champaign, IL 61826
(800) 637-1140

Medical Arts Press
P.O. Box 29200
Minneapolis, MN 55429
(800) 328-2179

Safeguard Business Systems
400 Maryland Drive
Fort Washington, PA 19036
(800) 542-2812

Bibbero Systems, Inc.
1300 North McDowell Blvd
Petaluma, CA 94952
(800) 242-2376

---

increasing profitability. The process of contacting various vendors should be done every 6 months in order to maintain cost containment measures. Most vendors have toll-free 800 numbers for customers to call. Don't hesitate to call these vendors to ask for pricing. Many will offer an additional discount to secure the business. Ask them . . . . you might be surprised by the answer!

FROM THE AUTHOR'S NOTEBOOK

If your office is located in an office building, you might want to check with other offices to see if they are interested in purchasing office supplies together. You can get a better price when buying in bulk.

References

Gerber, P., & Bijiefeld, M. "Medical Records: Make Sure Yours Are Trouble-Proof." *Physician's Management,* May 1993, pp. 57-76.
Gerber, P., & Bijiefeld, M. "The Medical Chart." *Physician's Management,* February 1992, pp. 42-51.
Gragg, E. "Filing Systems Evolve as Office Technology Advances." *The Office,* July 1993, pp. 12-14.
O'Donnell, W. "Your Patient Isn't the Only One Who Needs a Diagnosis." *Medical Economics,* May 18, 1992, pp. 119-123.

5

Health Insurance: Billing and Coding

Types of Insurance

Health insurance is one of the hottest topics of discussion these days. Even though national health care reform has been put on hold, an unprecedented wave of mergers, acquisitions, and alliances among health care providers, insurers, managed care organizations, and patients took place in 1994. The reasons for all this business activity in the health care field are spiraling medical care costs and the increasing burden of health care costs on the federal budget. As politicians struggle to find a solution to the growing health care crisis, the media reports on an almost daily basis the plight of the uninsured and the underinsured. A system that is equitable for all, as well as efficient, integrated, value-driven, and accountable, is needed. This is the challenge that will be faced in the future as the health care market continues to change and Act Two of the health reform debate begins, which it surely will.

The changes taking place in the health care industry are affecting medical offices in many ways. It is important for medical office managers to understand these trends so that they can make intelligent management decisions. Adapting to these changes as easily as possible will ensure the financial strength of the medical office. Twenty years ago, it was easy for physicians and their staff to know everything there was to know about the few available insurance companies. Today, there are countless insurance carriers, each offering more than one plan. This has created havoc in the business office of the medical practice and has made it impossible for medical office staff to know the extent of each patient's coverage unless they call each patient's insurance company and verify the patient's insurance.

The first health insurance company was founded in the mid-1800s. Now there are more than 3,000 health insurance companies in the United States, divided into six general categories:

1 Commercial insurance
2 Medicare
3 Medicaid
4 The Civilian Health and Medical Program for the Uniformed Services (CHAMPUS)
5 Managed care (health maintenance organizations [HMOs], preferred provider organizations [PPOs], and physician–hospital organizations [PHOs])
6 Blue Cross/Blue Shield

Years ago, companies covered 100% of the costs incurred due to illness or injury, and individuals received this insurance coverage in the way of a benefit from their employer. This benefit usually covered employees and their families. In most practices today, third-party payers (insurance companies) are responsible for 75% to 90% of the reimbursements. However, few insurance companies today cover the entire medical costs of a patient. In addition, there are more than 37 million people in the United States with no insurance coverage and many persons whose job provides insurance only for them, not for their families, and who must pay for insurance for their families.

Americans spend $23,000 a second on medical care, which computes to 2 billion dollars a day. Companies are finding themselves spending more on health coverage for their employees than on raw materials for their products. For instance, General Motors spent 3.2 billion dollars in 1994 for health benefits for their employees, which is more than they spent for the steel to produce their cars. Insurance payments comprise more than three-fourths of a physician's gross practice income. Understanding how the insurance system works is an important role of a medical office manager.

COMMERCIAL INSURANCE

There are many different commercial insurance companies in the United States. The following are some of them:

Aetna
Travelers
Prudential
Guardian
Metropolitan
Connecticut General

The list could go on and on. These insurance companies generally write policies for groups. Many employers use commercial insurances to provide insurance for their employees. Each employee group can have different regulations, so it is always necessary to call the number on the member's card to verify coverage and policies.

FROM THE AUTHOR'S NOTEBOOK

Many commercial insurance companies also have their own HMOs and PPOs. Be careful to check the member's card. For instance, in addition to basic commercial coverage, Prudential also offers a PPO called Prucare. Metropolitan Life offers a PPO called MetLife in addition to traditional commercial coverage.

MEDICARE

Medicare became available to older Americans in 1966 and consists of two parts: A and B. Part A Medicare covers the hospital expenses of the patient. The patient pays a deductible but does not pay a premium. Any individual who receives Social Security payments is automatically entitled to Medicare Part A. This is a benefit for senior citizens and is financed through the Social Security program. It is made up of monies provided through payroll taxes and self-employment taxes paid by all persons covered under the program. Employers are also taxed.

Part B Medicare covers 80% of outpatient and physician expenses and must be paid for by the patient in monthly payments. This part of Medicare is financed by contributions of the federal government in addition to the monthly premium paid by the patient. This is the Medicare part that the medical office deals with on a regular basis.

Many patients do not understand the difference between Medicare Part A and B. They also do not realize that they have to pay for Part B coverage. They assume that the card that is sent to them from the Social Security Administration covers all their medical needs. It is the office manager's responsibility to ensure that the medical biller in the office can adequately explain the difference between the two forms of coverage to these patients and advise them that they might want to carry some additional insurance to cover the 20% of expenses not covered by Medicare Part B. Many patients carry private supplemental insurance to pick up the 20% balance. Medicare Part B carries with it a yearly deductible of $100.00. This deductible is the patient's responsibility and must be paid by the patient every year. It is the responsibility of the office to make a serious attempt to collect this deductible; failure to do so can result in fines to the physician. Most of the supplemental insurances that patients carry do not cover the patient's deductible. A sample Medicare card is shown in Figure 5–1. It is important to note the difference on the card between hospital coverage (Part A) and medical coverage (Part B).

MEDICAID

In 1965, the federal government, in association with the individual state governments, established a health care coverage known as Medicaid. This insurance covers some of the costs of medical care and medicines for medically indigent individuals. There are guidelines that must be met to qualify for this insurance, and individu-

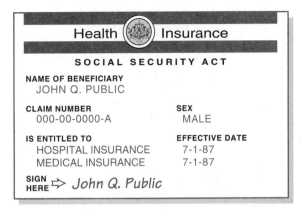

FIGURE 5–1. Sample Medicare card. (From Kinn, M.E. *Administrative Medical Assistant,* 3rd ed. Philadelphia: W. B. Saunders Company, 1993.)

als admitted to hospitals with no insurance benefits usually qualify for this service. Applications are made through the admissions office at the hospital in an attempt to aid the individual in their care. Medicaid is the fastest growing spending program in this country today. They spent $158 billion dollars in 1991 to cover the 27.3 million medically indigent people in our country.

CHAMPUS

In 1956, CHAMPUS was created to cover the medical needs of military personnel and their families. This insurance covered the fees of civilian physicians to treat any illness or injury of military dependents.

MANAGED CARE (HMOs, PPOs, AND PHOs)

In 1973, the HMO was created as the first managed care insurance concept. HMOs consist of members, who prepay for health insurance benefits. Most HMOs require a minimal payment at the time of service. This minimal payment ranges from $2 to $10, depending on the organization and the plan. HMOs require that their patients see a primary physician before setting up an appointment with a specialist. These primary physicians (called "gatekeepers") must authorize any referrals for testing or specialists. Their patients must *always* obtain a referral before seeing a specialist or seeking a test. A set fee is then paid to the physician for services rendered, and any balance must be written off.

A PPO is a group of hospitals, physicians, and/or pharmacies that contracts on a discounted fee-for-service basis with employers, insurance carriers, or third-party administrators. PPOs provide services to

---

BOX 5–1. RELEASE FORM TO BE SIGNED BY HMO OR PPO MEMBER WHO ARRIVES AT THE SPECIALIST'S OFFICE WITHOUT A REFERRAL FROM A PRIMARY PHYSICIAN

Date: _____

Name: _____

I understand that if I am not able to obtain a referral for this visit, I will be responsible for payment.

I also understand that I have two (2) weeks from this date to obtain this referral.

Signature: _____

---

subscribers at 10% to 20% below usual fees. A PHO is a legal entity that combines physicians and hospitals into a single organization for the purpose of obtaining payer contracts. In a PHO, the physicians remain owners of their practices, but they accept managed care patients under the terms of the contract.

HMOs and PPOs treated more than 40 million Americans last year, at a cost of 17% less than the traditional commercial insurance carrier. Any physician's office has the right to refuse treatment to an HMO or PPO member who arrives without a referral in hand. Many primary physician offices will not backdate a referral and they will tell a specialist's office to turn the patient away until the patient obtains a referral from them. A specialist who decides to treat a patient who does not have a referral would be wise to have the patient sign a release stating that if the patient cannot obtain a referral within one week, she or he will be responsible for this bill (Box 5–1). The patient may be billed only if she or he signs this release. Otherwise, the office, as a participating HMO/PPO office, cannot bill the patient for the service.

It is important for the medical office manager to check with each individual HMO and PPO to clearly understand its rules and regulations. Some plans allow the physician's office to bill the patient if she or he does not produce a referral. Some allow the office to bill the patient only if it has obtained the aforementioned signed release from the patient. The letter shown in Box 5–2 can be used in follow-up to the patient. In an attempt to avoid referral problems, the medical office staff can give each patient who has managed care insurance a letter explaining office policy on payment (Box 5–3).

BLUE CROSS / BLUE SHIELD

Blue Cross was established in the 1930s to cover the care of the patient in the hospital setting. In 1939, its sister coverage, Blue Shield, was established to cover physician and outpatient services. These insurance companies provide medical insurance under several different plans. Some plans are designed for patients with income limits, and others make the patient responsible for a small balance. If the physician's office is a participating office in Blue Cross/Blue Shield, any balance above the approved amount must be written off. Nonparticipating physicians are allowed to bill the patient for the balance.

FROM THE AUTHOR'S NOTEBOOK

Never attempt to guess which Blue Shield plan a patient has. There are many regional and local plans that have different requirements. Always look at the member's card and call the patient if there is any question as to which plan she or he belongs.

The Components of Insurance Coverage

MEDICAL

Medical insurance coverage pays the cost of services performed by a physician or outpatient service. Outpatient services can be performed in an independent facility, the physician's office, or the hospital. These services can be office visits, x-ray exams, laboratory tests, and physical therapy. Many plans will require second opinions, and the insurance company should always be notified before further treatment is given.

SURGICAL

Surgical insurance coverage pays the surgeon's fees for any surgical procedure that the patient might require, such as an appendectomy, resetting of a fractured bone, removal of a gangrenous limb, etc. Some plans require precertification on certain procedures. The medical office should call each insurance company to check on its rules.

HOSPITALIZATION

Hospitalization insurance coverage pays the costs incurred in a hospital setting. These are costs for room and board, pharmaceutical supplies, and medical supplies used by patients during their stay. Some plans have limitations on the number of days they cover. Each insurance plan is different and must be checked by the medical office before it admits a patient to the hospital.

MAJOR MEDICAL

Major medical coverage protects the patient from catastrophic medical bills. It is a supplement to the medical and surgical coverages and pays the balances for services rendered. This type of coverage keeps the patient's out-of-pocket expenses down.

PRECERTIFICATION / SECOND OPINION

Many insurance carriers require precertification of hospitalization and of certain procedures. The patient's insurance card generally spells out the type of plan the patient is carrying. It advises as to whether the patient is responsible for a co-pay, whether the plan calls for a second opinion, and whether the patient must obtain precertification. To save time on insurance billing, photocopy the front and back of the patient's insurance card and place the photocopy in the patient's chart or on the back of the patient's ledger card, if that is the type of system you are using. Many times, the physician will

---

BOX 5–2. **LETTER TO SEND TO UNREFERRED HMO OR PPO MEMBER REQUESTING PAYMENT FOR SERVICES**

March 24, 1993

Dear _____

Our records indicate that we have not yet received your promised referral. As you know, you must always obtain a referral from your primary physician before scheduling an appointment with our office.

According to your insurance plan, if you do not obtain a referral from your primary physician before coming to our office, it is then your responsibility to either obtain a referral within 10 days of your visit or pay for the visit yourself.

We have waited patiently for your referral to arrive in our mail, but, as of yet, we have not received it.

This bill is now your responsibility, and we expect payment of $ _____ in the mail to our office as soon as possible. Failure to pay will result in a transfer of your account to our collection agency.

Sincerely,

Jean Goralski
Office Manager

BOX 5–3. LETTER EXPLAINING OFFICE POLICY ON REFERRALS

To Our HMO Patients:

Your insurance company requires that when you are seeking care from a specialist's office, such as ours, you must first obtain a referral from your primary physician. You need to have this referral with you when you arrive at the specialist's office.

These referrals are essential to facilitate our billing process, and without them we cannot complete that process. Many of our patients forget to bring their referrals with them at the time of their visit, and this presents a problem. Most insurance companies are very strict regarding their policies and procedures, and many times they will not allow referrals to be backdated or to be issued after the time of the office visit.

We request that you help us to avoid this problem by remembering that referrals are required. Regrettably, we will have to reschedule your office visit if these forms are not presented to our receptionist at your time of check in.

We appreciate your cooperation in this matter, and if you have any questions regarding this letter, please feel free to contact our billing department located at our _____ office at _____ .
We would also like to take this opportunity to let you know that your business is greatly appreciated, and our staff enjoys working with you on your road to recovery and superior health.

Sincerely,

Carl Fortana

Billing Manager

FROM THE AUTHOR'S NOTEBOOK

When you are dealing with various different insurances, you might want to color-code either the patient chart or the file card. Using different colors for each insurance will help you easily keep track of all the plans.

instruct the office to admit to the hospital a patient who is not in the office at that time. This can be done quickly and efficiently if the photocopy of the card is in the office. The office personnel can easily check on eligibility and the need for precertification without having to have the patient there. If the plan requires either precertification or a second opinion and the physician's office does not obtain this, the physician will not be paid for her or his services. When calling the insurance company to obtain precertification, have available the following information:

- Patient demographics
- Treatment plan
- Signs
- Symptoms
- Diagnosis

"Superbills"

Many patients that a physician's office sees have to pay for their office visit and then bill their major medical insurance provider. To make this billing easier for the patient, the office should develop a "superbill" that lists the codes for all the procedures and services that the practice offers, with the specific ones performed for the patient checked off. The superbill is sent home with the patient. Some offices even print their most common diagnosis codes on these bills. The superbill should contain all the information required by the Physician's Information part of the insurance form. It should also list the following information about the practice:

- The name of the medical practice
- The address of the medical practice
- The telephone and fax numbers of the practice
- The physician's license number
- A space for the number assigned to the physician by the provider
- The practice's tax identification number
- The names of facilities where services may be performed

All superbills should be filed in the patient's chart or filed in an accordion file alphabetically. The latter is the best way to keep superbills. Make sure the date the claim is submitted is written somewhere on the superbill for easier tracking.

Computerized superbills are now available and are invaluable to a medical office. The superbill is compiled as before, with the exception of the way in which it is marked. It cannot be checked off or circled. A number two pencil must be used to blacken or fill in the designated circles. This form is then folded in half and fed through a scanner. The scanner is a small unit (approximately 4″ × 5″ that sits on the desk). Within 4 seconds, the information is scanned into the patient charge screen of the computer and any co-pay or deductible is then printed on the screen in front of the employee. By using this software and computerized superbill, the information is in the computer and ready for billing the same day. There are no possibilities of keystroke errors since the form is being scanned. This eliminates excessive data entry workloads and delays due to the time involved in entry of the information.

The Office Manager and Insurance Claim Submissions

The physician will probably expect the office manager to report to her or him on insurance submissions on a weekly basis. Some offices prefer to do this on a monthly basis. The office manager can keep a record of the total number of claims, and the total dollar amount of the claims, that were submitted to each payer. It would be helpful to separate these figures by the account class, in other words, by the various insurance groupings. An example is

- all Medicare claims together
- all HMO/PPO claims together
- all Blue Shield claims together

This record can be completed on a weekly basis and handed to the physician at scheduled meeting dates. This will give the physician an idea of the amount of services and billings that was generated that particular week.

Insurance submissions should be done on a daily basis. Many practices make the mistake of submitting them once a week. This causes unnecessary delays in turnaround times, and, depending on whether they are paper or paperless claims, the time required to submit a week's worth of claims together can be excessive. A medium to large practice can submit electronic claims to Medicare, Medicaid, Blue Shield, and HMOs/PPOs and paper claims to commercial insurance companies in approximately 1 hour. This can be done during the last 2 hours of the day and can be finished easily before the end-of-the-day backup has to be done. This system creates a flow of payments and shortens the turnaround time.

Patients and Their Insurance

Patients generally think they have total medical coverage, no matter what the problem. It is a rude awakening for many patients when they are told they are not covered for certain services or that they have a $500 deductible that must be met. Most patients do not take the time to read their insurance booklets and therefore have limited knowledge of their coverage. By asking to see their insurance card each time they visit, staff can clear up many problems before patients are seen by the physician. For instance, if they pay a co-insurance, it should be collected when they register at the front desk. Much of dealing with patients and their insurance involves patient education. Once patients understand the policy of the office, collecting deductibles and co-payments and obtaining referrals will become easier.

The *Patient Information Handbook* will come in handy for explaining office procedures involving fees and billing. The Insurance Verification Form that follows is another way of clarifying patients' insurance coverage while they are in the office. A letter giving patients instructions regarding insurance matters can also be helpful to some practices (Box 5–4). The letter may be handed to new patients when they arrive at the office. It is a warmer and more personal approach than the Insurance Verification Form. Many patients prefer this kind of personalized service.

FROM THE AUTHOR'S NOTEBOOK

Remember to get all the necessary insurance information from the patient during the office visit. It will save a lot of time later.

Coding

Medicare is most medical offices' largest source of income and the cause of their worst headaches. Trying to comply with all the new Medicare rules and regulations is not only confusing, but vexing. It is important that the office staff understand the new codes so that the office can maximize its reimbursement in a way that is not only fair, but profitable. Staff must be well acquainted with the *Physicians' Current Procedural Terminology (CPT)* and *International Classification of Diseases,*

BOX 5–4. LETTER EXPLAINING THE OFFICE'S INSURANCE BILLING POLICY TO PATIENTS

To All Our Patients:

We welcome you as a new patient to our office and are happy to extend to you every possible courtesy. To avoid billing and insurance problems, we would like to acquaint you with our office procedures. Service should be paid for when rendered. If for some reason this is not possible, please discuss other arrangements with me.

If you have health insurance, please read your policy so you know your coverage. Policies vary: some cover hospital care only, and others cover both office care and hospital care. Be sure to leave the name of your insurance company and your policy number and indicate which spouse is the insured or primary holder. If you change insurance companies, please NOTIFY OUR OFFICE AT ONCE.

Your insurance form is prepared by both of us. Each insurance form has a "patient side," which you must complete and sign. The copy of the receipt you receive from our office is all you need to bill your insurance. Attach our form to yours and mail both to your insurance company. A check will be mailed directly to you. I suggest that you note the date of mailing, so that you are able to follow-up if necessary. Always make copies of everything you send to your insurance company. This will save everyone time and aggravation if the claim is lost.

If you have insurance, who is responsible for your bill? Health insurance is designed to help you meet the cost of medical services. In most cases, it is not geared to pay the total fees. Your insurance contract defines your coverage. There is no contract between the company and your doctor. Therefore, the basic responsibility is yours. We would appreciate it if you pay your bill promptly, without waiting to "see what the insurance will pay," because our fees are not related to insurance coverage. Our office is interested in making you as comfortable as possible during your visits. Please feel free to call upon me for further information.

Sincerely,

Jane Doe

Office Manager

Ninth Revision, Clinical Modification (ICD-9-CM) codebooks. It is important to hire billing clerks who have experience with insurance billing and third-party regulations. Staff may know how to fill out the forms and where to send them, but do they really understand and use the information in the Explanation of Benefits that they receive from Medicare and other third-party payers? Given the complexity of the new Medicare regulations and the changing codes and fee structures, staff ignorance in this area is more of a threat to the livelihood of the medical office than it has ever been.

FROM THE AUTHOR'S NOTEBOOK

Many courses and workshops on coding are available to medical offices. They may last anywhere from 1 day to 3 days and can be very helpful in answering the everyday questions that arise. In addition, coding tips may be picked up from personnel from other offices present at the workshop.

Many publications are available to help a medical office keep informed of the various changes in the reimbursement area. It is important for the office manager to keep up with changes as they take place. The physician's specialty society will often send newsletters and publications that may also provide news of changes and requirements.

ICD-9-CM CODEBOOK

The ICD-9-CM diagnosis coding system has its roots in a bunch of statistical studies of diseases called "The London Bills Mortality" published in England in the seventeenth century. By 1937, these statistics had evolved into the manuscript called the *International List of Causes of Death*. Many more revisions of this list were made after this point, and eventually this work became the *International Classification of Causes of Death*. The World Health Organization (WHO) used this information in 1948, when it published its morbidity and mortality lists. These lists were revised many times over and finally became the *International Classification of Diseases (ICD)*.

In 1978, the WHO published its ninth revision of this list, and, at this point, this listing became internationally

known as the *ICD-9*. Once the *ICD-9* became recognized internationally, the U.S. National Center for Health Statistics (NCHS) addressed the need for a more precise clinical picture for its statistics. It added clinical information to the *ICD-9,* and thus the *ICD-9-CM* was born. In 1988, Congress passed the Medicare Catastrophic Coverage Act, which mandated the use of *ICD-9-CM* codes on all physician-submitted Part B claims. This system translates written medical terminology into numeric and alphanumeric codes. The *ICD-9-CM* codebook is published every year and consists of three volumes. Volume 1 contains the most specific information about diseases, symptoms, injuries, and conditions. It consists of code numbers presented in numerical order. Beside each code number is a diagnosis. In addition, each code is broken down into subcodes representing particular variations of that diagnosis. Volume 3 contains procedural information reserved for hospital use. Volume 2 is an alphabetical list of the diseases, symptoms, injuries, and conditions described in Volume 1 and their codes and is divided into three sections:

Section 1: Index to Diseases and Injuries
Section 2: Table of Drugs and Chemicals
Section 3: Alphabetic Index to External Causes of Injuries and Poisonings

Therefore, to code a diagnosis using the *ICD-9-CM,* you first use Volume 2 to find the diagnosis alphabetically. Beside the diagnosis will be a numerical code. You then look up that numerical code in Volume 1 to see the subcodes of that code and choose the specific subcode that represents the most specific diagnosis for the condition.

MANAGER'S ALERT

Try not to use any code in the *ICD-9-CM* codebook that has NEC after it. NEC means "not elsewhere classifiable" and indicates that the code should be used only when there is no alternative.

The service that was provided to the patient should correlate with the diagnosis code specified on the claim. Insurance companies reject claims in which the *CPT* service code specified does not match the *ICD-9-CM* diagnosis code specified. For instance, if a diabetic patient was seen in the office for a sore throat, it would be incorrect to use the diagnosis code of diabetes. Although the patient is a diabetic, the services she or he received on that particular day were for a sore throat and unrelated to the diabetes.

The *ICD-9-CM* disease codes are extremely precise and generally require some medical knowledge to understand them. Many medical office staff do not have the clinical background to be able to select the correct code for a particular claim. Regular staff meetings and explanations by the physicians will assist in the training of these staff members. It is best to involve the physician in this part of the billing process and ask for a diagnosis code for each patient. This will reduce incorrect diagnosis codings on claims.

FROM THE AUTHOR'S NOTEBOOK

Have the physician check each superbill or fee slip before the bill is sent. This will ensure that the bill is correct before it is sent.

Steps in Coding Using the ICD-9-CM Codebook

1 Identify the main diagnosis from the physician.
2 Secure any secondary diagnoses if available.
3 Choose the appropriate modifier if needed.
4 Locate the diagnosis in Volume 2.
5 Assign the diagnosis a tentative code.
6 Cross-reference the code in Volume 1 for specificity.

MANAGER'S ALERT

Be sure to code the diagnosis to the greatest level of specificity. Otherwise, the claim will be rejected. Be sure to note if it requires a fourth or fifth digit!

V Codes

V codes are *ICD-9-CM* to describe patients who are not ill but are seeking a specific health service, such as a screening, that could influence their health or have a special circumstance that could influence their health.

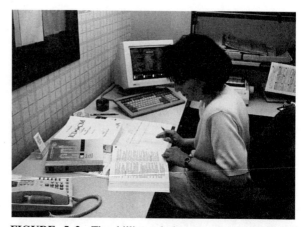

FIGURE 5–2. The billing clerk uses the *International Classification of Diseases, Ninth Revision, Clinical Modification* and *Physicians' Current Procedural Terminology* codebooks on a daily basis.

These codes are used in place of "rule out," which is no longer approved for coding. Examples of such services and circumstances are

- Measles vaccination
- Tissue or blood donation
- Follow-up visits
- Pregnancy
- History of colon cancer
- Annual pap smear
- Family history of hypertension
- Ruling out a gastrointestinal bleeder

E Codes

E codes are used to classify environmental events, circumstances, and conditions as the cause of injury, poisoning, and other adverse effects. Examples of E codes are

E 865.1 Accidental poisoning from shellfish
E 881.0 Fall from ladder
E 906.0 Dog bite
E 917.0 Struck by thrown ball

CPT CODEBOOK

The *CPT* codebook (Figure 5–2) is released on a yearly basis, with updates on coding and terminology provided throughout the year. This book contains all the codes necessary to report the services performed by a physician and was created in 1966 by the American Medical Association. This book's 400 pages are broken down by body part, itemizing the different services that can be provided by a physician. There is a five-digit numerical code for each service. This numerical code is the important part of submitting a claim for insurance reimbursement. If the office does not use the correct code, the claim will be either rejected or delayed in the carrier's processing department. Either way, the claim will be delayed, and reimbursement will be late arriving at the office. This can be a problem in offices that have no claim tracking system in place. If the office does not pursue a rejected claim, the payment may never be made.

FROM THE AUTHOR'S NOTEBOOK

Trying to contain costs by not buying the new *CPT* manual every year is a dangerous practice. Codes change and become deleted, and new codes are added every year! Make it a policy to order the new *CPT* manual every fall.

The specifics of the *CPT* codes should be carefully studied so that the physician and medical biller will recognize any changes in them from year to year. The *CPT* codebook is a must for the medical office and can be obtained from the American Medical Association. The address is

American Medical Association
Order Department
515 North State Street
Chicago, IL 60610

Magnetic computer tape and disk may also be purchased from the American Medical Association at the above address.

Choosing an Evaluation and Management Code

A methodical and logical thought process should be followed when attempting to choose the correct evaluation and management code. Following three simple steps will make the selection of an evaluation and management code less painful.

Step 1: Select a group of codes by determining
  1) The place of service
     a) Office
     b) Hospital
     c) Emergency room
     d) Nursing home
     e) Rest home
     f) Private home
  2) The type of patient
     a) Established patient
     b) New patient—haven't seen the patient for at least 3 years (if group practice, no one in group has seen the patient in the last 3 years)
  3) Whether the visit was a visit or a consult
     a) Consult—visit was requested by another physician
     b) Confirmatory consult—visit provided only advice or opinion
     c) Visit—face-to-face evaluation and management of the patient
Step 2: Analyze the level of service provided by using three key components:
  1) The history taking
     a) Problem focused
     b) Expanded problem focused
     c) Detailed or comprehensive
  2) The examination
     a) Problem focused
     b) Expanded problem focused
     c) Detailed or comprehensive
  3) The decision making
     a) Straightforward
     b) Low complexity
     c) Moderate complexity
     d) High complexity
Step 3: Choose the specific code by checking the level of service against the code listings in the *CPT* manual.

New Uniform Content Descriptors for Evaluation and Management Codes

The new content descriptors are uniform in describing each level of service for the evaluation and management codes. These descriptors contain seven components:

1 History
2 Examination
3 Medical decision making
4 Counseling
5 Coordination of care
6 Presentation of the problem
7 Time

History, examination, and medical decision making are

the key components in selecting a level of evaluation and management service. Counseling and coordination of care are not required in every patient visit. The time component is intended to assist physicians in selecting the most appropriate level of evaluation and management code. The designated uniform content descriptors for at least two, and sometimes three, key components must be used when selecting an evaluation and management code.

Definitions of the Uniform Content Descriptor

History

The evaluation and management codes consist of four types of history:

problem focused—*brief* history of present illness or problem; chief complaint

expanded problem focused—*brief* history of present illness or problem; chief complaint; problem-pertinent system review

detailed—*extended* history of present illness or problem; chief complaint; extended system review; *pertinent* past, family, and social history

comprehensive—*extended* history of present illness or problem; chief complaint; complete system review; *complete* past, family, and social history

Examination

The evaluation and management codes consist of four types of examination:

Problem focused—examination that is limited to the affected body part

Expanded problem focused—examination of the affected body part and other symptomatic or related organ systems

Detailed—extended examination of the affected body part(s) and other symptomatic or related organ systems

Comprehensive—complete single-system specialty examination or complete multisystem examination

Medical Decision Making

The complexity of establishing a diagnosis or management option is the main component of medical decision making and is measured by all of the following:

- The number of possible diagnoses or the number of management options that must be considered
- The amount or complexity of medical records; diagnostic tests; or other information that must be obtained, reviewed, and analyzed
- The risk of significant complications and/or morbidity associated with the presented problems, the diagnostic procedures, and the possible management options

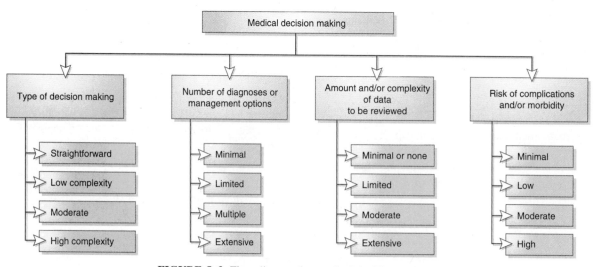

FIGURE 5–3. Flow diagram for medical decision making.

There are four types of medical decision making. For a decision to fit into one of the categories, it must meet two or three of the criteria in the category. Figure 5–3 will help you choose the proper type of decision making for each situation.

Counseling

Counseling consists of any conversation or discussion with the patient or family concerning one or more of the following areas:

- Diagnostic results and/or studies
- Prognosis
- Risks and benefits of management options
- Instructions for management or follow-up
- Importance of compliance with management option
- Risk factor reduction
- Education of patient and family

Presentation of the Problem

The *presenting problem* is the disease, condition, injury, symptom, sign, illness, complaint, or any other reason for the patient visit, with or without the diagnosis's being established at the time of the visit. There are five types of presenting problems:

Minimal—a problem that may not require the presence of the physician but is treated under her or his supervision

Self-limited or minor—a problem that runs a definite course, is transient, and is not likely to change the patient's general health permanently or has a good prognosis with management

Low severity—a problem with a low risk of morbidity without treatment, little or no risk of mortality without treatment, and full recovery without physical impairment

Moderate severity—a problem with moderate risk of morbidity without treatment, moderate risk of

mortality without treatment, and a prognosis of increased probability of physical impairment

high severity—a problem with a high risk of morbidity without treatment, a moderate to high risk of mortality without treatment, and a high probability of severe physical impairment

Time

The specific times expressed in the visit codes are averages and represent a range of times that vary with each clinical situation. The time devoted to counseling and coordination of care must be documented in the medical record. This documentation must include the actual time spent with the patient. During a hospital visit, time spent conferring with the nurses, reviewing the chart, and discussing the case with the care team can be included in the time documentation. On an outpatient basis, the time code must refer to face-to-face contact between the physician and the patient.

FROM THE AUTHOR'S NOTEBOOK

When counseling and coordination of care dominate more than 50% of the face-to-face physician–patient encounter, time is considered the key or controlling factor in selecting the level of evaluation and management code.

Documentation Required for Evaluation and Management Codes

The *CPT* evaluation and management codes were designed to classify the work of the physicians and require far more clinical documentation than the old visit codes. This documentation must include that a service was actually performed at the level that was reported and was medically necessary. In the evaluation and management system of coding, a new patient is defined as any patient who has not been seen by the physician or anyone in her or his group in the past 3 years. The three key components—history, examination, and medical decision making—and the nature of the presenting problem must be documented in the new patient's record. An established patient is a patient who has been seen by the physician or one of the members of her or his group during the past 3 years. Two of the three key components and the nature of the presenting

FROM THE AUTHOR'S NOTEBOOK

When physicians are covering hospital rounds for other physicians, they must code their visits as if the patient was already an established patient of theirs. They cannot use a new-patient code. They also cannot use an initial-visit code; they must use a hospital-subsequent-visit code.

problem must be documented in the established patient's medical record.

One area of grave misunderstanding is the consultation. One must be careful to differentiate between a consult and a visit when coding. The medical records must contain the following to justify a consultation code:

- The request for the consultation
- The consultant's opinion
- The services that were ordered or performed

FROM THE AUTHOR'S NOTEBOOK

A referral from another physician is not the same thing as a consult. A visit is not a consultation unless the office sends a written report back to the requesting physician. The words used in the documentation of a consultation MUST NOT include any form of the word "referral." This word, when used, indicates a "transfer of care," which is not a consultation.

FROM THE AUTHOR'S NOTEBOOK

Medicare reserves the right to downgrade the code if the consultation does not read as an opinion. Thus the wording the physician uses when writing the consultation report is extremely important. She or he must be sure to write "I recommend that text x should be done," instead of writing an order for the test. When the consultant *orders* the test, she or he is no longer considered a consultant, and the reimbursement may be lowered.

Proper documentation can mean the difference between downcoding and receiving the fee for the code billed for. During an audit, the office manager and the physician will come to realize the critical importance of proper documentation. Proper documentation is also helpful with liability. Staff should use a variety of codes when billing and carefully examine each visit to establish the proper code for it. This will require that the office manager have a conference with the physician to explain fully to her or him the evaluation and manage-

ment coding system. If the physician constantly uses the same codes for office visits, for example, this will raise a flag during processing and will automatically pinpoint the physician for an audit. The Health Care Financing Administration (HCFA) considers a practice's first year of using this system as a year of education. During the first year, constructive criticism in the form of letters and bulletins is sent to all physician offices advising them of errors in their coding. Once the HCFA feels the physician has had ample time to get aquainted with the system, fines will be levied and auditing will be conducted without hesitation.

From the professional liability standpoint, clear and concise medical records will often prevent an attorney from filing a claim. Any and every complication and unusual occurrence should be documented. Any issues that arise from a patient's family members should be documented. Noncompliance, informed consent, telephone calls, prescription renewals, etc. should be documented. In this era of cost-conscious health care, there is an increasing emphasis on documentation and quality of care. Keep this in mind: if you don't document it, you didn't do it! Box 5–5 provides documentation guidelines that will assist in accurate documentation of services provided. Failure to document services provided may affect the practice in a way that other practices have been affected—seeing themselves in the headlines (Figure 5–4)! A list of patient billing abuses commonly found by Medicare auditors is presented in Box 5–6. Is your office guilty of any of them?

FROM THE AUTHOR'S NOTEBOOK

Type the various categories and descriptor definitions on a 3×5 card and have it laminated for durability. The card will easily fit into the coat pocket of the physician, so that she or he can refer to it when coding patient visits.

MANAGER'S ALERT

Physicians who consistently use higher codes than their colleagues will definitely hear from their carriers. Abusers will face fines.

BOX 5–5. GUIDELINES FOR DOCUMENTATION THAT SUPPORTS HIGHER LEVELS OF SERVICE

Relevant Diagnoses, Symptoms, and Conditions

When these affect the medical decision making, document them! The guidelines relate to *possible* diagnoses. For example, a patient with chest pain could have a number of possible diagnoses—myocardial infarction, angina, pneumonia, rib fracture, etc. It often helps to list some of the things you have to rule out, even if the final diagnosis is indigestion.

Treatment Options

If a patient has shoulder pain, document the treatment that you considered: medications, hot packs, exercise, joint injections, etc.

Test Results Reviewed (or To Be Reviewed)

Document all test results that you reviewed: laboratory tests, x-rays, electrocardiograms, etc. It is a good idea to initial each result after reviewing it. If you order additional studies based on the results that you reviewed, write them down on the chart.

Consulting the *Physician's Desk Reference (PDR)*

Document when you look up medications in the *PDR* or search a database for information.

If Another Physician Is Called

Document all calls to other physicians, the radiologist, the cardiologist, etc.

Past Medical Records

If you reviewed past medical records from a hospital or another physician, document this.

Communication with Family

Document any conversations with nursing home personnel, family members, etc., regarding the care and medical decision making for the patient.

Risk Factors

Document any risk factors or multiple symptoms that justify a higher level of service.

Statements To Avoid

Avoid using phrases such as "Patient feels fine," "Patient has no complaints today," and "No change."

Medical Necessity

Medical necessity for all diagnostic tests should be clear. Indications include symptoms, monitoring of drug therapy, follow-up of abnormal test result, toxicity to certain medications.

Family and Social History

Both the family history and the social history must be included in notes to support a Level 4 or 5 visit.

Review of Systems

Document the review of systems well. Document even normal findings.

Choosing a Surgery Code

Major Surgery

The initial evaluation by a surgeon is not included in the global surgery package. The initial evaluation or consultation may be billed for separately. The "global payment" is a "package payment" that the physician receives that encompasses several services and charges, including

- Preoperative visits
- Postoperative visits
- Complications after surgical procedures
- Intraoperative services
- Postoperative pain control
- Medical supplies
- Miscellaneous services

Preoperative visits include the visits 1 day before surgery. Postoperative visits include all visits within 90 days of the surgery. A postoperative visit for an unrelated problem does not fall into this category. If the patient is seen for an unrelated problem that requires an additional and separate course of treatment, the visit is billed for separately. Any complication that arises from the surgery that does not require an additional trip to the operating room is included in the global package. Any additional intraoperative services that are usually necessary and part of the original procedure are included in the global fee. Postoperative pain control is included in the postoperative visits and cannot be billed for separately. All medical supplies with the exception of tray fees are included in the original service. Surgical tray fees can be billed for separately. Any miscellaneous treatment, such as suture or staple removal, wound care, catheters, intravenous solutions, and removal of naso-gastric and tracheostomy tubes, generally qualifies for the billing of a surgical tray fee.

Minor Surgery and Endoscopy

Minor surgeries and endoscopies are also tied into global fees. The global payment for these procedures includes

- Patient visits
- Postoperative visits
- Minor surgery
- Endoscopies

Patient visits on the same day as the surgical procedure are always included in the global payment, whether they are on an outpatient or inpatient basis. For minor

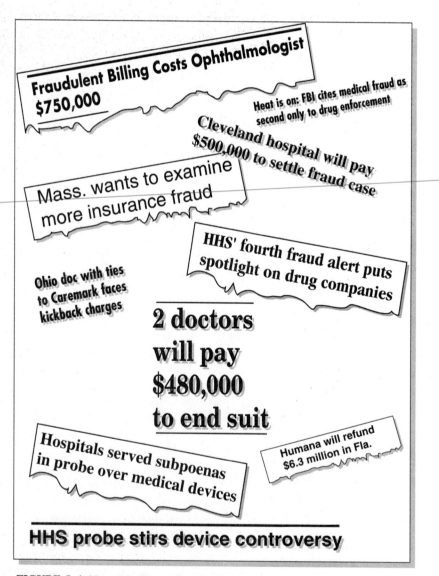

FIGURE 5–4. News headlines reflect the importance of documentation of services.

BOX 5–6. MEDICARE ABUSE HIT LIST

Anesthesia—standby anesthesia services (most often done in ophthalmology)

Ambulatory surgery centers

Cataract surgery—excessive preoperative visual acuity services

Coding—excessive use of higher level codes, such as billing for all comprehensive visits

Colonoscopy—billing for this service when medical documentation does not support the indication for a colonoscopy

Consultations—billing for consultations on established patients, for minor diagnoses that do not support this level of service, and when referral is from the same specialty

Cryosurgery—excessive coding of the lesion as 3 cm (the size of the freeze area) when the lesion is much smaller

Cystoscopy—billing separately from other endoscopic procedures

D&C—billing on same date as hysterectomy or other certain pelvic surgeries

Endoscopy—performing this procedure instead of less costly studies, such as x-ray studies

Facelifts—billing as removal of fatty tumors

Keratosis—excessive billing for removal of sebaceous keratosis

Laboratory tests—billing for excessive repetition of tests when results are normal

Lesions—billing for excision of physically impossible lesions, that is, those that are too large to be removed in a physician's office

Office visits—upcoding; overutilization billing, particularly when services rendered were deemed not medically necessary

Urine culture and sensitivity—unnecessary billing for follow-up care

Courtesy of United Communications Part B Answer Book.

surgery, the postoperative days vary from 1 to 10 days, based on the procedure. The Federal Register contains all of the information necessary for the office manager to check the procedures that apply to the physician's specialty.

Modifiers to CPT Codes

A modifier is a numerical or an alpha character that is added to a *CPT* code to indicate that the service or procedure was altered for that specific circumstance. The modifier does not change the definition of the *CPT* code reported. Modifiers may be used to report

- An unusual event
- That only part of a service was performed
- That the service was only a technical, not professional, component of a procedure (for example, the taking of an x-ray is the technical component but the intrepreting of an x-ray is the professional component)
- That the service was increased
- That the service was decreased
- That the service had to be performed more than once
- That the service had to be performed by more than one physician

The following are modifiers that can be used to explain services further:

–20 Microsurgery

The services performed required microsurgery, requiring the use of a microscope. This modifier cannot be used when the physician is using a magnifying surgical loop attached to a headband or glasses. This modifier has no effect on payment.

–21 Prolonged Evaluation and Management Service

The services provided were prolonged or greater than those usually required for the highest level of evaluation and management within a given category. This modifier can be used only with the highest level of care for that category. It has no effect on payment.

–22 Unusual Procedural Service

The services provided were greater than usually required for the procedure reported. Use of this modifier may result in an increased payment if the claim has sufficient documentation attached. This can be accomplished by attaching a copy of the operative note to the claim.

–23 Unusual Anesthesia

The services required general anesthesia, as opposed to usually not requiring any anesthesia or just local anesthesia.

−24 Unrelated Evaluation and Management Service

The services required an additional unrelated service by the same physician during the postoperative period. This modifier can be used only on an evaluation and management code. It has no effect on payment.

−25 Significant, Separate Evaluation and Management Service

The services required a significant, separately identifiable evaluation and management service above and beyond the usual care associated with that service. This modifier can be used only on an evaluation and management code. It has no effect on payment.

−26 Professional Component

Certain procedures performed are a combination of a physician component and a technical component. This modifier is used when only the physician component is being reported. Use of this modifier can affect payment. The fee schedule contains various different payment amounts for professional components.

−32 Mandated Services

The services related to a mandated consultation and/or related service. This has no effect on payment.

−47 Anesthesia by Surgeon

Regional or general anesthesia was provided by the surgeon. This modifier is not covered by Medicare.

−50 Bilateral Procedure

Unless otherwise identified, bilateral procedures performed during the same operative session should be billed by reporting the first procedure with its five-digit code and then reporting the second procedure using the modifier. Payment on this modifier is based on 150% (200% for radiology) of the fee schedule payment amount. This modifier can be used only on certain codes.

−51 Multiple Procedures

When multiple procedures were performed on the same day or at the same session, the major procedure should be reported using the five-digit code. The second procedure is then reported using the modifier. Payment is adjusted for multiple surgeries according to standard percentages (100% for the highest fee schedule allowable, 50% for the second highest, and 25% for the third through fifth highest). Special rules apply to dermatologic, endoscopic, and anesthetic procedures.

−52 Reduced Services

The service performed was either partially reduced or eliminated at the surgeon's request. For exams that are considered global, use of this modifier will not affect payment. For other situations, such as aborted procedures, a reduction in payment may be made. Documentation explaining the reduction should accompany the claim.

−54 Surgical Care Only

One physician performed the surgery, and another provided preoperative and/or postoperative care. Payment is limited to the allotted time spent on preoperative and intraoperative services only.

−55 Postoperative Management Only

One physician performed only the postoperative care, and another surgeon performed the surgery. Payment is limited to the allotted amount of postoperative care only.

−56 Preoperative Management Only

One physician performed only the preoperative care, and another surgeon performed the surgery. Payment is included in the payment allowed for surgery. Do not use this modifier with Medicare claims.

−62 Two Surgeons

The skills of two surgeons were required. Use this modifier when reporting both surgeons' procedures. This modifier will usually increase payment by 25%, split equally between the two surgeons. Documentation of the necessity of both surgeons must accompany claim.

−66 Surgical Team

A team of physicians was required to perform a specific procedure. Use this modifier for each team physician's procedure. Different carriers pay differently on this modifier. Documentation for the necessity of the medical team is necessary for payment on this claim.

−76 Repeat Procedure by Same

The service needed to be repeated.

−77 Repeat Procedure by Another

The service needed to be repeated by another physician. This modifier provides no additional payment and is used for informational purposes only.

–78 Return to Operating Room for Related Procedure

The physician needed to return the patient to the operating room for a related procedure during the postoperative period. Payment for use of this modifier is limited to the amount allotted for intraoperative services. Use this modifier only with surgery codes.

–79 Unrelated Operating Room Procedure by Same Physician

The patient required an additional unrelated procedure during the postoperative period. This modifier has no effect on payment and can be used only on surgery codes.

–80 Surgical Assistant

Surgical assistant services may be identified by adding this modifier to the surgical *CPT* code. During certain operations, one physician assists another physician in performing a procedure. The physician who assists the operating surgeon would report the same surgical procedure the operating surgeon reports. However, the operating surgeon *would not* append any modifier to the procedure she or he reports. The modifier –80 would be reported only by the assistant surgeon.

–81 Minimum Assistant Surgeon

Minimum surgical assistant services are identified by adding this modifier. For example, the operating physician begins a surgical procedure alone, but during the operation, a minor problem is encountered that requires the service of an assistant surgeon for a short period of time. The services provided by the surgeon who provided this minimal assistance during the surgery would be reported with Modifier 81 appended to the code for the surgical procedure.

–82 Assistant Surgeon

Services required the need for an assistant surgeon. When a resident surgeon was unavailable, use this modifier. Payment is based on 16% of the fee schedule payment amount for the service rendered.

–90 Reference Laboratory

When a service was performed by an outside laboratory other than the treating or reporting physician. This modifier has no effect on payment.

–99 Multiple Modifiers

Under certain circumstances, one or more modifiers may be necessary to report a service.

Global Surgery Modifiers

A modifier is a numerical or an alpha character that is added to a service or procedure to indicate that the service or procedure was altered for that specific circumstance. The modifier does not change the definition of the code reported.

Split-Care Modifiers

Split-care modifiers are used when the surgeon performs less than the global package reported. These modifiers are as follows:

–56 This modifier is used for preoperative care only.

–55 This modifier is used to report postoperative care only. The information necessary to use this modifier should be reported in Box 19 of the HCFA 1500 Form. The information should include the date of the surgery and the surgical procedure.

–54 This modifier is used to report intraoperative care only. It includes 1 day of preoperative care.

Modifiers Identifying Additional Services

–24 This modifier is used to report an unrelated evaluation and management service that was performed by the same physician during the postoperative period.

–25 This modifier is used to report a condition of the patient that called for a separate evaluation and management service that was greater than the care that is normally associated with the specific service or procedure reported.

–78 This modifier is used to report a return visit to the operating room for a related procedure. For this modifier to be used, the second operating room visit had to fall within the postoperative period.

–79 This modifier is used to report an unrelated procedure or service that was performed by the same physician during the patient's postoperative period.

FROM THE AUTHOR'S NOTEBOOK

The modifier –25 can be used to report an eligible patient visit that may have been performed on the same day as a minor surgery or endoscopic procedure.

There is an area of confusion in reference to the patient who is admitted to the hospital. If the specialist is the admitting physician, she or he should bill for the initial hospital visit. The attending physician should bill for a subsequent hospital visit. Only if the attending physician admits the patient is she or he entitled to use the initial-hospital-visit code.

The Medicare Coding System: A Rationale for Change

On January 1, 1992, Medicare traded in its existing coding system for a new evaluation and management coding system. These evaluation and management codes make up approximately 35% of all Medicare Part B payments to physicians. The American Medical Association *CPT* Editorial Panel developed these new codes that replaced the *CPT* coding system previously used. Their goal in making this change was to develop a coding system that would take into consideration geographic localities and physician specialties. The previous system coded services in a uniform way that was not always appropriate for all physicians. This previous system accommodated various physician coding practices by using a "reasonable charge" payment methodology coupled with a prevailing charge, which was calculated in each locality for each physician specialty. The new (resource-based relative value scale) (RBRVS) payment system does not allow for any variation in physician coding. The nationwide relative value units were mandated by Congress and prohibited adjustments based on specialty or locality.

Coding Tips

The following tips may help the office manager and physician in dealing with the new codes:

- Routinely check the patient's charts for proper documentation.
- Order the *CPT* and *ICD-9-CM* codebooks on an annual basis.
- Have the physician take an active role in the coding process.
- Read all the Medicare special bulletins and any other bulletins from third-party payers.
- Learn to use properly the modifiers available to you.
- No distinction is made between a new and an established patient in the emergency room.
- Use nursing facility service codes for patients in a psychiatric residential treatment center.
- Two office visits on the same day for the same patient may be reported if the problems were unrelated and the correct modifier is used.
- A new patient is one who has not been seen by anyone in the practice in the past 3 years.

Companies That Provide Coding Services

Several companies publish books and newsletters on coding procedures (Box 5–7). The companies listed in Box 5–8 provide on- and off-site personnel to fill temporary staff vacancies or to clear coding backlogs; some also offer coding education and consulting services.

Is the Medicare Appeal Appealing?

Few medical offices have ever filed an appeal to Medicare or, for that matter, have ever even thought about doing so. Most offices are intimidated by the process and are unsure how to handle such a task. A recent statistic released from Medicare shows that more than 50% of all claims sent for appeal have had their initial decisions reversed. This statistic should make the appeal process more appealing!

There are a few steps that must be taken before starting the appeal process. First, it is best to resubmit the claim, if it hasn't already been resubmitted. This often eliminates the need for an appeal and is easier to do than an appeal. This can be done only if the claim is whole and not partial. Rejected partial claims must be submitted for an appeal. There are five steps in the appeal process:

1 Informal review
2 Fair hearing

BOX 5–7. **WHERE TO TURN FOR CODING HELP**

American Health Information and Management Association
Suite 1400
919 North Michigan Avenue
Chicago, IL 60611
(800) 621-6828
Publishes coding manuals and other resources.

American Hospital Association
840 North Lake Shore Drive
Chicago, IL 60611
(312) 280-5900
Publishes *ICD-9 Coding Manual* and markets video teleconferences on coding issues.

American Medical Association
P.O. Box 109050
Chicago, IL 60610
(800) 621-8335
Publishes *Current Procedural Technology, CPT 1993* and *CPT Assistant.*

Aspen Publishers, Inc.
7201 McKinney Circle
P.O. Box 990
Frederick, MD 21701
(800) 638-8437
Publishes *CPT Coding Made Easy.*

Berman & Associates
P.O. Box 292918
Dayton, OH 45429
(800) 442-1554
Publishes *The Physician's Medicare Authority.*

Healthcare Information Services
Attn: Mary Frances Milking
Suite 3
882 Middle Avenue
Menlo Park, CA 94025
(415) 315-3527
Publishes *CodeXpert,* an index to *ICD-9* coding resources.

Medi-Index
5225 Wiley Post Way, No. 500
Salt Lake City, UT 84116
(800) 999-4600
Publishes coding books and other resources and provides consulting services.

PMIC
4727 Wilshire Blvd
Los Angeles, CA 90010
(800) 633-7467
Publishes and distributes coding resources.

St. Anthony Publishing, Inc.
Suite 700
500 Montgomery Street
Alexandria, VA 22314
(800) 632-0123
Markets a variety of coding products, including a monthly newsletter entitled *Coding for Physician Reimbursement.*

---

3 Hearing by the administrative law judge
4 Review by the Appeals Council
5 Federal district court hearing

There are various time limits and monies involved in each step of the process. Every office is given a Medicare carriers' manual. Referring to the section on appeals can be very helpful during this process.

Informal Review. All requests for informal review of a claim must be made within 6 months and 5 days of the date on the Explanation of Medicare benefits. A claim for any dollar amount can be made at this point. At this point, the medical office may want to file an HCFA-

1964 Request for Review Form; however, this is not required. All that is necessary to start this process is to write a letter asking for a formal review of the claim (Box 5–9). This letter should include the following information:

- the patient's name
- the patient's Medicare number
- the dates of service in question
- the procedure codes

Most offices find that it is best to attach a copy of the Explanation of Benefits to the letter. It is also a good idea to attach any additional information that might help to justify the services rendered. Remember to be specific. You have complete control over what you submit to Medicare. There is no such thing as too much information.

BOX 5–8. COMPANIES THAT PROVIDE CODING SERVICES

ARTS, Inc.
Suite 113
100 Corporate Pointe
Culver City, CA 90230
(310) 641-7446

Bottomley & Associates, Inc.
Suite 108
2434 Highway 120
Duluth, GA 30136
(800) 969-4503

Care Communications, Inc.
101 East Ontario
Chicago, IL 60611
(800) 458-3544

Lexicode
Suite H
2821 Ashland Road
Columbia, SC 29210
(803) 798-0453

MRT & C, Ltd.
Suite 208
1350 East Arapaho
Richardson, TX 75081
(800) 544-1752

Fair Hearing. If only part of the claim was denied, the office can request a fair hearing. A fair hearing is given by an experienced reviewer designated by Medicare. It can be requested only within 6 months of the informal review decision. There is also a restriction on the amount of the claim in question. Each fair hearing must be on a claim in the amount of $100 or higher. Again, there is a form, HCFA-1965, that can be used to request this hearing. The office may also request this hearing by writing a letter. The office must be aware that there are three different types of fair hearings:

1 Telephone hearing
2 On-the-record hearing
3 In-person hearing

The HCFA requires that all telephone and in-person hearings be granted. When preparing for these hearings, the office must have the same information as gathered for the informal review. Any additional documentation is a must!

FROM THE AUTHOR'S NOTEBOOK

The office may request a copy of all the information regarding the requested appeal from the Medicare carrier. This will help in reviewing the case before the hearing. This is one of Medicare's best kept secrets!

Hearing by the Administrative Law Judge. If the claim is denied at the fair hearing, the office may request a hearing by an administrative law judge. This hearing must be requested within 60 days of the final fair hearing decision, and the claim must be worth at least $500. At this step in the appeals process, there is no longer a Medicare employee making the decisions. A hearing officer decides at this point whether a reversal of the previous decision is warranted. If the hearing officer reverses the decision, the office wins!! If the hearing officer agrees with the previous decision, the request is forwarded to an administrative law judge. These reviews take place in the Office of the Hearings and Appeals at the Social Security Administration. The scheduling of this hearing can take as long as 1 year.

Review by the Appeals Council. The next step is a review by the Appeals Council. This council is also a division of the Social Security Administration. A request for a review by this council should be made through the Social Security Administration and must

---

BOX 5–9. LETTER FROM THE PHYSICIAN'S OFFICE REQUESTING AN INFORMAL REVIEW OF A REJECTED CLAIM

Medicare Part B
Department of Review
P.O. Box 890413
Camp Hill, PA 17089-0413

Dear Sir or Madam:

Please refer to the attached Medicare Explanation of Benefits form. We are challenging Medicare's denial of our daily visits, rejected as unnecessary concurrent care.

On _____ , our practice was asked to see the above-listed patient in consultation by the patient's primary care physician for a condition that required the consultative expertise of a gastroenterology specialist. We completed this consultation and furnished a report to the attending physician.

Due to the unique nature of this patient's condition, which related to his diagnosis of _____ _____, we agreed to continue to follow the patient along with the attending physician, specifically as it related to the patient's diagnosis. After a thorough evaluation, additional advice was rendered in the medical record relative to ongoing patient progress. The attending physician continued to serve as overall manager of

the patient's care; however, the diagnosis of _____ was well beyond the scope of the attending physician's expertise, thereby necessitating our resources.

Medicare's denial of our daily care based on too many physicians for the reported condition should in this case be overturned. The unique condition required the services of a board-certified subspecialist of internal medicine—a gastrointestinal specialist. Failure to have provided these services would certainly have compromised the patient's clinical outcome.

We ask that you reconsider this claim for payment and forward the reimbursement to our office at your earliest convenience. Thank you for your attention to this matter.

Sincerely,

Betty Shipton

Billing Manager

---

be made within 60 days of the administrative law judge's decision. The claim must be in the amount of $500 or more. Once the appeal process reaches this step, it is wise for the office manager to step down and enlist the help of an experienced health care attorney. An attorney is required should the appeals process go to the next step, so it is generally a good idea to engage one at this level.

Federal District Court Hearing. Should the claim be denied by the Appeals Council, a civil action must be filed in a federal district court. This claim must be filed within 60 days of the mailing date of the Appeals Council decision. To be eligible for this action, the claim in dispute must be worth $1,000 or more. Any claim under $1,000 cannot be tried at this level. The two additional requirements at this level are that the office be represented by an attorney and that the claim be filed in the federal district in which the office is located.

Submitting Clean Claims

A clean claim is one that has been submitted with no errors. It contains the necessary information regarding the patient's coverage and diagnosis and the services rendered. It contains all the necessary information regarding the treating and referring physician. A clean claim is one that can be processed electronically; it has no error that requires the services of an individual. Claims that arrive at an insurance processing center with errors must be transferred to an individual for processing. This delays the claim processing and therefore payment to the physician. It is critical for the office manager to stress the importance of a clean claim and to ensure that the billing process in the office promotes clean claims. The errors most commonly made on the HCFA 1500 Form are listed in Box 5–10.

Electronic Claims

By using electronic claims submission, the office spends less time preparing the claim for submission and receives reimbursement than if a paper claim was submitted. This paperless processing of claims goes by several names: *electronic media claims, electronic data interchange,* and *electronic claims processing.* Medicare and Blue Cross/Blue Shield have had electronic claim submission systems in place for many years now. Larger HMOs, Medicaid, and commercial insurance company clearinghouses are now also going electronic. There are several reasons why electronic claims submission is preferable to paper claims submission:

- Payment is faster.
- Paperwork is reduced.
- Staff time and costs are reduced.

Submitting claims electronically makes payment dramatically faster. The checks are automatically deposited into the practice's bank account, and the Explanation of Benefits is either printed out on the office's printer or mailed to the office. In any case, the turnaround time for a claim is much faster. Faster claim turnarounds translate into improved cash flow. The average physician's office submits approximately 80% of its gross earnings to third-party insurances; therefore, the cash flow improvement can mean substantial increases in revenue. There is no need for postage, and thus there is a reduction in paperwork and staff time and costs. It has been estimated that by using an electronic claims submission system, a medical office saves between $1 and $4 on each claim submitted. There is no need for an employee to print the claim form, fold it, place it in an envelope, and stamp and mail it.

Electronic claims are submitted to the insurance carrier from the computer via the telephone lines and take only a short time to transmit. The software of the computer translates, edits, and formats the data according to the rules of each insurance carrier. When considering whether to purchase electronic claims submission software, you should

- Ask neighboring practices if they have any experience with electronic claims. Ask if you can come and see their system in operation.
- Contact the carriers whom you bill and ask for the names of qualified software vendors.
- Consider attending the next professional meeting to speak with software vendors and look at their displays.
- Ask your office's health care consultant, if you have one, to recommend a qualified vendor.
- Ask the vendor how long it has been involved with electronic claims submissions.
- Ask the vendor for references, that is, the names of offices for whom the vendor has installed systems.
- Ask the references about the vendor's service and support.
- Ask the vendor about charges associated with electronic claims packages.
- Ask the vendor about the cost of service contracts.
- Ask the vendor about updates on the software.
- Ask the vendor whether training for the staff and physicians is available.

BOX 5–10. ERRORS COMMONLY MADE ON THE HCFA 1500 FORM

1 Health insurance number is incorrect or missing.
2 Provider number is incorrect or missing.
3 UPIN is missing.
4 Place of service is incorrect.
5 Guarantor information is incomplete.
6 Date of service is incorrect.
7 Form is addressed to incorrect carrier.
8 Modifiers are incorrect or missing.
9 Diagnosis codes are truncated.
10 Number of units billed is incorrect.

Medicare Audits

There is a very simple way to avoid Medicare audits—learn exactly what the auditors are looking for when they review a practice's claims. Every insurance carrier has a manual on payment procedures, supplied by the HCFA. This manual states that each carrier must select at least 7 per 1,000 physicians for comprehensive medical reviews. Reviewers will look for patterns and abnormal practices. The HCFA manual includes a section titled "Post Payment Alert List," which describes types of abuse that have been detected across the nation. Some of these abuses are as follows:

Laboratory tests—numerous repetitions of a test, even though previous results were within normal limits

Consultations—repeated use of the same high-level consultation code

Office visits—repeated use of the same high-level office visit code and frequent use of the office visit code for stable maintenance patients

Repeated use of a single code or level

Pre- and postoperative care—for visits not included in global fees

Transfer of Patients

When a patient is transferred from one hospital to another, selecting the proper billing codes can be tricky. When a patient is in Hospital A and is transferred to Hospital B, Medicare will pay for discharge-day management from Hospital A and for hospital admission to Hospital B. Generally, the hospital admission service is a lower level code, since the patient is already an established patient of the physician.

References

Beard, P. L. "What the Medicare Fraud Squad Looks for in Claims." *Medical Economics,* July 12, 1993, pp. 42-46.

Petrie, K. J. "How To Set Your Fee Schedule." *Physician's Management,* March 1993, pp. 106-109.

Medicare Special Bulletin, June 25, 1993.

6

Medical Billing, Credit, and Collections

Billing
- *The Return Envelope*
- *Professional Courtesy: How Much Does It Really Cost?*
- *Medical Office Registration and Billing*
- *Billing and Statement Types*
- *Payment at the Time of Service*
- *Development of a Billing Cycle*
- *How the Billing Cycle Works*
- *Overpayments*
- *When the Office Makes a Mistake in Billing*
- *The Financial Disclosure Letters*
- *Undelivered Mail*
- *Credit Cards—Friend or Foe of the Medical Office?*

- *Are Billing Services the Answer to Your Prayers?*

Collections
- *Collections Policy*
- *Develop an In-Office Collections System*
- *Stay within the Law: Some Collection Don'ts*
- *Telephone Collections*
- *Collection Letters*
- *The Dreaded Collection Agency*
- *Collection Percentages*
- *Collecting from an Estate*

Educating the Staff and Patients about Payment for Services

Billing

THE RETURN ENVELOPE

The return envelope is a very important tool of the billing office, but it is often dismissed as an unneeded expense. It is a proven fact, however, that individuals pay bills that include a return envelope before they pay bills for which they have to provide their own envelope. Whether the reason is that it is convenient for them or they feel they are getting something for free, customers pay a bill faster when it is accompanied by a return envelope. It works for the utility companies; why not for the doctor? Some offices prefer to use a colored envelope for their return envelope, so they can detect it easily in the mail. Colored or plain white, the return envelope is well worth the few cents it costs to enclose it.

PROFESSIONAL COURTESY: HOW MUCH DOES IT REALLY COST?

"Professional courtesy" means providing a service for free, and in a recent survey, about 97% of physicians said they offer some type of professional courtesy. A substantial sum of money may be lost to professional courtesy. Where does it stop? With colleagues and their families? With hospital employees? With pharmacists and dentists? With members of the clergy? Letting professional courtesy get out of hand can cause an office financial difficulties. The physicians polled in the survey said that the percentage of their patients who received professional courtesy from them ran from 2% to 15% per year. To determine whether the office is losing too much revenue to professional courtesy, the office manager might want to keep track of all the services provided to courtesy patients for one month and assign the proper dollar figures to these services. Showing the physician the total is a good way to convey the dollars that are being lost to courtesy patients.

If the physician decides that change is in order regarding write-offs, she or he and the office manager should sit down and develop a firm policy regarding professional courtesy and instruct the office staff to use it. The following are some guidelines that may help in developing this policy:

- If the patient has insurance that will cover some or most of the services rendered, use it! This applies even to patients who are physicians and their families.
- If the patient who is a physician does not have health insurance, 100% professional courtesy is customary and expected.

- Professional courtesy applies to professional services only, not laboratory studies, injections, x-ray exams, etc.
- A fee schedule can be created to handle professional courtesy to patients who are professionals but are not physicians. The following is an example:

- Hospital employees 25%
- Nurses 25% to 50%
- Clergy 25% to 50%
- Pharmacists/dentists 25%

How do you tell another professional that you will no longer be granting professional courtesy to her or him? It can be done simply and professionally. Obtain a list from the computer with the names and addresses of patients currently receiving professional courtesy. Highlight the names of those who are affected by the change in policy. Have the staff send letters to these patients explaining this policy change and why it was necessary. The letters should follow the example shown in Box 6–1. Letters should be sent as soon as the policy has been created. Don't wait until patients show up at the office for an appointment to tell them they will no longer be receiving the physician's services for free!

Some medical offices use reciprocity as a form of professional courtesy. For instance, the physician may grant professional courtesy to a dentist, who in turn provides the physician's family with free dental care. The most important thing to remember about professional courtesy is that there must be a policy in place and all staff members must be aware of it.

MEDICAL OFFICE REGISTRATION AND BILLING

The following is the core of information needed from each patient, regardless of her or his financial class, at the time of registration:

- Insurance information—photocopy both sides of the insurance card
- Driver's license number
- All demographic and financial information
- Employment information
- Consent/authorization signatures

All patients should be reminded of their financial responsibility, be it a $10 co-pay or a $100 deductible (Figure 6–1). Each individual payer requires different information, as the following lists indicate:

- Medicare
  - Policy number

BOX 6–1. LETTER TO COLLEAGUE EXPLAINING THAT HE OR SHE WILL NO LONGER BE RECEIVING SERVICES FOR FREE

August 4, 1995

Dear Dr. Conklin:

In the past, we have not been charging you for our services. As you know, the cost of providing services to patients continues to rise, creating a situation whereby our paying patients are responsible for incurring all the increased costs of our practice. To keep down costs and prevent an increase in our fees, we find it necessary to discontinue our courtesy policy to patients who are receiving courtesy at this time. Because we expect you to pay normal fees in the future, we are also willing to submit to your insurance company for these services. Any fee collected from your insurance company will be accepted as payment in full if you have the appropriate coverage.

Your understanding and cooperation are important to us. We value you and your family as patients and will continue to provide you with the very best of medical care. If you have any questions regarding this policy change, please feel free to contact me.

Sincerely,

Dr. Carolyn Vail

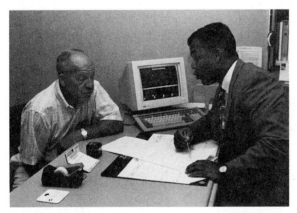

FIGURE 6–1. The office manager explains the insurance deductible to a patient.

- Spouse's employment
- Patient's retirement date
- Whether the patient has been in the hospital in the last 60 days
- Medicare questionnaire
- Secondary insurance information, if any, and card copy, if applicable
- Medicaid
  - Current monthly card
  - Address

- Birthdate
- Card holder's name
- Secondary insurance information, if any, and card copies
- Workers' Compensation
  - Date of injury
  - Address of place of injury
  - Letter from employer
  - Workers' Compensation form
  - Workers' Compensation number of previous injury
  - Secondary insurance information and card copy
- Health maintenance organization (HMO)/preferred provider organization (PPO)
  - Name of primary care physician
  - Referral number for visit
- Commercial/Blue Cross
  - Plan code
  - Correct policy number
  - Correct group number
  - Name as written on card

BILLING AND STATEMENT TYPES

Various billing and statement types are available for use by medical practices.

Computerized Billing

Many offices today are computerized and run their billings from their computer system. This can be done in two ways: data mailers and statements.

Data mailers are composed of several sheets of paper that are arranged in such a way that when the computer prints, it imprints the patient bill and the mailing envelope at the same time (Figure 6–2). Some data mailers may also contain a return envelope for the patient's convenience. This is an efficient way to bill patients; however, it can be costly. The office manager should evaluate the time it takes employees to fold, stuff, and address these bills. This can be weighed against the cost of the data mailer to determine the most cost-effective way in which to bill patients.

Statement billing is a computer printout of a patient's statement. An example of a "pinfed" patient statement is shown in Figure 6–3. These statements are continuous and must be separated, folded, and stuffed into envelopes to be mailed. This bill may contain such information as

- Service rendered
- Charge for service
- Date submitted to insurance company
- Date paid
- Balance due

Some computers can be programmed to print specific notes on these bills, such as:

"This bill is now 30 days past due. Please send payment."
"This bill is now 60 days past due. Please remit!"
"This bill is now 90 days past due. Avoid collection proceedings by remitting today!"

There might be a limitation as to the number of characters the computer can print in such a note, so some abbreviations might need to be used.

Manual Billing

Offices that are not computerized use manual billing systems. For instance, large offices may use a ledger system, in which a ledger card is kept for each patient or family. This card is photocopied at the end of each month, placed into a window envelope, and mailed to the patient. These cards are generally used with a pegboard system.

Typewritten statements may be used by smaller, less busy offices. These statements are generally typed on

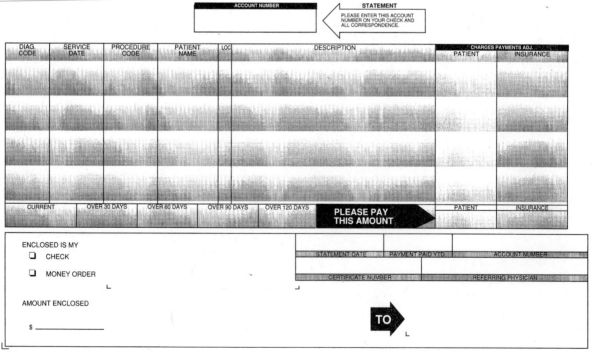

A

FIGURE 6–2. Example of a data mailer for a patient statement. **A** shows the patient bill, and **B** shows the envelope. (Courtesy of VERSYSS, Inc.)

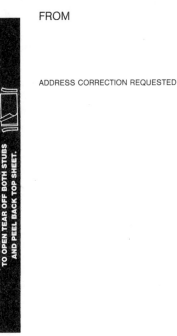

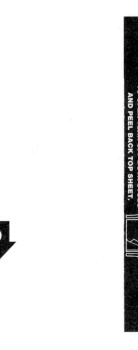

B

FIGURE 6–2. Continued

"continuous form" paper so that the typist can type one statement after another without having to put new paper into the typewriter. The statements are then separated, folded, and placed into billing envelopes.

As discussed in Chapter 5, many medical offices use a "superbill," a form that serves as a charge slip, patient receipt, patient billing statement, and insurance reporting form. Superbills are imprinted with the physician's name, office address, and phone number. They also contain the space necessary for the information required by the various different insurance companies. Today's superbill may look quite different from superbills in the past. There are companies today that offer a computerized superbill that can be used with a scanner to input the charges and diagnoses directly into the patient's computerized account. The superbill is fed through a scanner that immediately prints the information on the computer screen. This saves the office valuable time and is less likely to contain errors because no keystrokes are involved in the data entry process.

Offices using non-computerized billing systems can apply brightly colored pressure-sensitive labels with collection warnings on them to the front of patient statements. Box 6–2 shows some warnings that may be printed on the labels.

PAYMENT AT THE TIME OF SERVICE

Another part of patient education is training patients to pay for their services at the time of their office visits. The front-desk staff should be trained to ask for payment at this time. When patients schedule office visits, they should be informed of the office's collection policy and told that payment is expected at the time of service. Staff should be trained to expect the common responses: "I forgot my checkbook," "I always get billed," "I just wrote my last check before coming here," "I'll mail the check to you," "They always bill my insurance." Instruct the staff to be firm but courteous when dealing with patients who delay in paying.

DEVELOPMENT OF A BILLING CYCLE

It is important to have a billing policy in place. Patient statements should be mailed in a timely manner. If the number of statements to be mailed each month is large, it might be easier to mail them in a cycle. In cycle billing, patient statements are split into quarters of the alphabet and billed on a weekly rotation. The first week of the month, all patients with last names that begin with the letters A–F are billed. The second week of the month, all patients with last names that begin with the letters G–L are billed. The third week of the month, all patients with last names that begin with the letters M–R are billed. The fourth week of the month, all patients with last names that begin with the letters S–Z are billed.

HOW THE BILLING CYCLE WORKS

Step 1

The patient calls to schedule an appointment with the physician and is reminded to bring her or his insurance card to the office at the time of the appointment. While the patient is on the phone, her or his demographic and insurance information is obtained. If the patient has a managed care plan, she or he is reminded to bring a referral for the visit from a primary physician.

In addition, it is important that patients know exactly what is expected of them in the office before they schedule an appointment. The educated patients of today often call and ask a series of questions regarding procedures of the office before they will schedule an appointment. If they do not like what the office is telling them, they will simply call another. The office should not be concerned about turning down patients who do not seem willing to pay its fees and follow its payment guidelines. This policy should be discussed with the physician before it is instituted.

Some physicians still believe that a medical practice is not a business. However, more and more physicians are changing their view on this issue. When prospective patients call to schedule an appointment, they

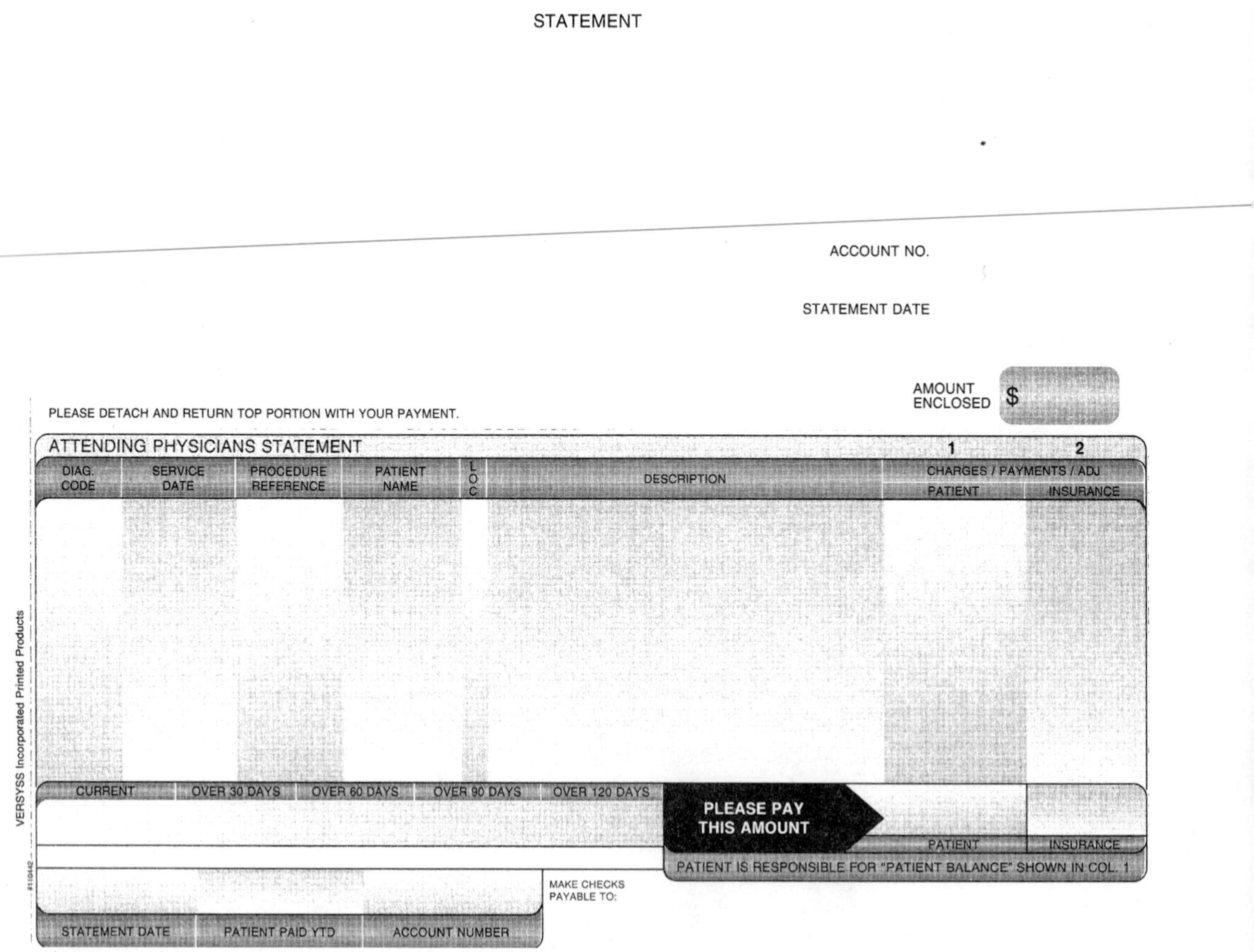
STATEMENT

ACCOUNT NO.

STATEMENT DATE

AMOUNT ENCLOSED $

PLEASE DETACH AND RETURN TOP PORTION WITH YOUR PAYMENT.

ATTENDING PHYSICIANS STATEMENT

DIAG. CODE	SERVICE DATE	PROCEDURE REFERENCE	PATIENT NAME	LOC	DESCRIPTION	1 CHARGES / PAYMENTS / ADJ PATIENT	2 INSURANCE

CURRENT	OVER 30 DAYS	OVER 60 DAYS	OVER 90 DAYS	OVER 120 DAYS	PLEASE PAY THIS AMOUNT	PATIENT	INSURANCE

PATIENT IS RESPONSIBLE FOR "PATIENT BALANCE" SHOWN IN COL. 1

MAKE CHECKS PAYABLE TO:

STATEMENT DATE	PATIENT PAID YTD	ACCOUNT NUMBER

VERSYSS Incorporated Printed Products

#110442

FIGURE 6–3. Pin-fed patient statement form. (Courtesy of VERSYSS, Inc.)

BOX 6–2. COLLECTION WARNING LABELS

Please remit promptly to avoid collection agency action.

PAST DUE

Please contact our office immediately if there is a problem.

We accept VISA and MC. Do you wish to apply your overdue balance on them?

YOUR ACCOUNT IS 90 DAYS PAST DUE! PAY NOW!

No payment has been received from your insurance company. This bill is now payable by you!

This bill is your RESPONSIBILITY!!

SERIOUSLY OVERDUE ACCOUNT!!

Your insurance company has paid its share of this bill. The balance is now your responsibility!

FINAL NOTICE

FINAL NOTICE: If we do not hear from you within 10 days, this account will be turned over to our collection agency.

FINAL NOTICE
This is the last statement you will receive from this office. The next notification will be from our collection agency!

should be instructed that the fee for an office visit is $ _____. They should also be told that follow-up visits are only $ _____. It is best to explain that this fee does not cover any diagnostic workup that they might also have to have done, if the physician deems it necessary. Most offices submit these diagnostic tests to the patient's insurance company for payment. This is a courtesy and should not be abused. There will always be the patient who refuses to pay for an office visit before submitting the claim to her or his insurance company. Train the staff to explain to the patient that this is not the policy of the office and that payment for the visit must be made at the time of service. The staff should give the patient a receipt that she or he can send to the insurance company for reimbursement.

Step 2

The patient arrives at the office for the appointment. Her or his demographic information is obtained, if it was not obtained on the phone. The patient is asked for her or his insurance card, and the front and back of the card are photocopied. If the patient is a Medicare patient, a Medicare authorization is signed. If the patient has insurance other than Medicare, a general medical authorization is signed. If the patient is a managed care patient, in a specialty office, a valid referral is collected. If the patient is responsible for a co-pay, the co-pay is collected at this time.

All patients who belong to an HMO must be told that they cannot be seen without a referral from their primary physician. Most physicians will not backdate a referral, so it is extremely important that patients have the referral at the time of their visit. The physician who treats the patient without a referral runs an excellent chance of not getting paid. It is the front-desk person's responsibility to establish whether the patient has a referral for her or his visit. It is also important to check the referral to see what services have been approved for your office to do at that visit. Any service performed without the primary physician's permission will not be paid for by the HMO.

If the physician for whom you work has established a policy that she or he will not participate in any insurances, it is important for the office staff to make this policy clear to patients. The staff can be helpful in assisting patients with their insurance forms. Financial arrangements can be made with the office manager regarding payment plans. Some offices hand out financial arrangement sheets to all new patients. This financial agreement sheet can be tailored to fit any practice and its policies. When patients are given this sheet, they will have a full understanding of the policy of your office, and payment should be smoother.

Step 3

The patient leaves the examination room and goes to the front desk, where follow-up appointment and testing are scheduled, if appropriate. Payment is collected for the physician's service on that day. Insurance information is confirmed.

Step 4

Services are billed to the appropriate insurance companies.

Step 5

The patient statement is mailed to the patient on the normal monthly billing cycle.

OVERPAYMENTS

Occasionally, patients overpay on their accounts. Before the check is entered on a daily sheet or into the computer, it should be returned to the patient with VOID written across the front of it. However, because of the system used in some offices, it is difficult to intercept the check before it is entered into the computer as a credit. When this occurs, an office check is written for the amount paid and is sent to the patient. The adjustment is made in the computer on the day the office check is mailed to the patient.

It is wise to keep a log of overpayments for tracking purposes. This can be done simply by writing them in a spiral notebook. The entry should contain the following information:

- The patient's name
- The number of the patient's check
- The number of the return check
- The amount of the return check
- The date the check was received from the patient
- The date the office check was sent to the patient
- The reason for the refund
- The initials of the employee requesting the refund

The staff member requesting a refund check should fill out a Patient Refund Form (Box 6–3) and submit it to the bookkeeper or office manager for reimbursement.

BOX 6–3. PATIENT REFUND FORM

Date: _____

Refund Check Payable To: _____

Address: _____

_____

Reason for Refund:

_____

_____

_____

Name of Person Requesting Refund:

_____

Approved By: _____

Date of Refund: _____

The form should have a copy of the patient's check attached to it.

Overpayments made by third-party payers are handled in the same manner. A form for third-party payer refunds similar to the Patient Refund Form can be designed and should contain the following additional information:

- The name of the patient and/or guarantor
- Identifying agreement number or Social Security number
- Patient's date of birth for proper identification

A copy of the check from the insurance company should accompany the refund request form and should also accompany the refund check sent to the third-party payer.

WHEN THE OFFICE MAKES A MISTAKE IN BILLING

Always admit any mistakes the office may have made in billing. Patients often tell the office that they think there is a mistake on their bill. This is sometimes a stall tactic so that they do not have to pay their bill. However, if the office did make a mistake, it should be admitted and rectified immediately. This shows the patient the integrity of the office and the staff members.

FROM THE AUTHOR'S NOTEBOOK

When the office has made an error in billing to an insurance company, it is important to notify the insurance company immediately and ask how to go about correcting the situation. Some insurance companies ask that you wait to send a reimbursement check to them until they send you the necessary paperwork. Others will ask for a check in the amount they paid, accompanied by a copy of the Explanation of Benefits.

THE FINANCIAL DISCLOSURE LETTERS

It is important to realize that not everyone will pay her or his bills. It is impossible to collect certain accounts, not because the collection system in place is faulty or the staff are not doing their job, but because some patients present to the office with true economic hardship. However, there should be a policy in place for these occasions. A copy of the patient's first complete tax return (Form 1099) should be requested in every case of hardship. In 1994, the U.S. poverty levels were updated. The poverty level for one individual is $7,360. For a family, this figure increases by $2,480 for each additional person. This level refers to all income sources before taxes. The Financial Disclosure Form shown in Box 6–4 can be used to determine the financial stability of a patient. Any patient who claims hardship should be asked to fill out this form. It is sent to the patient with a cover letter and is followed by either an acceptance letter or a rejection letter, as shown in the box.

UNDELIVERED MAIL

The U.S. Post Office offers a service whereby any mail sent from a professional office can be located by the use of "Address Correction Requested." All of the medical office's envelopes should have these words printed on them. If these words are either printed or stamped on the envelope sent to the patient who has moved, the Post Office will automatically research and locate the new address of that patient. It will send the office a form with the new address stamped on it. (However, if the patient did not arrange to have her or his mail forwarded, it will not be possible to obtain the new address.) This tool is very helpful when offices are attempting to send statements to patients who are no longer in the area.

Some mail will be returned with various phrases handwritten on the front of the envelope. This is usually the work of patients attempting to avoid paying their bills. Such phrases as "Not here" or "Refused" are generally written by the patient, family member, or friend. The Post Office uses a stamp to explain the undelivered mail.

If the mail is returned and the U.S. Post Office cannot help, there are a few other methods to locate lost patients. The following is a list of possible means of obtaining patients' addresses or phone numbers:

- Call the patients' employers for updated information.
- Check the telephone book—it can come in handy sometimes.
- Call emergency contact or relative of the patient.
- The hospital billing department may have the information.
- A referring physician may have updated information on a mutual patient.

CREDIT CARDS—FRIEND OR FOE OF THE MEDICAL OFFICE?

Health care providers are constantly looking for more effective ways to collect patient fees. If the medical office accepts credit cards, patients can pay for services

---

BOX 6–4A. FINANCIAL DISCLOSURE COVER LETTER

Date: _____

Re: _____

Amount: _____

Dear

Per our telephone conversation, you stated that you could not afford to pay the above balance.

Enclosed you will find a **Financial Disclosure Form** for you to fill out. Please return this form to my attention at the address above, and a determination regarding your financial situation will be made.

If you fail to return this form, we will have no choice but to start legal collection proceedings for this account. If you have any questions, please feel free to contact our office at (222) 222-4444.

Sincerely,

Jan Mikels
Billing Manager

BOX 6–4B. FINANCIAL DISCLOSURE FORM

Patient Name: _____

Social Security #: _____

Guarantor: _____

Relationship: _____

Address: _____

_____

_____

Phone # _____

Are you currently employed? _____ Y _____ N

Disabled? _____ Y _____ N

Employer, if applicable: _____

Employer's address: _____

_____

Other sources of income: _____

Spouse's name: _____

Employed? _____ Y _____ N

Total monthly income: _____

Number of dependents: _____

Total monthly expenses: _____

Mortgage: _____ Rent: _____

List other significant monthly expenses (car loans, medical, personal, etc.)

1. $ _____

2. $ _____

3. $ _____

Please attach a copy of the following:

_____ Prior year's income tax form

_____ Prior year's W-2 form

_____ Payroll stubs

I understand that if my request for waiver of co-insurance charges is approved, it will apply as long as my primary insurance carrier's reimbursement is as stated above. I also understand that I am responsible for all deductibles and denial charges.

I, _____ , certify that the facts set forth in this Financial Disclosure Form are true and correct to the best of my knowledge.

Date: _____

Patient's signature: _____

BOX 6–4C. NONAPPROVAL LETTER

Date: _____

Re: *Sussex County Internal Medicine Associates Serious Past Due Balance of:* $ _____

Dear

I am in receipt of your **Financial Disclosure Form** regarding your financial situation pertinent to the above outstanding balance. After thoroughly researching your form, I have determined that you are financially capable of paying the above balance of $ _____ .

I am willing to set you up on a payment plan of at least $ _____ by the _____ of each month. You will receive a monthly statement showing your payments.

If this account goes 60 days with no payment, it will be necessary to turn it over for legal collection proceedings. Thank you in advance for your cooperation. I'm looking forward to the resolution of this account.

Sincerely,

Jan Mikels
Billing Manager

BOX 6–4D. APPROVAL LETTER

Date: _____

RE: *Sussex County Internal Medicine Associates Serious Past Due Balance of:* $ _____

Dear

We have received your Financial Disclosure Form regarding your financial situation pertinent to the above balance.

After thoroughly researching your form, I have decided to waive your portion of the bill.

If you have any questions, please feel free to contact our office at (222) 222-4444.

Sincerely,

Jan Mikels
Billing Manager

even if they do not have the cash to do so. VISA and Mastercard are busily visiting medical offices in an attempt to get them to accept credit card payments. According to VISA credit services, more than 172,000 health care facilities throughout the nation accept major credit cards for payment of services. More than 44,000 medical offices are part of these facilities wishing to offer patients more flexible and convenient payment terms by the use of these cards. Many patients simply do not have the funds available for payment at the time of the office visit. If the office itself has a cash flow problem, the accountant may urge the office to accept credit card payment. This payment method decreases the office's billing expenses and increases its cash flow.

Patients who have major medical insurance find that using a credit card gives them the flexibility to pay for medical services at the time of the visit and then submit the bill to their major medical payers. In most cases, by the time the patient receives the credit card statement, the payer has issued a check to the patient for reimbursement of services. It has been found that medical practices that accepted credit cards in order to decrease their accounts receivable reduced the average time for overdue accounts by 9 days. One of the most common reasons credit cards are accepted by medical practice is so that accounts receivable can be collected over the telephone. This decreases the number of accounts that need to be placed with outside collection agencies.

The credit card option gives patients an alternative way to clear their balances. Patients who always have an excuse as to why they cannot pay for their visit at the time of service now have the option of putting it on their credit card. If a practice chooses to accept credit cards, it is best to advertise this, so that the patients are aware that this is now an option available to them. This can be done by installing a sign that is provided by the credit card company (which is tastefully done with a caduceus on it, for those physicians who still cringe at the thought of patients' using credit cards), by having the credit card insignias printed on the patient statements, and by placing the insignias on collection notices as an option for payment. Some practices have great success with the credit card option of payment, and can honestly report that their collections have improved since the implementation of credit cards.

Group practices constitute 86% of all large practices in the United States that accept credit cards, and 22% of all solo practices accept credit cards. Even though credit card acceptance is high in the medical field, the percentage of patient payments made with credit cards

is only 6%. Most patients, 81%, still prefer to write a check for the medical service they received. It has been found that practices that are frequently paid with credit cards receive payment in full from their patients 2.5 times more often than practices that are only occasionally paid with credit cards.

There are drawbacks to this system, however. Credit card companies charge anywhere from 2% to 10% on each transaction. This fee can be kept to a minimum, depending on the volume of use and the size of the bill. There are application fees to pay and equipment fees to consider. Some offices purchase the equipment outright, whereas others lease it. Some offices use electronic "point of service" machines, whereas others use the less expensive manual imprinting units. The office should understand that it is responsible for the verification of each card on charges over $50 or more. In addition to these costs, some banks will also charge the practice for the charge slips used in the imprinters. It is necessary to evaluate the type of clientele the practice has. Are they generally older patients who would not use credit cards? Are they young and middle-aged professionals who live in a world of credit? The type of clientele the practice serves is an important consideration when deciding whether to accept credit cards.

Credit cards are becoming increasingly accepted by physicians, such as dermatologists and plastic surgeons, whose services are not always covered by insurance plans. When this happens, many patients choose to use their credit cards as a form of payment. The 24-hour care center, or "Doc-in-a-Box," as some people call it, also often encourages patients to pay by credit card, so that it is assured payment by these walk-in patients it will likely not see again.

ARE BILLING SERVICES THE ANSWER TO YOUR PRAYERS?

Many offices have difficulty maintaining an efficient billing department. The billing process is sloppy, and the rules and regulations of the insurance companies boggle the mind. Is an outside billing service the answer?

A billing service is just what it says it is: a service that contracts with you to provide you with insurance billing. It will handle all bookkeeping and patient billing for the practice. It is the billing service's job to be up to date on the latest in Medicare and insurance company regulations. If you have decided the office could use the help of a billing service, contact several such services and obtain information regarding their services and fees. Inquire about the frequency of insurance claim submissions and whether or not they are submitting claims electronically.

One area to research when considering a billing service is the way it collects the claims from your office. Some billing services have representatives who arrive at the office at certain intervals to collect the claims. Other services use a courier or ask that the claims be sent via overnight mail. Some sophisticated services have their computer dial into your office computer to retrieve the information. When and how often the claims are sent is also valuable information for the office to have before signing a contract with a billing service.

Their fees are generally negotiable, and fee should be a major factor in hiring the right billing service for your practice. Some billing services charge the practice by selling it vouchers and charging a certain amount per voucher. Others take a percentage of what they collect.

It is also important to discuss patient confidentiality with the billing service and ask how it maintains privacy when working with these claims.

Collections

COLLECTIONS POLICY

The words "prompt payment" are not often heard in a medical office. Many offices have accounts that are seriously overdue, thus creating a large accounts receivable balance that negatively affects the practice.

It is extremely important for the medical office to have a collection policy in place. Many offices are lax in the organization of their overdue accounts. However, the smart office has a specific process for collecting overdue accounts. It is a good idea to include this policy in the patient handbook that is given to patients at the time of their first visit. If the office does not provide a patient handbook, a written explanation of billing and collection procedures should be given to all patients as they register at the office. This "patient education" is a necessary part of the collection process.

DEVELOP AN IN-OFFICE COLLECTIONS SYSTEM

The office should determine the actions it will take to follow up on delinquent accounts and what times it will take them. Many offices do not have a policy in place and therefore have a large percentage of their accounts receivable sitting unattended. The collection process described above will be beneficial in setting up this

system. Having a plan in place helps to educate the patient to the fact that the office expects to be paid.

Once you have a plan in place, you must stick to it and not let emotions guide actions. Sometimes, staff members will let a bill slide because they feel the patient will eventually pay it. In all but a few of these cases, these employees have been taken, and no payment is ever received. All this does is delay the collection process. Many patients pay their doctor last, feeling that the doctor has a lot of money and doesn't need it. Box 6–5 shows a sample Billing Status Report that can be used to document follow-up actions taken regarding delayed payment.

STAY WITHIN THE LAW: SOME COLLECTION DON'TS

There are two governing bodies that the medical office should be aware of when doing collections: the federal government and the state government. In some states, the physician's office must follow the same guidelines that the collection agencies in that state follow. Negligence of the rules can inadvertently negate the debt. Serious repercussions can result from not following these guidelines, so it is imperative that they are strictly followed. Be wise—stay within the law! The following are some guidelines to help you do so:

Develop an in-office collections procedure. The billing department, along with the office manager, should develop a system for handling overdue accounts. An example of such a system is as follows. At 30 days, the patient receives a phone call from a staff member, who says that she or he is following up to make sure that the statement arrived at the patient's home. At 60 days, the statement is sent printed or stamped with a message advising the patient that the account is now 60 days past due and remittance should be immediate to avoid collection proceedings. A "Final Notice" is sent at 90 days, a week after the billing statement. This "Final Notice" advises the patient that if payment is not received within 7 days of the receipt of the notice, legal collection proceedings will be started. It is advisable to make one last call to the patient before sending her or his account off to the collection agency. Have the staff state that the patient's account has been pulled for legal collection proceedings and that they are making a courtesy call before the account is sent.

- Most state collection laws allow telephone collections only between 8:00 AM and 9:00 PM. Do not call at any other time of the day or night. Call the

BOX 6–5. BILLING STATUS REPORT

Patient Name	Issue	Action taken

state Bureau of Collections and ask for information regarding collection laws.

- Do not call a patient's place of employment unless it is absolutely necessary, because some employers prohibit personal phone calls at work. Check your state's law. The number of calls that can be made to a patient's place of employment varies from state to state.
- Do not use a postcard as a collection tool.
- Do not misrepresent your identity.
- Do not misrepresent the office by using a form designed to create a false belief.
- Do not use a misleading letterhead.
- Do not accuse the patient of fraudulent behavior.
- Do not engage in continuous or repeated phone calls,
  - continuous meaning making a series of phone calls, one right after another,
  - repeated meaning calling with excessive frequency under the circumstances.
- Do not shame a patient into payment.

TELEPHONE COLLECTIONS

Patients do not like to be reminded of their outstanding debts. A series of telephone calls to them regarding these debts can be very beneficial to the collections process. However, as already mentioned, telephoning must be done with the hours designated by state law. In addition, staff should be trained to be professional at all times and not to respond to anger with anger.

Some patients are easily reached at dinnertime. Staff should be instructed that when a phone call fails to find the patient at home, they should note the time the call was made and should do this after subsequent unsuccessful attempts to contact the patient. A pattern in the patient's absence will often appear. For instance, if staff are calling at dinnertime, late afternoon, or early evening and finding no one at home, it might be concluded that the patient works evenings. By placing that account on the morning calls list, staff might catch the patient at home.

Instruct staff to *always* be sure that the person they are speaking to is the patient. If it's not the patient, they should leave a message, but not the reason for the call. A patient's outstanding debt can be discussed only with the patient in some states; the patient's debt cannot be discussed even with her or his spouse. The office must obtain the state regulations regarding this before making calls. Thus a collections call should take place as

follows. When someone picks up, staff should say, "Hello, Mrs. Brenner?" If the person identifies herself as Mrs. Brenner, it is permissible to discuss the outstanding debt. If the person says, "No, this is her daughter. Can I help you?", staff must simply give their own name and the name of the physician's office and leave a message for Mrs. Brenner to call the office at her earliest convenience. Staff must be trained to never state to anyone except the patient that they are calling in reference to an overdue account.

A "pregnant pause" placed at the right time in the conversation will sometimes evoke a response from patients regarding their nonpayment. For instance, after identifying themselves and stating the name of the physician's office, staff can say, "I'm calling about your overdue account balance of $45.00." A pause at this point in the conversation generally works! In most cases, it is best for staff to take a positive stand and say that they know the patient intends to pay this overdue account, but that perhaps she or he needs some type of payment arrangement. The patient should be given a time frame in which to work; for example, "Can we expect your monthly payment of $20.00 by the end of the week?" If the payment does not reach the office by that date, a reminder call should be made. Failure to follow up on these situations will result in nonpayment and a lackadaisical attitude on the part of the patient. Follow-up is extremely important when making collection calls.

> ### MANAGER'S ALERT
>
> Never threaten a patient with a debt collection action that you have no intention of pursuing. Under the Fair Debt Collection Practices Act, it is a violation to threaten to take action that is not intended to be taken. The office that makes such idle threats can be sued for harassment.

COLLECTION LETTERS

Some offices have found the use of collection letters to be helpful. You can design a series of collection notices and letters for the office similar to that shown in Box 6–6. Many offices buy brightly colored paper and, with the use of the computer and photocopier, print professional-looking notices. The use of a letter format as opposed to a form for the first contact with the patient has been found to be beneficial.

BOX 6-6A. COLLECTION NOTICE FOR MEDICARE DEDUCTIBLE

March 24, 1995

Name: _____

Amount Due: $ _____

Account #:   _____

The above amount of $ _____ has been applied to your Medicare deductible. This charge results from your visit with the doctor on _____ .

We would appreciate it if you could forward a check in the amount of $ _____ to our office as soon as possible. A self-addressed envelope is enclosed for your convenience.

Thank you for your cooperation in this matter.

Sincerely,

William Scott
Billing Manager

BOX 6-6B. OVERDUE ACCOUNT LETTER

June 16, 1995

Kathleen Keiper
P.O. Any Box
Anytown, USA

Dear Mrs. Keiper:

Our records indicate that you have a seriously overdue account balance of $ _____ and that **no** payment has been made.

We would appreciate **immediate** payment to avoid any further collection proceedings.

If you have any questions, please feel free to call our office.

Thank you for your cooperation in this matter.

Sincerely,

Ann Gentz
Billing Manager

BOX 6–6C. 60-DAY COLLECTION LETTER

February 14, 1995

Samuel Miller
270 Wendell Street
Big City, USA

Dear Mr. Miller:

Our records indicate that your account balance is 60 days past due. We have submitted this balance of

$ _____ to your insurance company, but we have not received any payment as of this date.

Your insurance policy is a contract between you and your insurance company. Unfortunately, we do not have the personnel to continue to pursue this matter.

This unpaid balance of $ _____ is now your responsibility. Please mail a check to our office in this amount and contact your insurance company for payment to reimburse you. Thank you for your prompt attention to this matter.

Sincerely,

Charles Whalen
Office Manager

BOX 6–6D. 90-DAY COLLECTION NOTICE

FINAL NOTICE

DATE: _____

ACCOUNT NUMBER: _____

NAME: _____

YOUR ACCOUNT IS NOW SERIOUSLY PAST DUE—FAR BEYOND OUR USUAL LIMITS.

UNLESS YOU MAKE IMMEDIATE ARRANGEMENTS TO PAY YOUR ACCOUNT, WE WILL HAVE NO CHOICE BUT TO REFER IT TO OUR COLLECTION AGENCY.

REMIT PAYMENT WITHIN 10 DAYS TO ABOVE ADDRESS.

BALANCE DUE: $ _____

BOX 6–6E. **SOFT COLLECTION LETTER**

November 16, 1995

Dolores Safin
1600 Park Hill Street, Apt. 3
Any City, USA

Dear Mrs. Safin:

Your account with our office is long past due, but I don't believe in sending collection letters to receive payment for my services.

I believe most people are fair, and want to pay their bills as soon as possible. So, instead of harassing you with dunning letters, may I appeal to your sense of fairness:

If money is tight for you right now, please pay any other bills that are older than ours. We will wait for any patient who makes an effort to meet his obligations. But, if it's our turn, please send a check to us soon.

If you want more time to pay your bill or want to set up a payment plan, just call us and tell us how we can help you. We will appreciate this courtesy, and it will save both of us a lot of worry.

Sincerely,

Bill Crawford
Accounts Supervisor

THE DREADED COLLECTION AGENCY

The best way for medical services to collect fees is through in-office collection processes, which is the way some offices handle their severely overdue accounts. Most offices, however, do not have the resources and personnel to handle these accounts past a certain point. They focus their efforts on collecting overdue accounts up to and including 90 days and at that point refer overdue accounts to collection agencies, the "pros." If the patient hasn't paid in 90 days, it is clear that the patient does not intend to pay this bill. The likelihood that in-office collection methods will succeed greatly decreases after the 90-day period. According to the Commercial Collection Agency Section of the Commercial Law League of America, 25% of the accounts that are delinquent for 3 months are not recovered (Box 6–7 shows the death of the value of a dollar after time). At 6 months, there is a 40% account mortality rate, and at 12 months, 75% of the accounts must be charged off and forgotten.

To choose a competent and efficient collection agency, the office manager might want to call other offices to see which agencies they use. It is wise to hire a collection agency, on the basis of a solid referral. Some offices choose to request a list of collection agencies from the local medical society or hospital.

Once information is secured from the prospective agencies, it is very important to analyze their collection methods and find out the fees they charge for the accounts collected. The collection agency chosen should be ethical and provide services in a manner in which the office feels comfortable. After all, the collection agency is a reflection of the office. Collection agencies charge for their services in a variety of ways. Some take a percentage (33.3% is the norm), and some collect a flat fee for each account handed over to them. These fees are certainly negotiable, and it has been found that the flat fee is not a favorable way to pay a collection agency. Many collection agencies use vouchers to obtain information regarding the account being

---

BOX 6–6F. **SOFT REMINDER LETTER**

October 31, 1995

Zachary Alberts
10 Darby Street
Any Town, USA

Dear Mr. Alberts:

After two reminders, we still haven't received your check for the balance of your overdue account.

Perhaps there is some question in your mind about this balance. If so, please contact us at once; I am certain we can straighten the matter out immediately.

However, if you have no questions, and our figures agree, why delay payment any longer? Even partial payment will be greatly appreciated. We shall expect a prompt reply. Thank you.

Amount Due: $ _____

Sincerely,

Bill Jansen
Billing Department

BOX 6–6G. **FRIENDLY REMINDER LETTER**

August 1, 1995

A Friendly Reminder . . .

It is entirely possible, Mrs. Andrews, that you have already settled this account and that our letters have crossed in the mail.

If so, please disregard this notice.

If, however, you have not yet paid your account balance of $ _____ , will you please do so today? We appreciate your attention to this matter.

Thank you.

Sincerely,

Faith Connor
Billing Manager

BOX 6–6H. OVERSIGHT COLLECTION LETTER

September 18, 1995

Walter March
RD 2
Lake Town, USA

Dear Mr. March:

Our accountant has brought to our attention that you have an overdue account balance of $100.00. We are sure that this is just an oversight on your part, and that payment will be made within the week. However, if there is a problem, we are sincerely interested in helping. If you require us to set up a payment plan for you, please call our office and our billing clerk, Donna, will be happy to help you.

If there is a problem that needs special attention, we invite you to come to our office to discuss this problem. Should you wish to do so, please call our office to set up an appointment with Donna. We would like to help with any special arrangements that might be necessary.

If this has just been an oversight on your part, please drop a check in the mail so that we may credit your account as soon as possible. We thank you for your cooperation in this matter, and look forward to hearing from you.

Sincerely,

Sherry Huber
Office Manager

---

placed. Some agencies charge for these vouchers (Figure 6–4), and some include it in the price of the collection service. Investigate all methods to ascertain which is best for your practice.

> ► **MANAGER'S ALERT**
>
> Have the practice attorney review any contract with a collection agency before you sign it.

The office manager should always have the last say regarding whether an account should be turned over to the collection agency. There may be extenuating circumstances regarding one or two of the patients that the biller might not be aware of. *No* accounts should be placed into collections before they are reviewed. Review helps to prevent any counterallegation that

could come up. The normal period of time an account should remain in collections is 6 months. After that time, the account should be returned to the office and a decision should be made as to the next course of action. At this point, many offices simply write off these accounts and place a sticker on the patient's chart regarding this action.

Some offices cease to provide care for patients who have neglected to pay for their services. They send termination letters to the patients after the collection agency returns the account. This action eliminates any liability that might arise in the future with these patients. A few offices will have either the billing manager or the office manager file in small-claims court for the balance on the bill. This is costly and many times is just throwing good money after bad.

All accounts should be logged into a loose-leaf book when they are placed in collections. This creates a paper trail of these accounts and allows the success of the

---

BOX 6–6I. **COLLECTION DEPARTMENT NOTICE**

COLLECTION DEPARTMENT
FINAL NOTICE

DATE: _____

ACCOUNT NUMBER: _____

NAME: _____

BALANCE DUE: _____

WE HAVE CORRESPONDED WITH YOU ON SEVERAL OCCASIONS REGARDING YOUR CHARGES FOR SERVICES PERFORMED BY OUR PHYSICIANS. BECAUSE OF YOUR FAILURE TO PAY THIS ACCOUNT OR TO MAKE SATISFACTORY PAYMENT ARRANGEMENTS, WE MUST TAKE FURTHER ACTIONS.

WE DO NOT DESIRE TO INITIATE ANY ACTIONS THAT WOULD HARM YOUR CREDIT RATING. HOWEVER, WE MUST INSIST THAT THE BALANCE DUE ON YOUR ACCOUNT BE PAID WITHOUT FURTHER DELAY. IF WE DO NOT RECEIVE YOUR CHECK WITHIN *TEN (10) DAYS,* THE NEXT COMMUNICATION YOU RECEIVE WILL BE FROM OUR COLLECTION AGENCY.

BOX 6–7. **TIME MARCHES ON . . .**

How many times have you heard the value of the dollar decreases quickly??

In looking at accounts receivables, the value of the dollar decreases at the following rate:

Current Value	$1.00
After 2 months	$ .90
After 6 months	$ .66
After 1 year	$ .45
After 2 years	$ .23
After 3 years	$ .16

This is an important factor to keep in mind when collecting overdue account balances in a medical office. Calculate the cost of collecting accounts when they are severely overdue. In many cases, it is simply more cost-effective to write them off than to pay office staff to collect them.

---

collection agency to be tracked. The monthly reports sent by the collection agency should be compared with the book in the office for evaluation of the collection agency's services. Many collection agencies want the patients to pay the monies directly to them and not to the medical office. This is also a negotiable point. If the agency wants the business, it will do anything to satisfy the customer—you!

COLLECTION PERCENTAGES

Statistics show that new physicians have a lower collection rate than established practices. Type of communities, geographic location, and age of physician are also important statistics in collections.

Collection Rates by Years in Practice

1–5	85.5%
6–10	88.6%
11–20	90.0%
21–30	90.7%

Collection Rates by Physician Age

30–34	85.9%
35–39	87.0%
40–44	88.4%
45–49	90.0%
50–54	90.5%
55–59	90.6%
60–64	91.0%
65–69	90.7%
>70	90.3%

Collection Rates by Community Type

Urban	90.1%
Suburban	90.4%
Rural	88.9%

Collection Rates by Geographic Areas

Far Western states (including Alaska and Hawaii)	89.8%
Rocky Mountain states	88.9%
Plains states	90.5%
Great Lakes states	90.7%
Southwestern states	90.2%
Mid-Southern states	88.7%
South Atlantic states	90.1%
New England states	88.0%
Mid-Eastern states	90.3%

COLLECTING FROM AN ESTATE

Collecting payment for service to the deceased requires great tact, because the family of the deceased is already on an emotional rollercoaster. This is not the time to offend the family by sending threatening letters and collection notices. The best way to start collections on a deceased patient is to be sure to collect all that is appropriate from the third-party payers involved. Once these payers have reimbursed their share, the balance must be treated with care. A simple call to the family to obtain the name and address of the executor who will be handling the estate is the next step. Estates usually close within 12 months of the date of death, so it is imperative to follow through in a timely manner. Contact the executor involved and provide the proper documentation to support the outstanding debt. The executor will then add you to the list of creditors for payment. The executor of the estate can be a lawyer, family member, or friend. It is necessary to keep in constant contact with that person to check on the status of the claim.

A claim can also be filed at the local courthouse with Registrar of Wills. This claim is filed against the estate, and if the estate is solvent at the time of probate, the bill is paid. Should the estate not be solvent, the state establishes a priority system to determine who is paid and in what order. The first three bills to be paid from an estate are

1 Funeral costs
2 Expenses of settling the estate
3 Claims due for the deceased person's last illness

> ### FROM THE AUTHOR'S NOTEBOOK
>
> The claims submitted by the billing service are only as good as the information that is provided to them by the office. The office is responsible for all claims and actions by the billing service, so check them out before hiring them!!

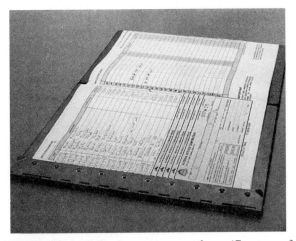

FIGURE 6–4. Collection agency vouchers. (Courtesy of National Revenue Corporation.)

Laws vary from state to state, so be certain to check with your practice's attorney on policy. Some offices have their attorney collect this fee for them; however, it is best to pay office personnel rather than an attorney for this service.

Educating the Staff and Patients about Payment for Services

No matter how successful a practice is, if it is not making a profit, no one wins. It is as important to the office staff as it is to the physician that all monies owed are paid in a timely fashion. The factors in successful collection are simple:

- Listen carefully to the patient's explanation for nonpayment. Sometimes, the staff must interpret what the patient is saying.
- Communicate clearly.
- Show consideration for the patient.
- Develop a policy.

If a medical practice has a difficult time with overdue accounts it is often because the office has not established a payment policy that the patient must follow. Much success can be attributed to proper education of the patient about your billing procedures and policies.

It is better for patients to be aware of your payment policies before they come to the office; however, many physicians think it is unprofessional to have their office speak of fees before the visit. This is slowly changing, and the future will bring more and more office policy changes as cutbacks in reimbursement from insurance carriers and government agencies hit each individual physician's office. Of particular importance is that the employees know the rules and regulations of each insurance company. It is better to know ahead of time what is and is not covered by the insurance company than to provide a specific service and later find out that the office will not be paid for this service. The office staff must understand that there are three entities involved in patients' care: the physician, the patient, and their insurance company.

Both the physician and the staff must be aware of the collection rules. It is essential for office personnel to be aware of the internal workings of all insurance companies. Medicare, Blue Shield, and many major HMOs and PPOs are now sending bulletins on a regular basis to keep physicians' offices aware of changes in regulations. It is important that not only the insurance clerk, but also the receptionist/secretary, is aware of all the regulations and changes taking place with insurances. It is the office manager's duty to oversee these rules and regulations and to conduct office meetings on a regular basis to explain and answer any questions the office personnel might have.

Many collection seminars are given throughout the country at various times of the year. It is usually good practice to send the collection staff to one or two of these seminars. They can be costly, but the money can come back to the office in efficient collections. Some offices send copies of Medicare bulletins to their patients to show that the office is harassed just as much as, if not more than, patients. This also points out to patients that it is not the office's rule, it is the insurance companies.

References

American Collectors Association. Fair Debt Collection Practices Act. Minneapolis, MN: American Collectors Association, Department of Education, 1988.

Clark, L. "Why It's Getting Tougher To Collect Your Fees." *Medical Economics,* December 19, 1988, pp. 127-132.

Comeau, J. F. "Collection Systems That Deter Lawsuits." *Physician's Management,* February 1992, pp. 113-118.

Lewin, R. "The Touchiest Billing Situation You'll Ever Face." *Medical Economics,* August 23, 1993, pp. 117-123.

White, O. "Seven Ways To Make Insurers Pay You Quicker." *Medical Economics,* June 1993, pp. 39-41.

7

Ethical and Legal Issues in Health Care

Properly Trained Staff: A Legal Necessity

Before the patient meets the physician for the first time, she or he progresses through several steps, steps that are direct reflections on the physician in the patient's mind. These steps are as follows. The patient

1 Makes telephone contact with the medical office to make an appointment.
2 Travels to the office.
3 Finds a place to park.
4 Locates the office if it is in an office building.
5 Arrives at the waiting room.
6 Is greeted by the receptionist.
7 Has a preliminary visit with the office nurse.

While progressing through these seven steps before meeting with the physician, the patient is arriving at conclusions about the practice. Many things can go wrong before the patient ever meets the physician. Some of these steps, such as the distance from the patient's home to the office or the lack of close parking on the day of the appointment, cannot be changed. However, some steps can be controlled by the office manager and the staff. The importance of a properly trained office is greater than most realize. The patient views the staff's attitude as the attitude of the office as a whole. If the patient is greeted by an unfriendly receptionist or a cold and uncaring nurse, the entire visit is off to a bad start. Remember, most patients are unhappy about being at the doctor's office to begin with. Unhappy patient experiences can be translated into a lawsuit.

Under the legal principle of "vicarious liability," the physician is ultimately responsible for the actions of her or his staff. This principle means that not only are employees legally responsible for their actions, but also the physician is responsible for their actions. Thus the office manager should carefully choose and train all employees. The selection and training process is discussed from a human resource point of view in Chapter 2. From a strictly legal standpoint, there are a few basic areas in which staff training is extremely important: patient satisfaction, medical records, telephone tactics, confidentiality, and billing and collections.

The Contented Patient

There are a number of "hot spots" in the medical office, that is, areas where patients frequently become dissatisfied with the physician or the office staff. If the office manager is aware of these hot spots, she or he can work to ensure that problems in some, if not all, of these areas are avoided.

Ten Medical Office Hot Spots

1 The answering service
2 The appointment time frame
3 Return telephone calls
4 Avoidance of telephone medicine
5 The waiting room
6 The wait in the waiting room
7 Protection of patient confidentiality
8 Office billing department
9 The medical record
10 Curbing of after-hours prescription renewals.

The Answering Service. The after-hours answering service is a direct reflection on the physician and the office. What the answering service staff say, their attitude toward the patient, and how they process the patient's information can cause unhappiness that may lead to lawsuits. The office manager should sit down with the supervisor of the answering service to establish a policy of how they are to handle calls. Once this has been established, the answering service staff are accountable for any deviation from this policy. The office manager should make an effort to find a good service, since this is an important function of the office.

Appointment Time Frame. The amount of time a patient waits for an appointment can also be a sore point. If patients have a problem that they feel cannot wait but are unable to secure an appointment in a reasonable amount of time, things can get ugly! If the patient is an established patient, the abandonment issue (discussed later) could very well come into play. Always attempt to give patients appointments in a reasonable amount of time. If there are no available appointments, have the receptionist ask the physician how to handle the situation.

Return Telephone Calls. Another issue that may lead to an abandonment lawsuit is not returning patient's calls. Patients who continually call with problems and do not receive calls back from the physician will leave the practice and seek the care of another physician. This not only is a legal issue, but borders on an ethical issue and affects the growth of the practice. Most physicians do not want unhappy patients.

Not Practicing Medicine over the Telephone. Many patients want to be treated over the phone. They try to eliminate going to the physician's office, because they don't want to be bothered or don't want to pay for an office visit. Avoiding telephone medicine is one of the most important policies an office can make, and it should be stuck to no matter how insistent the patient is. Keep in mind the basic principle that the patient must be seen before treatment is rendered. Practicing telephone medicine gives the practice a severe handicap and leaves it open to liability. Simply don't do it!

The Waiting Room. Having an unfriendly waiting room is one sure way of making patients unhappy. Up-to-date magazines, soft music, or even a television can help to ease the anxious patient. Having educational reading material available can also be helpful. The "waiting room blues" are discussed in Chapter 3. The waiting room should be warm and inviting, not cold and sterile. Make it as comfortable an experience as it can be.

The Wait. Even if the waiting room is cozy, patients do not want to spend a lot of time there! Most patients in a waiting room are sick; they just want to be seen and go home. It is important for the patients to know that the office is concerned about their time, as well as the office schedule. If situations arise that disrupt the schedule, the staff should be trained to advise the patients that there has been a problem. Some offices offer coffee and tea at times like this. Others ask if the patient wishes to go out for coffee and return in a half hour.

Confidentiality. Remember, voices carry! Office staff should be reminded that gossip is ugly and not appropriate in a medical office. Any talk regarding a patient should be private, quiet, and strictly on a professional level. Sitting in the waiting room and hearing staff talking about another patient's hairdo is a sure turnoff. This sounds like a commonsense issue; however, some suits have stemmed from just such an instance!

Billing Department. The dreaded billing department . . . where all the nasty people work! It is good to concentrate on the bottom line, but, in many cases, billing and collection problems are the source of legal actions against the physician. There needs to be a balance between hardnosed and easygoing. Many patients have problems with billing and insurance. Train the staff to start off on the right foot by asking, "How can we help you?"

Medical Records. There are some common areas where the medical record can become a liability. Be careful not to release records without proper authorization. Do not allow staff to use abbreviations that they have made up. If abbreviations are necessary, staff should use standard abbreviations. **Do not** allow staff to use cute or smart-aleck phrases or abbreviations to describe the patient's disposition. This can create problems for the physician should a lawsuit arise, not to mention that it is totally unprofessional. Also, when staff have made a mistake in documentation, do not let them try to help by altering a patient's medical record. This could spell disaster!

Prescription Renewals. Institute a policy that all prescription renewals must be documented in the patient's chart. As discussed in Chapter 4, a stamp can be made for this purpose and is a neat way to record this information. Train the staff to let the physician know if they think there is a problem with a patient's prescription. A pharmacist may call to question a particular prescription or to advise the physician that the patient had that prescription refilled last week by another physician. This is very important information and must be *immediately* passed on to the physician. This information should also be documented in the patient's chart. There should be a policy for staff to follow regarding situations such as this. Beware of patients who just want prescriptions and not an appointment to see the physician.

The Department of Health and Human Services

The Department of Health and Human Services (DHHS) is a part of the executive branch of the federal government. The secretary of the DHHS reports directly to the President regarding issues of health, welfare, income security plans, policies, and programs. There are five divisions of the DHHS:

1 Social Security Administration
2 Health Care Financing Administration
3 Human Development Services
4 Public Health Service
5 Family Support Administration

Social Security Administration (SSA). The SSA is the division that is directly responsible for the nation's Social Security program. The Social Security fund is supported by employees and employers across the nation. When the earning capacity of an individual decreases because of disability, the fund pays benefits to assist the employee, and when an individual's earning capacity ceases because of death, the fund pays benefits to the individual's family.

Health Care Financing Administration (HCFA). The HCFA is responsible for administering the Medicare and Medicaid programs and the medical care and quality assurance that goes with them. This division develops policies and procedures related to program recipients, such as hospitals, nursing homes, physicians, and insurance contractors. The HCFA is also responsible for working with the state governments regarding the needs of medically indigent people.

Human Development Services (HDS). HDS directs programs for children, the elderly, Native Americans, persons with disabilities, and individuals living in rural areas. It develops programs, controls equal employment opportunity and civil rights policies, and supervises research. HDS also directs public affairs.

Public Health Service (PHS). The PHS was developed to help protect the nation's health, both physical and mental. It coordinates with each state the national health policy, associated programs, research, alcohol and drug abuse, and enforcement of laws regarding medical devices, safe foods, and safe cosmetics. One of the agencies that is a part of the PHS is the Food and Drug Administration (FDA). The FDA supervises and controls the introduction of new drugs, foods, cosmetics, and medical devices. Every food and drug product found on store shelves today is regulated by the FDA.

Family Support Administration (FSA). The FSA advises the secretary of the DHHS on the needs of children and families. It directs family support programs in federal, state, and local governments. It directs and coordinates programs for the Secretary of Labor regarding employment and training.

The A List of a Medical Practice

ABANDONMENT

Abandonment is a physician's severance of the professional relationship that existed between her- or himself and the patient without reasonable notification and during a period when the physician's services were needed by the patient.

Once a physician assumes the care and treatment of an individual, a physician–patient relationship is established. During this established relationship, the physician may not withdraw from the patient without giving the patient enough notice to obtain a new physician.

FROM THE AUTHOR'S NOTEBOOK

A physician–patient relationship is created when a referring physician refers a patient to another physician, and this physician agrees to assume the care of the referred patient.

It is the office manager's responsibility to ensure that when the physician is absent from the practice, another physician provides care to the practice's patients. If there is not adequate coverage for the patients during the physician's absence, the physician could be charged with abandonment.

ABORTION: THE CONTROVERSY

Abortion is the termination of a pregnancy at a time when the fetus is incapable of sustaining life on its own.

Medical professionals today are faced with a twofold problem regarding abortions. They may incur civil liability for refusing to perform abortions, and they may incur criminal liability by performing abortions when they are prohibited by the state's laws. Many states have placed indirect restrictions on abortions by cutting off state funding for clinics in which abortions are performed. You will find in dealing with this very controversial issue that the U.S. Supreme Court often passes the burden of judgment to the states. Any physician who is considering performing abortions should monitor closely the judicial proceedings in their state and should consult with an attorney before making any decisions. Some states require that gestational age be determined, that medical necessity be determined, that informed consent be obtained, and that a spouse or parent be notified. Each state has its own laws regarding abortion, and even on a federal level, these laws change rapidly.

There may be a personnel problem should your physician decide to perform abortions. Many states issue the "Right of Conscience," a document that informs medical personnel of their right to refuse to participate in abortions, to the employees of physicians who have decided to perform abortions. As an office manager, you must be aware that no civil, criminal, administrative, or disciplinary action can be taken against an individual who refuses to aid in an abortion.

Should your physician opt to perform abortions in her or his facility, you must contact the Department of Health in your state to check on the regulations regarding such a facility. Some states require that an Abortion Facility Registration Form be signed and various reports be filed, such as

- A quarterly facilities report
- A report on induced termination of pregnancy
- A report on pathological examination
- A report on maternal death
- A report on complications during or following abortion

AIDS: THE PLAGUE OF THE 1990s

Acquired immune deficiency syndrome (AIDS) is a collection of specific, life-threatening infections that are a result of an underlying deficiency in the immune system of infected individuals. AIDS is not the cause of death; it is simply the catalyst of death, in that it destroys the body's capacity to ward off viruses and bacteria that it would ordinarily fight off. Infection with the virus that causes AIDS (the human immunodeficiency virus) is highly contagious and is found in high numbers in

- Homosexual males
- People who use intravenous drugs
- Prostitutes (both female and male)
- People with hemophilia

This disease has caught the attention of the World Health Organization, and there are now educational programs in place in every nation in the world today. At the time of this writing, 1 in every 250 Americans has been diagnosed with AIDS. There are 36,000 health care workers who have contacted AIDS through the workplace, according to the Centers for Disease Control and Prevention (CDC). Everyone who has AIDS dies. No cure has yet to be found for this quickly spreading plague.

The medical office's liability for the transmission of this disease lies in the realm of transmission through transfusions of HIV-infected blood, accidents involving needlesticks, and failure to take the appropriate precautions when dealing with AIDS patients. States have set up laws governing the health care setting and the AIDS virus.

The federal government, through its Occupational Safety and Health Administration (OSHA) regulations, is attempting to protect the physician and health care worker from unnecessarily becoming infected by the AIDS virus.

Because of the social stigma associated with AIDS, it is thought that the incidence of the disease is being underreported. It is the responsibility of all physicians and hospitals to report their patients with AIDS to their county office of the state Department of Health. It is the office manager's responsibility to see that the reporting requirements are fullfilled.

Each state has its own legislation regarding AIDS testing. Some states require pretest counseling, some require posttest counseling, and some require both. Office managers should be educated in their state's regulations regarding AIDS testing and should educate their staff concerning these regulations.

Generally, physicians and their employees are required to maintain the confidentiality of all AIDS-related information. This rule applies whether the information was obtained on a voluntary basis or on an involuntary basis. This information can be disclosed only to the following:

- The patient
- The physician who ordered the test
- Any person designated by the patient to receive such information
- The Department of Health and the CDC
- An individual with a court order
- A funeral director
- A health care worker directly involved in the care of the individual
- Peer review organizations

No health care worker can refuse to treat a patient with AIDS. It is necessary, however, for health care workers to take the proper steps in protecting themselves and other office patients from the transmission of the virus. The OSHA regulations regarding barrier methods and employee AIDS testing are discussed in detail in Chapter 10.

ANTITRUST LAWS: STILL GOING STRONG AFTER 100 YEARS

The antitrust laws, first developed when America's businesses were forming alliances in order to reduce competition, were practically nonexistent in the health care field until 1975. With health care expenditures on the rise, the demand for economical approaches to the delivery of health care is increasing. The growing number of health care professionals and the various alternatives to health care delivery have become major issues today. The Sherman Antitrust Act is the federal law that has come into play in the health care field. The Sherman Antitrust Act has two parts:

1 Every contract, combination in the form of trust or otherwise, or conspiracy in restraint of trade or commerce among the several states . . . is declared to be illegal.
2 Every person who shall monopolize, or attempt to monopolize, or combine or conspire with any other person or persons to monopolize any part of the trade or commerce among the several states . . . shall be deemed . . . guilty of a felony.

In plain English, Part 1 deals with the type of conduct that may be encountered in the health care industry. Part 2 deals with monopolies.

Areas of concern for health care include price fixing, limiting new entrants into the area, preferred provider arrangements, exclusive contracts, and so on. Physicians are more likely to be confronted with private, nongovernmental antitrust actions than with governmental actions. The recent antitrust actions by the federal government have focused on physicians' conduct. In an extended meeting in 1988 between the American Medical Association and the U.S. Department of Justice, it was decided that the government would stop intervening in medical practice to force competition among physicians.

Exclusive Contracts

Physicians practicing in certain specialties often become involved in exclusive contracts for their services with hospitals and insurance companies. These physicians are generally pathologists, anesthesiologists, cardiologists, and radiologists, whose services cannot be provided by other physicians.

Price Fixing

As a general rule, physicians practicing in one geographical area should not agree on what prices to charge for services, unless they are partners. The physician and the office manager should be cautious when discussing the pricing of medical services with competitors.

> **MANAGER'S ALERT**
>
> Be very careful when discussing prices with other office managers. It is easy to get caught up in a friendly conversation and to forget that you are giving away trade secrets. It is best to avoid the subject of money altogether.

Moratoriums

Hospitals often institute staff moratoriums, which means that they do not allow any further appointments to the staff. These moratoriums are generally only for a specific time period and are lifted at a later date, at which time applications are accepted. Moratoriums must be applied in a nondiscriminatory manner. If your physician is just moving into an area where the hospital has a closed staff, it is imperative that she or he obtain counsel for representation of this issue.

AUTOPSIES

A licensed physician, usually a pathologist, may perform an autopsy or postmortem examination on a deceased patient within 36 hours after death. Autopsies are done for the following four reasons:

1 To establish the cause of death.
2 To educate.
3 To serve legal purposes (in which case, they are usually done by the coroner).
4 To maintain quality assurance regarding hospital care (i.e., to make sure the death was not due to error at the hospital).

It is mandatory that the physician or office manager obtain the appropriate authorization before the autopsy is performed. Authorization may be given by the following persons in order of preference:

1 The deceased patient, with spousal consent
2 Written authority by the deceased
3 The spouse of the deceased
4 Any adult children of the deceased
5 Any adult grandchildren of the deceased
6 The parents of the deceased

7 The brothers or sisters of the deceased
8 The nephews or nieces of the deceased
9 The grandparents of the deceased
10 The uncles or aunts of the deceased
11 The adult cousins of the deceased
12 The adult stepchildren of the deceased
13 A relative who is next of kin of a previously deceased spouse
14 Any other relative or friend with written authorization from the deceased

A coroner does not need to obtain the necessary authorization to perform an autopsy. He or she must, however, investigate the circumstances surrounding the death to establish whether the death was the result of a criminal act.

MANAGER'S ALERT

There is never a time that an attending physician can order an autopsy without the necessary authorization!

The Death Certificate

A medical office should contain a file with blank death certificates. Often, a patient will die in a hospital while the physician is having office hours. The funeral director must obtain a death certificate before picking up the body. She or he will call the office and ask to stop by to pick up the death certificate. If your office does not have a death certificate, the funeral director generally carries them and will provide you with one. The funeral director will fill out the necessary information on the certificate; however, the physician must write the cause of death on the certificate and sign it. The attending physician at the hospital usually supplies the funeral director with the death certificate. This certificate must be filed with the local registrar of vital statistics within 96 hours.

Good Medical Records . . . A Legal Asset

The importance of good medical records becomes evident in cases of malpractice. A study has shown that 30% of malpractice cases are due to problems with the patient's medical record. Documentation is a very important part of the defense against a malpractice charge and should not be taken lightly. The medical record is one of the most important pieces of evidence in any malpractice case. Most people find it difficult to remember last week, let alone 5 years ago. This is where a good, complete medical record is invaluable. If it contains proper documentation, a medical record can jog the memory of a physician and help her or him to recall the events of the patient care.

Any strange behavior or personality traits should be documented in the patient's chart. The complexity of the problem coupled with the therapeutic plan of action should be carefully explained in the medical record.

All medical records should be kept by using the RALTIC method (Box 7–1). That is, it is important for the information in a medical record to be *r*elevant (that is, containing nothing superfluous), *a*ccurate (clear and free of error), *l*egible (neat, and preferrably typed), *t*imely (dated and in proper sequence), *i*nformative (documenting treatment, prognosis, diagnosis, etc.), and *c*omplete (that is, with no ommissions).

The Legal Life of Financial Records

Retention of financial records is an important issue and should be followed closely by the office manager. The following guidelines will assist the office manager in deciding how long to maintain certain financial records in the medical office. They should be reviewed with the practice accountant for verification.

Records to Be Kept Indefinitely

1 General ledgers
2 Financial statements
3 Capital assessment records

BOX 7–1. THE RALTIC METHOD FOR KEEPING MEDICAL RECORDS

Relevant
Accurate
Legible
Timely
Informative
Complete

Records to Be Kept 10 Years

1 Payroll register

Records to Be Kept 7 Years

1 Accounts receivable ledger cards
2 Remittance advices (Explanations of Benefits)
3 Cancelled payroll checks

Records to Be Kept 5 Years

1 Bank statements/cancelled checks
2 Records on uncollectible accounts
3 Time cards or time sheets

Records to Be Kept 4 Years

1 Payments and reports to the government (IRS, state government, etc.)
2 Vendor contracts
3 All dealings with Medicare

Records to Be Kept 2 Years

1 Purchase orders

Records to Be Kept 1 Year

1 Accounts receivable trial balances

The Physician–Patient Relationship

Medical care is not an inalienable right that is guaranteed to every individual. The physician has control over the patients she or he chooses to treat. However, once the physician–patient relationship has begun, the patient has the right to expect it to continue unless the physician gives her or him suitable notice that it is going to end. Making an appointment does not constitute a physician–patient relationship, but once the patient arrives in the office, the relationship begins. Since there are no specific laws regarding the beginning of this relationship, most cases are decided by the court. For example, depending on the court, it is possible, though not probable, that the woman to whom the physician gave medical advice to during open house at their children's school could view that encounter as a physician–physician relationship. It is important for the office manager to train the staff regarding giving advice to patients. When a staff member offers advice to a patient, the law views this as advice from the physician's agent, creating a duty on the physician's part to treat this patient.

There are a limited number of instances in which the physician can see the patient without being considered to have entered into a physician–patient relationship. They are

- Examining a patient for life insurance purposes.
- Giving expert opinion for a Workers' Compensation or disability carrier.
- Performing a preemployment physical.
- Performing a court-ordered examination.

Keep in mind that any emergency treatment that a physician offers must be carried through by the physician. In other words, once a physician accepts an undertaking in an emergency situation, she or he is obligated to this patient. The physician may not neglect or withdraw her or his services unless there is another physician available to continue treatment of the patient.

Termination of the Problem Patient

One of the major considerations when dismissing a problem patient is the effects of a relatively new law protecting discrimination against people with disabilities. This law, the 1990 Americans with Disabilities Act, was designed to prevent discrimination due to a disability. A disability is any physical or psychological problem that makes the individual unable to perform daily life activities. The term *psychological* is defined legally as any emotional or mental illness. Some physicians have patients with severe psychological problems whose behavior creates problems in the medical office. If the physician decides to terminate the physician–patient relationship with such a patient, she or he could be liable under the 1990 Americans with Disabilities Act. This law specifically addresses professional health care offices. Any noncompliant or disruptive patient with psychological problems that could be regarded as a disability is protected by this law. If this patient is interfering with the care of others, however, and it can be proven, it is possible to terminate the physician–patient relationship under the new law without complications. The office manager should be aware of the law; however, if paper trails are created, and documentation of disruptive acts and verbal abuse to the staff and physician is carefully entered into the patient's medical record, there should be no problems with dismissal.

Cases have been brought to court for just this reason, but, to date, these cases have been found in

---

BOX 7–2A. SAMPLE PATIENT TERMINATION LETTER

Dear Ms. Crane:

We are no longer able to provide care to you and request that you find another physician within [time period designated by office policy] of the date of this letter. If you have an emergency, we will continue to provide you with medical care for the time period stated above, or you may seek medical care in the nearest emergency room. Once you have obtained a new physician, we will be happy to forward a copy of your medical records to this new physician. It will be necessary for you to either sign a Records Release Form or send us a note with your signature and the address of the new physician.

Sincerely,

Dr. William Scott

BOX 7–2B. SAMPLE PATIENT TERMINATION LETTER

Dear Mr. Callon:

I find it necessary to inform you that I will no longer be able to serve as your physician or prescribe medications for you. The reason for this decision is _____.

Because you may need medical attention in the future, I recommend that you promptly find another doctor to care for you. You may want to contact the medical society or local hospital for the names of physicians near you who are accepting new patients.

I will be available to provide you with emergency care until _____.

This will give you time to obtain a new physician. I will be happy to forward a copy of your medical records to your new physician upon receipt of a signed Records Release Form from the physician.

Sincerely,

Dr. Joseph M. Babinetz

---

favor of the physicians. A 2-week to 1-month notice is recommended for patients to secure a new physician. An attorney will generally recommend that if the physician is terminating a patient for psychological reasons (noncompliancy, disruptions, etc.), the office should not give the patient the exact reason for the termination. Some sample termination letters can be seen in Box 7–2. Any of these letters can be copied or changed to fit the needs of the practice. The office

manager should meet with and evaluate these letters with the physician to be sure that the correct format for the office is used.

It has been found that patients who are noncompliant and disruptive, miss appointments, and have drug problems are the most likely to sue a physician. This type of patient should be terminated as soon as a problem develops, because continued care only increases the possibility of liability. The office manager should be consulting with the office staff who are involved in the care of the patients. They can point out problems with this patient to the office manager. If the physician is not aware of the problems with this patient, it is the office manager's job to list the past problems and state feedback from the staff.

The office manager will find that many of these patients do not pay their bills and can sometimes be gently nudged out of the office by continued pressing for payment. These patients do not want to pay, so they dismiss the physician when asked for payment. This eliminates the need for the office to instigate such an action.

Good office staff will often recognize a problem patient in the first call for an appointment, and this feedback from the staff should not be ignored! Listen to them! The office does not have to take every patient who calls.

BOX 7–2C. **SAMPLE PATIENT TERMINATION LETTER**

Dear Mr. Miller:

Since you have refused to follow our medical advice by signing out of the hospital, we find it necessary to terminate our physician–patient relationship. We feel that we can no longer have a beneficial, therapeutic relationship with you and would be pleased to send your records to the physician of your choice.

If you require medical attention before securing a new physician, we urge you to seek care in the nearest hospital emergency room. We do urge you to seek a new physician as soon as possible.

Sincerely,

John H. Doe, M.D.,
for Cardiovascular Specialists

BOX 7–2D. **SAMPLE PATIENT TERMINATION LETTER**

Dear Mrs. Walters:

I find it necessary to inform you that I am withdrawing from further professional attendance upon you for the reason that you have persisted in refusing to follow my medical advice and treatment. Since your condition requires medical attention, I suggest that you place yourself under the care of another physician without delay. If you so desire, I shall be available to attend to you for a reasonable time after you have received this letter, but in no event for more than 5 days from the date of this letter.

This should give you ample time to select a physician of your choice from the many competent physicians in this area. With your approval, I will make available to this physician your case history and information regarding the diagnosis and treatment that you have received from me.

Sincerely,

Lawrence Conklin, M.D.

BOX 7–3. **LETTER RECOMMENDING COURTESY TREATMENT**

Dear Mr. Jones:

As we discussed during your recent office visit, your condition is still undiagnosed and lies in an area outside my circle of expertise. It could be nothing, or it could be very serious. I will continue to serve as your physician, but you must understand and take responsibility for the fact that you are making it impossible for me to provide you with the kind of care you require. I would like to take this opportunity to refer you to a charity hospital where you might obtain the testing that is necessary for your care.

Should you wish to follow through with this suggestion, please call my office and my staff will aid you in making the proper arrangements for your testing.

Sincerely,

Dr. Jennifer Waldron

CERTIFIED MAIL DELIVERY—A MUST

A termination letter should be sent by certified mail, with a return receipt requested. One copy of the letter should also be sent regular mail, and another copy should remain as a permanent part of the patient's medical record. There is a fee for certified mail delivery, but it provides the sender with a receipt on which is written the name of the individual who received the letter. This receipt should be kept in the patient's chart and should be attached to the copy of the letter.

To send the letter, you must attach to the envelope a white receipt for the certified mail. You need to fill it out with the recipient's name and address. You also need to complete a green delivery receipt with the recipient's name and address on one side and your name and address on the other. The green delivery receipt will be returned to you as a postcard with the recipient's signature on it. An example of this type of mail service is shown in Chapter 3.

FROM THE AUTHOR'S NOTEBOOK

Ask the postal clerk to stamp the front of the envelope with "addressee only/restricted delivery." This ensures that no one else but the patient or designee is allowed to sign for the letter.

Often, the certified mail will be returned to your office stating that it was not picked up. Many individuals have so many debts that creditors are looking for them on a regular basis. They generally will not pick up certified mail for this reason. That is why you should send a copy of the letter by regular mail also. The returned envelope should also be placed in the patient's medical record.

ALTERNATIVES TO TERMINATION

There are other ways in which the medical office can care for patients who should be terminated but the physician feels need care. Difficult patients who require extensive amounts of testing can be referred to a charity hospital or enrolled in a courtesy patient plan at the local community hospital. Any hospital that receives monies from the federal government must provide a certain amount of free and charitable care to individuals with hardships. Many difficult patients are difficult because they do not have the funds to obtain further testing. More and more individuals refuse testing because they are unemployed or uninsured. These patients can be sent a letter that explains the alternatives to their care. An example of such a letter is shown in Box 7–3.

Informing patients that they are possibly going to be terminated from the physician's practice is another alternative to actually taking the action. When a physician tells patients that they are being considered for termination from the practice because they refuse to take their medicines, is sometimes enough to motivate the patient into compliance.

Boomerang Patients

If the practice is old enough, there might be occasion to deal with the "boomerang" patient. Many physicians find themselves in the predicament of being on call in the emergency room and having a dismissed patient appear and require treatment. The physician, not being able to refuse treatment, should explain to the patient at the time of service that this emergency treatment is on a one-time basis only. The physician should carefully explain that this *does not* reaffirm their physician–patient relationship. It is good for the office manager to check the bylaws of the hospital before this type of situation arises to be sure that the physician's actions are in line with them.

Ethics: The Gray Ghost

Many philosophers, teachers, and theologians will agree that there is no objective method of arriving at an ethical decision. When it comes to ethics, there is no right answer, there is just a range of acceptable actions that can be taken. Most hospitals now have ethics committees that guide physicians and other staff members through various situations. These committees can minimize many conflicts between physicians, staff members, and families. They can help defuse volatile situations when they arise.

Physicians face many difficult ethical choices in today's world of high-tech medicine. Some of the dilemmas in the stew pot of ethics are

- End-of-life decisions
- Confidentiality
- Mapping of genomes
- HIV detection and notification
- Beginning-of-life technologies

END-OF-LIFE DECISIONS

There is now a law in the United States that guarantees individuals the right to decide for themselves the limits they wish to set on the use of life-sustaining therapy on them when they are terminally ill or in a vegetative state. This law, the Patient Self-Determination Act, came into effect in December 1991. It requires that hospitals, nursing homes, personal care facilities, hospices, home health care agencies, and health maintenance organizations ask patients whether they have prepared an advance directive, that is, a Living Will or a Durable Power of Attorney for health care.

To date, less than 15% of all individuals in the United States have living wills. In one survey, 70% of seriously ill patients said they wanted to discuss their end-of-life decisions, but only 6% had actually taken the steps to do so. The medical office can help patients by understanding the Patient Self-Determination Act and having blank Living Wills and Durable Power of Attorney forms in their offices. In fact, the law requires that institutions educate both their staff and the community about the law. The office manager should instruct the staff on the law and its ramifications in a workshop or seminar. It can be very helpful if all staff are familiar with the law and can aid the physician in educating patients. With all the attention this topic has received in television programs, radio talk shows, newspapers, and magazines, it is unusual for individuals to know nothing of these directives. Still, a good medical office will not wait until the last minute to speak to their patients about the Patient Self-Determination Act. It is a good practice to have it discussed before it is actually needed, so that emotions do not cloud the decision making (Figure 7–1). The office manager may want to designate one staff member to finish with the patient after the physician has begun the education process. It is easier if the patient brings up the subject, and this can be nudged by keeping booklets about the Patient Self-Determination Act in the waiting room for the patients to read (Figure 7–2). Many patients will become interested in speaking with someone about the act. Each state has developed booklets and forms that can be obtained for use by patients. Box 7–4 shows one state's Living Will. One of the most important things for the medical office to remember is that

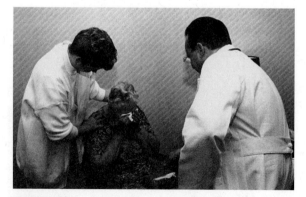

FIGURE 7–1. Discussing end-of-life decisions can be emotional.

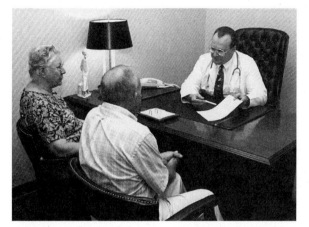

FIGURE 7–2. The physician explains the living will to patients.

Doctors Advise–Patients Decide

When a patient has prepared an advance directive, the medical office and the physician can make treatment decisions regarding the aggressiveness of the patient's care.

Many community centers and church groups are also becoming involved in educating people about the Patient Self-Determination Act.

Some states do not honor the Living Will. The office manager must contact the practice's attorney to check on state regulations. The office might be located in a state that honors a Durable Power of Attorney but not a Living Will. Be it a Living Will or a Durable Power of Attorney, some form of advance directive is now necessary. Health care providers who comply with valid advance directives are immune from civil and criminal liability. That is, withholding or withdrawing life-sustaining treatment in compliance with a valid advance directive does not constitute a suicide or a homicide.

This immunity notwithstanding, health care providers are not forced to comply with the advance directive. The advance directive can be revoked at any time and in any manner by the patient, regardless of the patient's physical or mental condition at the time it is revoked. This revocation becomes a part of the patient's medical record.

A different format of Living Will from that shown in Box 7–4 is shown in Box 7–5. It may be changed to follow specific guidelines issued by individual states. Living Will and Durable Power of Attorney forms may be obtained from the local medical society.

CONFIDENTIALITY

Information that is shared between a physician and a patient for the purpose of medical treatment is considered confidential communication. Any unauthorized disclosure of this information breaches this contractual obligation between the physician and the patient. The vast majority of states have strict regulations regarding the confidentiality of the information physicians receive from their patients. Most state physician–patient statutes are similar to the following:

"No physician should be allowed, in any civil matter, to disclose any information which he acquired while attending the patient in a professional capacity, which enabled him to act in that capacity, which shall tend to blacken the character of the patient, without consent of the patient except in civil matters brought by such patient for damages on account of personal injuries."

If any of the above elements are met in the physician–patient relationship, the physician is barred from disclosure of any information without the patient's permission.

The purpose of adopting a physician–patient privilege was to create an atmosphere in which patients could feel secure enough to disclose any information that might pertain to their medical problems. The Principles of Medical Ethics that have been laid out by the American Medical Association (AMA) establish a broader statute of confidentiality than is found in the judicial codes. The AMA code of ethics advocates the confidentiality of all contacts between the medical office and the patient.

There are a few exceptions to the state Duty of Confidentiality statute that are pertinent to daily operations in a medical office. A patient's medical information may be released when

- The patient files a lawsuit for personal injuries.
- Consent has been obtained.
- The court orders it.
- A third party has requested it.

The patient who files a lawsuit for personal injuries waives the physician–patient relationship by filing suit. This suit allows consent of disclosure of medically related injuries/illnesses. It is not uncommon for patient records to be requested by third parties for the purpose of insurance, employment physicals, etc. A court may order a patient's medical information in cases of communicable diseases, child abuse, etc.

BOX 7–4. **ONE STATE'S LIVING WILL**

LIVING WILL DECLARATION

As authorized by the Commonwealth of Pennsylvania "Advance Directive For Health Care Act", April 1992.

I, _____ , being of sound mind, willfully and voluntarily make this declaration to be followed if I become incompetent. This declaration reflects my firm and settled commitment to refuse life-sustaining treatment under the circumstances indicated below.

I direct my attending physician to withhold or withdraw life-sustaining treatment that serves only to prolong the process of my dying, if I should be in a terminal condition or in a state of permanent unconsciousness.

I direct that treatment be limited to measures to keep me comfortable and to relieve pain, including any pain that might occur by withholding or withdrawing life-sustaining treatment.

In addition, if I am in the condition described above, I feel especially strong about the following forms of treatment:

    I ☐ do or ☐ do not want cardiac resuscitation.
    I ☐ do or ☐ do not want mechanical respiration.
    I ☐ do or ☐ do not want tube feeding or any other artificial or invasive form of nutrition (food) or
          hydration (water).
    I ☐ do or ☐ do not want blood or blood products.
    I ☐ do or ☐ do not want any form of surgery or invasive diagnostic tests.
    I ☐ do or ☐ do not want kidney dialysis.
    I ☐ do or ☐ do not want antibiotics.

I realize that if I do not specifically indicate my preference regarding any of the forms of treatment listed above, I may receive that form of treatment.

Other instructions:

    I ☐ do or ☐ do not want to designate another person as my surrogate to make medical treatment decisions for me if I should be incompetent and in a terminal condition or in a state of permanent unconsciousness. Name and address of surrogate (if applicable): _____

    _____

    Name and address of substitute surrogate (if surrogate designated above is unable to serve):

    _____

    _____

I made this declaration on the _____ day of _____ (month, year).

Declarant's signature: _____

Declarant's address: _____

The declarant or the person on behalf of and at the direction of the declarant knowingly and voluntarily signed this writing by signature or mark in my presence.

Witness's signature: _____

Witness's address: _____

Witness's signature: _____

Witness's address: _____

Compliments of the Delaware Valley Geriatrics Society

Each state has a law regarding the confidentiality of AIDS testing. The smart office manager obtains copies of state guidelines regarding AIDS testing and distributes them to the staff during an office meeting when discussing procedures and guidelines.

In today's high-tech world, we use fax machines for a multitude of purposes. Many offices fax test results, medical records, and so on to hospitals. Insurance companies will even request that medical records be faxed. Confidentiality is a serious issue when using a fax machine to transmit information. It is very important to add a confidentiality notice to the fax transmission cover sheet. This will protect the faxed information from being disseminated or photocopied. A sample confidentiality notice is shown in Box 7–6.

HIV DETECTION AND NOTIFICATION

A wide range of ethical and moral issues surround the HIV epidemic. The following are issues that need to be addressed by the AMA and health care regulatory agencies:

- Mandatory testing of health care workers
- Mandatory screening of patients for HIV
- Confidentiality
- Discrimination

GENOME MAPPING AND BEGINNING-OF-LIFE TECHNOLOGIES

A genome is a complete set of the genes of an individual. In one of the most exciting scientific

---

BOX 7–5. **THE LIVING WILL**

This declaration is made this _____ day of _____ being of sound mind, willfully and voluntarily make known my desires that my moment of death shall not be artificially postponed.

If at any time I should have an incurable and irreversible injury, disease, or illness judged to be a terminal condition by my attending physician who has personally examined me and has determined that my death is imminent except for death-delaying procedures, I direct that procedures that would only prolong the dying process be withheld or withdrawn and that I be permitted to die naturally with only the administration of medication, sustenance, or the performance of any medical procedure deemed necessary by my attending physician to provide me with comfortable care.

In the absence of my ability to give directions regarding the use of such death-delaying procedures, it is my intention that this declaration shall be honored by my family and physician as the final expression of my legal right to refuse medical or surgical treatment and accept the consequences from such refusal.

Signed _____

City, County, and State of Residence _____

The declarant is personally known to me, and I believe him or her to be of sound mind. I saw the declarant sign the declaration in my presence (or the declarant acknowledged in my presence that he or she had signed the declaration) and I signed the declaration as a witness in the presence of the declarant. I did not sign the declarant's signature above for or at the direction of the declarant. At the date of this instrument, I am not entitled to any portion of the estate of the declarant according to the laws of intestate succession or, to the best of my knowledge and belief, under any will of declarant or other instrument taking effect at declarant's death, or directly financially responsible for declarant's medical care.

Witness _____

Witness _____

BOX 7–6. CONFIDENTIALITY NOTICE FOR FAXED INFORMATION

This facsimile message and the document(s) accompanying
this telefax transmission may contain confidential
information
which is legally privileged and intended only for the use
of the
addressee named above. If the reader is not the intended
recipient or the employee of the intended recipient, you
are
hereby notified that any dissemination, copying, or
distribution
of this communication is strictly prohibited. If you
received this
communication in error, please notify us immediately by telefax
or telephone and return the original documents to us via
the U.S.
Postal Service at the above address. Thank you for
your help.

---

endeavors going on today, some scientists have been making radical attempts to alter the basic building blocks of the body and personality by altering genomes. If they have patients' genomic information, physicians could perform interventions and alteration of the genetic structure prior to the development of symptoms. The concern, however, is that some physicians may use genomic information simply to change people's behavior, not prevent disease.

More pressing for society at this point are the issues that our increasing reproductive technology has presented us. The following is a list of issues that the medical office should be aware of:

- The gift procedure
- Fetus harvesting
- Sperm donors
- Egg donors
- Surrogate motherhood
- Abortion of the problem fetus

Beginning-of-life issues and issues related to the mapping of genomes are not issues that most medical office staff will have to face. They are mentioned here merely to make the office manager aware of them and to provide a very basic understanding of them. Awareness of these issues must now be part of medical practice.

Informed Consent

Consent is the voluntary agreement by a person who has sufficient mentality to make an intelligent choice to allow something proposed by another. It can be either express or implied. *Express consent* is a verbal or written agreement to undergo a medical procedure. *Implied consent* is consent implied by some type of action or inaction by silence that leads to the presumption that consent has been given. Consent must be obtained from the patient, or from a person authorized to be a delegate of the patient, before any medical or surgical procedure can be done. Touching a patient who has not given consent to be touched could be considered battery. It is necessary to give patients sufficient information, in a form that they can understand, before asking them to make health care choices. Informed consent requires that patients have full understanding of that to which they have consented.

Negligence

HOW TO LOWER YOUR CHANCES OF BEING SUED

Negligence is the commission or omission of an act that a reasonably prudent person would or would not do under any given circumstance. This conduct is caused by heedless or carelessness that is a deviation from the standard of care as we know it. There is no sure way to guard against a lawsuit. Even the best physicians are threatened at some time in their career with a lawsuit. Why do patients sue? Unhappiness . . . that's a clue! Maintaining good relations with patients is a way to minimize malpractice suits. Many suits arise from emotional problems, whereby the patient feels the physician doesn't care or the staff was rude.

Patients want a physician who is available, who cares about them, and who listens to them. They want office staff who are warm and caring, efficient, and professional in every way. All patients think their problem is an emergency, whether the staff agrees or not. Well-trained office staff always listen, never giving patients the impression that they are not important or their problem is not urgent. Often, the decision to sue is made by the neighbor across the street, a family member dealing with guilt, or a person with a financial crisis in the family. Chapter 15 discusses the many ways the office can promote patient satisfaction. Many suits can be prevented by simply making it a point to have good relationships with patients. Box 7–7 lists the states' statutes of limitation for malpractice and wrongful death charges. The following are *seven ways to prevent malpractice suits:*

1 Maintain good medical records.
2 Have a risk management plan.
3 Have good, solid foundations for all medical care given.
4 Have good rapport with patients.
5 Have prescription renewal policies in place.
6 Have respect for patients and their families.
7 Strive for good treatment outcomes.

The legal importance of keeping good medical records has already been discussed in this chapter. In addition to keeping good records, it is necessary for the office to develop a good risk management plan and stick to it! Solid foundations for medical care and good rapport with patients are a must! This can alleviate many nasty situations from the practice. The need for a good prescription policy has already been discussed. However, it's not enough simply to have a policy written. You must abide by it . . . no exceptions! Having respect for patients and their families is one of the most important things the office can do to prevent malpractice suits. Treat patients and their families as you would want to be treated, and you can never go wrong. Good outcomes, of course, are what everyone wants. They are

not always possible. Everyone must recognize this, while continuing to do the very best they can.

FORMS OF NEGLIGENCE

Negligence can take the following forms:

- Malfeasance
- Misfeasance
- Nonfeasance
- Malpractice
- Criminal negligence

Malfeasance is the execution of an unlawful or improper act. *Misfeasance* is the improper performance of an act, resulting in injury to another. *Nonfeasance* is the failure to act, when there is a duty to act, as a reasonably prudent person would act. *Malpractice* is the negligence or carelessness of a professional person, such as a nurse, pharmacist, physician, lawyer, or accountant. *Criminal negligence* is the reckless disregard for the safety of another. It is the willful indifference to an injury that could follow an act.

DEGREES OF NEGLIGENCE

Ordinary negligence—Ordinary negligence is the failure to do what a reasonably prudent person would do under the circumstances or the doing of that which a reasonably prudent person would not do under the circumstances.

Gross negligence—Gross negligence is the intentional or wanton omission of care that would be proper to provide or the doing of that which would be improper to do.

Deposition Demands

The time might come when the office manager is called on to provide a deposition in a lawsuit between a physician and a patient. Other members of the staff might be summoned also, so it is important to understand the few basic steps to giving a deposition.

Before giving the deposition, prepare an updated copy of your resume, in case it is required by the legal counsel. Review any documents in which you had a hand. This would include any telephone logs, medical records, financial statements, etc. Meet with the practice attorney or malpractice insurer's attorney who will be representing you. Review the plaintiff's complaint and the defendant's answer, so you are clear on the issues.

BOX 7–7. STATES' STATUTES OF LIMITATION FOR ALLEGING MALPRACTICE OR WRONGFUL DEATH

STATE	MALPRACTICE	WRONGFUL DEATH
ALABAMA	2 yrs	2 yrs
ALASKA	2 yrs	2 yrs
ARIZONA	2 yrs	2 yrs
ARKANSAS	2 yrs	3 yrs
CALIFORNIA	1 yr	1 yr
COLORADO	2 yrs	2 yrs
CONNECTICUT	2 yrs	2 yrs
DELAWARE	2 yrs	2 yrs
DISTRICT OF COLUMBIA	3 yrs	1 yr
FLORIDA	2 yrs	2 yrs
GEORGIA	2 yrs	2 yrs
HAWAII	2 yrs	2 yrs
IDAHO	2 yrs	2 yrs
ILLINOIS	2 yrs	2 yrs
INDIANA	2 yrs	2 yrs
IOWA	2 yrs	2 yrs
KANSAS	2 yrs	2 yrs
KENTUCKY	1 yr	1 yr
LOUISIANA	1 yr	1 yr
MAINE	2 yrs	2 yrs
MARYLAND	3 yrs	2 yrs
MASSACHUSETTS	3 yrs	3 yrs
MICHIGAN	2 yrs	2 yrs
MINNESOTA	2 yrs	3 yrs
MISSISSIPPI	2 yrs	2 yrs
MISSOURI	2 yrs	3 yrs
MONTANA	5 yrs	2 yrs
NEBRASKA	5 yrs	2 yrs
NEVADA	2 yrs	2 yrs
NEW HAMPSHIRE	6 yrs	2 yrs
NEW JERSEY	2 yrs	2 yrs
NEW MEXICO	3 yrs	3 yrs
NEW YORK	2½ yrs	2 yrs
NORTH CAROLINA	3 yrs	2 yrs
NORTH DAKOTA	2 yrs	2 yrs
OHIO	1 yr	2 yrs
OKLAHOMA	2 yrs	2 yrs
OREGON	2 yrs	2 yrs
PENNSYLVANIA	2yrs	2 yrs
RHODE ISLAND	3 yrs	3 yrs
SOUTH CAROLINA	6 yrs	6 yrs
SOUTH DAKOTA	2 yrs	3 yrs
TENNESSEE	1 yr	1 yr
TEXAS	2 yrs	2 yrs
UTAH	4 yrs	2 yrs
VERMONT	3 yrs	2 yrs
VIRGINIA	2 yrs	2 yrs
WASHINGTON	3 yrs	3 yrs
WEST VIRGINIA	2 yrs	2 yrs
WISCONSIN	3 yrs	3 yrs

At the deposition, wait until the question has been asked in full before attempting to answer it. Answer only the question that was asked. Don't give any extra information. If you do not understand the question, ask the attorney to rephrase it. Tell the attorney that you are not sure you understand the question. If you become tired or feel confused, ask to take a break to confer with your attorney. Never answer a question with a guess. If you do not know the answer, say so. Be honest!! The practice attorney will be able to guide you in the areas that are critical to the case. The key to giving a good deposition is to be accurate and truthful at all times.

Delegation of Duties

The office is more efficient when various duties are delegated to paraprofessionals; however, by doing this, the office could make itself vulnerable to various liabilities. The delegation of routine duties can sometimes become a headache for both the office manager and the physician. One way to prevent this problem is to stay well within the limits of the law. Any time the office manager or physician asks an employee to perform a task that is in the gray area, such as running an errand to pick up the physician's special surgery eyeglasses from the optician, the office exposes itself to trouble.

Sexual Harassment

It is not uncommon to pick up a newspaper and read about a sexual harassment case in the medical field. This seems to be a problem that is running rampant in medicine. A 1991 Harvard University Medical School survey showed that 27% of Massachusetts' female physicians had experienced at least one incident of sexual harassment in the previous year. A poll conducted by the National Association of Female Executives in New York showed that 64% of individuals who said they had been sexually harassed did not report the incident and that 83% of the people polled believed that harassment occurs more often than is reported. Some physicians are being charged with sexual harassment in the medical office setting. There must be a policy in place to prevent sexual harassment and sexual harassment charges from ever happening. This policy should be that a medical assistant, nurse, lab technician, or any other clinical personnel accompanies the physician into the exam room when examining a patient (Figure 7–3).

Sexual harassment comes in various forms and the office should be prepared with a written policy regarding patients and sexual harassment. Always remember, do not exhibit any type of behavior that could misconstrued. It is the office manager's job to protect the physician by the proper handling of patients while in the office.

Complying with the Americans with Disabilities Act

Many small businesses are trying to comply with the regulations resulting from the relatively new Americans with Disabilities Act. Many times it is just a matter of common sense, business sense, and money. This act came into effect in 1992, but its scope was broadened in July 1994, requiring that any company with 15 or more employees comply with its regulations. It replaces the Rehabilitation Act of 1973 and protects the rights of the more than 35 million people in this country who have physical and mental disabilities, by requiring that changes be made in restrooms, that tables accommodate patients in wheelchairs, and that several other changes be made throughout the office (Figure 7–4). In some buildings, the timing must be changed on the elevators to accommodate wheelchair entrance and exit. This law requires Braille signage and interpreters to be available if needed (discussed in detail in Chapter 11). Changes in mindset must also take place; there can be no discrimination against individuals with disabilities who

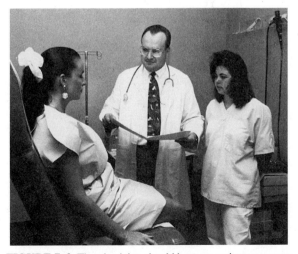

FIGURE 7–3. The physician should have an assistant present in the examination room.

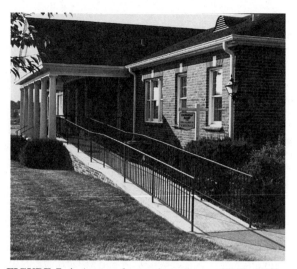

FIGURE 7–4. A ramp for use by patients with disabilities.

are applying for positions in the office. These individuals are protected from discrimination regarding hiring, firing, and benefits. Seminars are offered by social service agencies and hospitals to increase sensitivity to patients and workers with disabilities.

The Job Accommodation Network is available to provide advice and solutions for small businesses and large corporations trying to comply with these regulations. Some changes that must be made can be costly. If the office is being leased, the landlord should be contacted to determine what percentage of these changes are her or his responsibility. Ramps, widened doorways, and removal of barriers should be the responsibility of the landlord.

The Family and Medical Leave Act

The Family and Medical Leave Act went into effect in August 1993. This law includes facilities with 50 or more employees working in different offices within a 75-mile radius of each other. It requires employers to allow employees to take up to 12 weeks of unpaid leave during any 12-month period because of the birth of a child; the adoption of a child; the serious illness of a child, spouse, or parent; or the serious illness of the employee. This law does require that employees give at least 30 days notice before taking the leave, if possible. Employers are required to hold the employee's position or provide the employee with a position that is of like status, pay, and responsibility. However, a salaried

employee who is one of 10% of the highest paid employees at a given worksite would be denied this job guarantee, but not the leave. The employer may require a medical certification to support an employee's request for leave. This is allowed under the law.

The employer is allowed to require an employee to use her or his accrued paid leave, such as vacation or sick leave, at the beginning of the leave and take the balance of the 12 weeks as unpaid leave. Planning for how the work of the employee is going to be done while the employee is gone is crucial! It is important for managers to know how to handle different situations that might come up. Managers become frustrated when trying to accommodate the needs of everyone, but it must be remembered that any decisions made will affect everyone—the physician, the staff, the patient, and themselves!

The Legal Aspects of Labor Relations

The relationship that exists between an employer and an employee is regulated by both federal and state laws. The National Labor Relations Act was enacted in 1935 and defines certain conduct of both employees and employers as unfair labor practices. It provides for hearings on complaints when such practices have occurred. The National Labor Relations Act has jurisdiction over any medical office with gross revenues of more than $100,000 per year.

The Fair Labor Standards Act of 1938 establishes minimum wages and a maximum of hours of employment. This law permits an established work period of 14 consecutive days as an alternative to the usual 7-day week. If the 14-consecutive-day pay period is chosen in the medical office, overtime rates need only be paid for hours worked in excess of 80 per pay period. Administrative and supervisory personnel are exempt from overtime wages. The Equal Pay Act of 1963 is an amendment to this act and addresses wage disparities based on sex. This act simply means "equal pay for equal work."

The Equal Employment Opportunity Act of 1972 prohibits employers from discrimination on the basis of race, color, religion, sex, or national origin.

The Age Discrimination in Employment Act of 1967 prohibits age-based employment discrimination against individuals between 40 and 70 years of age. The purpose of this law is to promote employment in the aging population when the ability of the individual permits employment.

Workers' Compensation laws give employees a legal way to receive funds for injuries on the job. Any employee who is injured while performing job-related duties may sue the employer for injuries sustained. This law is based not on negligence, but rather on the employee–employer relationship. This law is a state law and therefore varies from state to state.

The Practice Attorney

Because our society is litigious, it is important to have a qualified, knowledgeable attorney on staff. The practice attorney should be well informed in the field of health care, in addition to business. This lawyer should be called on for advice regarding employment issues, tax issues, business issues, government regulation in regard to health care, and insurances. If the lawyer chosen is not familiar with an issue she or he is asked to handle, she or he might call on a partner to handle that particular issue.

The task of the medical office manager is to help the office obtain this professional by carefully evaluating various legal firms, their fees, and their knowledge of health care issues. The following is a short list of areas in the medical practice where an office attorney could be needed:

- Physician contracts
- Retirement and profit-sharing plans
- State and federal legislation
- Health insurance plans
- Partnership and corporation formation
- Office and equipment leases
- Managed care contracts
- Representation of the physician in "collection" cases
- Representation of the physician in hospital matters
- Employment issues

Ask about their fees and their areas of expertise. Attorneys' fees can be an unpleasant surprise if the office is not quick to establish a foundation for charges. Most attorneys negotiate their fees; they are not carved in stone. Demand the parameters of payment at the outset and carefully watch all charges. Today's lawyers tend to be flexible. Beware of being told that a fee agreement is "iron-clad"; you may find that the attorney meant "what we agreed upon, plus expenses."

Ask what the firm charges for making photocopies, filing documents, and doing research. Interview several attorneys before hiring the one for the job. After all, this individual will be making decisions and giving advice that will affect your business.

References

Clark, L. "When and When Not To Protect Patient Privacy." *Medical Economics,* May 1991, pp. 99-109.

Crane, M. "The Medication Errors That Get Doctors Sued." *Medical Economics,* November 1993, pp. 36-41.

Delmar, D. "Be Wary of Legal Pitfalls When Dismissing Problem Patients." *Physicians Financial News,* June 1991, pp. 1, 31.

Kanoti, G. "The Toughest Ethical Choices Encountered by Physicians." *Physician's Management,* May 1992, pp. 71-79.

Kirschner, M. "How Advance Directives Can Ease Your Burden." *Medical Economics,* April 1992, pp. 75-87.

Luxenberg, S. "How To Tell When Your Lawyer Is Overcharging." *Medical Economics,* September 1993, pp. 92-97.

Mabon, R. "How To Do a Discovery Deposition." *Group Practice Journal,* November/December 1993, p. 49.

Murray, D. "Dismiss a Patient, Invite a Lawsuit?" *Medical Economics,* August 1993, pp. 57-70.

Pozgar, G. *Legal Aspects of Health Care Administration.* Rockville, MD: Aspen Publishers, 1990.

Schorr, B. "The National Practitioner Data Bank: A Case of Overkill?" *Physician's Management,* January 1993, pp. 109-121.

Sopko, S. "Complying with the Disabilities Act." *The Office,* July 1993, pp. 31-32.

Tannenbaum, R., & Berman, M. "Why Even Patients Who Like You Will Sue You for Malpractice." *Physician's Management,* April 1993, pp. 85-97.

Wold, C. "The Art of Malpractice Risk Management." *Physician's Management,* February 1993, pp. 57-68.

8

Computers in the Health Care Environment

Why Do I Need a Computer?

Computers affect almost all of us in our daily lives and are changing our lives today just as the telephone changed people's lives in the past. Computers help us gather, organize, store, and process information. It is important for a medical office manager to be computer literate, because we live in an information age of high technology and fast pace. Buying the right computer is much like buying the right battery for a car. If it fits right, it will run more efficiently. By now, everyone has realized that in the health care environment, the computer and all its peripherals are a way of life. It has become an indispensable tool in the field of medicine.

The past 10 years have seen greater emphasis placed on the management aspects of a medical office. More and more medical offices are finding that they can become more efficient with the use of a computer, and with the costs of health care increasing every year, it is imperative that the medical office be managed efficiently (Figure 8–1). Computers allow office managers to do just that!

There are many uses for a computer system in medical office, and once you have one in place, more and more uses will arise. If you have any doubts remaining as to whether you need a computer in your office, the following list of some of the uses for a computer system in the medical office should take care of them! The computer is used for

- Billing
- Age analysis of accounts
- Claims processing
- Collection letters
- Reminders
- Appointment scheduling
- Recall lists
- Accounting functions
- Employee vacation schedules and sick days
- Inventory
- Ability to generate reports
- Word processing
- Access to national data banks
- Access to hospital computers
- Drug interactions
- Research
- Patient education
- Medical records
- Policies and procedures
- Referring physician lists
- Continuing Medical Education (CME) programs
- Label and envelope printing
- Check writing
- Prescription writing
- Electronic claims
- Preparation of the deposit slip
- W-2 forms
- Hospital records
- Profiles by patient demographics
- Profiles by diagnosis and procedure
- Literature retrieval
- Retirement plans
- Interoffice memos
- Correspondence

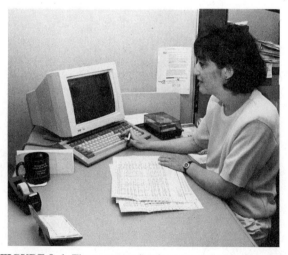

FIGURE 8–1. The computer has become an invaluable asset to the employees of a medical office.

Computer Talk

To buy a computer system that is right for the practice, it is necessary to understand the language of computers.

Hardware—The hardware is all the physical parts of the computer system. The physical parts are
- the processor
- the monitor
- the hard drive
- random access memory (electronic chips)
- modems
- the printer
- the keyboard
- disc drives

Software—Software is the set of instructions without which the computer can do nothing. When you type an instruction on the keyboard, the software interprets that instruction and follows it, giving you the information that you requested. Many different software programs are available that meet the needs of the medical office.

Processor—The processor is the circuit chip that gives the computer the ability to process information. There are several generations of processors on the market today, and each generation is faster than the one before it. A computer with a 486 processor is much faster than a computer with a 386 processor. Faster chips mean more efficiency.

Monitor—The monitor is the screen. Monitors are available in monochrome (gray and white) or color. A color monitor reduces eye strain. A common color monitor is the Super VGA, or SVGA. The tiny dots that form the graphics of a computer are called *pixels*. The higher the number of pixels, the clearer the graphics of the computer.

Hard drive—A hard drive is a must for a medical office computer system. It is a small box inside the computer that contains discs that provide long-term information storage and allow retrieval of this information. It comes in sizes of 20, 40, 60, 80, and 120 megabytes of memory.

Megabyte—A megabyte is one million bytes of computer storage.

Byte—A byte is a group of eight bits that is used to represent a single letter, number, or symbol in a computer. The *bit,* short for binary digit, is the fundamental unit of storage in all digital computers.

Random access memory—Random access memory, or RAM , is the primary set of memory chips used to store data or instructions that can be altered by the user. It can be likened to short-term memory in humans, as the hard drive is likened to long-term memory. RAM comes in sizes ranging from 256 kilobytes to 16 megabytes. The higher the number, the more memory, and the faster your computer will perform computations and do what software programs tell it to do. For most medical offices, 4 megabytes are adequate.

Keyboard—The keyboard is the equipment that is used to type the information into the computer. Keyboards are basically all the same, with the exception that some have more special-function keys than others. The needs of your office will dictate the type of keyboard you need.

Modem—The modem is a device that allows the office to send and receive information over the telephone line. Modems open many doors for the medical office; for instance, they allow satellite offices to exchange information, they allow the office to access hospital billing departments for information, and they allow offices to submit insurance claims electronically. Modems are offered in 1200-, 2400-, and 9600-baud rates. For the purposes of a medical office, the 2400- and 9600-baud rates are found to be most appropriate.

Baud—A baud is the number of signal changes in a communications channel per second, which controls the speed at which communication are transferred.

Printer—Printers come in assorted shapes, colors, and sizes (Figure 8–2). The printer's function is to produce a hard copy (document) of the information that is in the computer. The laser printer is the top-of-the-line printer and produces a finely finished product. The laser printer, however, is very expensive. Most medical offices find that a dot matrix printer more than meets their needs. It can be loaded with various types of forms and statements to handle the printing responsibilities of the medical office. Some larger offices and clinics purchase a laser printer to use for all correspondence and a dot matrix printer to print insurance forms and statements. When considering whether to buy a laser printer, find out the number of pages it prints per minute and the resolution. How much RAM your computer has is an important factor when purchasing a laser printer. To work, laser printers must hold an entire page of information before printing it. Your computer must have enough RAM to meet this demand. If your office is thinking of buying a laser printer, your computer should have 2 to 4 megabytes of RAM.

Disc drives—Disc drives are used for loading programs, which come on floppy discs, onto the hard drive of the computer and for using a floppy disc that has information on it without loading it onto the hard drive. Even if you have a hard drive, you will still have need for disc drives. The two sizes of floppy discs are 5 1/4 inch and 3 1/2 inch. Most offices use the latter. Larger professional offices outfit their computers with both sizes to allow for greater flexibility.

Backup tape—A final and crucial part of the computer system is the backup tape. This allows for all of the computer files to be copied onto a tape drive so that they will not be lost if there is ever a problem with the hard drive. Backup tape drives

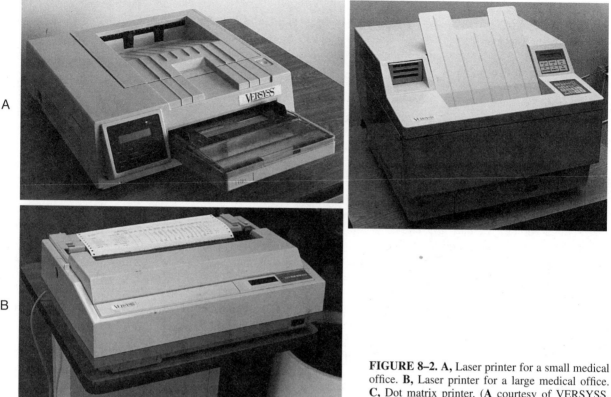

FIGURE 8–2. A, Laser printer for a small medical office. **B,** Laser printer for a large medical office. **C,** Dot matrix printer. (**A** courtesy of VERSYSS, Inc.; **B** and **C** courtesy of Xerox Corporation.)

are viewed as a safety net so that valuable information is not lost. They use a tape similar to the tape in an ordinary tape recorder and can hold from 60 megabytes to 5 gigabytes of information. The tape that you select should be large enough to hold the entire contents of your hard drive. If your hard drive is 120 megabytes, the backup tape should be 120 megabytes. Tapes come in different sizes, from a standard-size cartridge to a 4-mm cartridge. Speed and easy use are major factors in this decision. Because backup should be done at the end of every day, the tape should be fast and convenient.

Computer Security

"Our computer system is very updated. It gives no information to those who need it, and plenty to those who do not!"

—Anonymous

Security is a very important aspect of the computer system that many don't think of until it is too late.

Computer misuse is on the rise in today's society. Many types of computer abuse do not have a bearing on the medical office; however, some do. For instance, an employee who wishes to know the salaries of all the staff, including the physician, or an employee who is disgruntled about the lack of a raise and wishes to retaliate may access sensitive information and use it to cause trouble. The best defense against computer fraud is a password system. Employees who need to have access to certain programs can be given passwords so that entry is possible. Those without passwords who try to gain access would be denied. Passwords can be permanent, or they can be changed on a monthly basis, whereby they expire after a certain date and time. New passwords would need to be issued the following working day.

Negotiating the Contract

Each computer vendor will use a standard sales agreement when selling the computer system. Computer companies are competitive and hungry for your business. Keep this in mind, as well as the following ground rules, and negotiate yourself a good price.

- Always involve your attorney and listen to her or his advice!
- Make sure all promises are written out and signed by the vendor.
- Push for a delay in payment. Don't agree to make the final payment on the system until the system has been in place for 1 month. This will give you time to get the bugs out!
- Hold the vendor to a specific date by which the computer should be up and running. If this date arrives and the computer hasn't been completely set up, you want to be able to walk away from this deal to purchase another computer.
- Specify damages for which your vendor should be responsible should the computer not perform to your liking. It is best if you can negotiate a clause that states that the vendor is responsible for legal fees should it come to that.
- Ask the vendor to specify in writing that the system proposed has not been sold to anyone else for less money.

Purchasing the Computer

PURCHASING SOFTWARE

Determining the *software package,* or group of software programs, that you will need to perform the many tasks of your office is the first thing you do when buying a computer system. To determine what software programs the office needs, discuss with the physician what she or he wants the computer to do. Make a list of these tasks and a list of the tasks you want the computer to do and shop around to check out the various medical software packages available. Several medical software companies are listed in Box 8–1. Before you purchase a computer system for the office, make sure that you have researched all the software companies and their medical programs. Insist on in-office demonstrations so that everyone can listen and ask questions. It is a good idea to involve the office's computer operator in the decision making at this point.

Software Options

Medical software programs perform a multitude of functions. Some of these functions are as follows:

- Appointment scheduling (Boxes 8–2 and 8–3)

- *International Classification of Diseases, Ninth Revision,* coding
- *Current Procedural Terminology* coding
- Patient information
- Billing
- Insurance form generation
- Envelope and postcard addressing
- Label addressing
- Electronic submission of claims to insurance companies
- Missing insurance information (Box 8–4)
- Generation of deposit slips and audit trails (Box 8–5)
- Practice analysis (Boxes 8–6 and 8–7)
- Hospital/physician interface
- Recall and letter notices (Box 8–8)
- Clinical and drug histories
- Word processing
- Credit and collections packages (Boxes 8–9 and 8–10)
  Patient ledger accounts
- Chart tracking
- Payroll
- E-mail (electronic mail)
- Inventory control
- Medical records transcription
- Office management packages
- Patient Encounter Form printing
- Year-end statements (Box 8–11)
- Tracking packages
- Practice marketing
- Medical records (Boxes 8–12 and 8–13)

The most important of these functions are the patient billing and insurance functions. The software you purchase should be able to track accounts, age accounts, edit accounts, and resubmit them. It should also be able to submit insurance claims electronically. There was a time when electronic submission was simply an option. It is not an option any longer. Medicare will be starting to fine offices that submit claims on paper. Paperless claims are preferred and, sometimes required, by insurance companies today. Medicare, Blue Cross/Blue Shield, Medicaid, and many health maintenance organizations/preferred provider organizations are requesting that their claims be submitted electronically. There are even certain commercial insurance companies that offer this service.

Like many specialty packages, the aforementioned options have been offered for years and can be tailored to fit the needs of each individual medical office. Companies can customize packages to be convenient and easy to use. When thinking about having a program customized for your office, always check on the cost of this service; it can be quite expensive. With a little shopping around, you might be able to find a system that closely parallels your office's needs without the added expense of customization.

Software Support

When purchasing software, it is vitally important to have good support. The software company you select should always be available and should be extremely knowledgable about the software program that you have selected. Not everyone is computer literate, and this must be kept in mind when purchasing a software

package. It is an easier task to computerize the office if the software is user friendly.

Your software support people will become your best friends. Before purchasing a system, ask for references for the support people and check with these references on the quality of the support provided. It is important that they are accessible. Some companies have their phone support system divided into two types. The Hot Line is available to help with immediate and emergency situations, for instance, when your system freezes and, no matter what you do, won't budge! The second type of phone support allows you to leave a message, and someone will get back to you within a reasonable amount of time (Figure 8–3). A reasonable amount of time is within 4 hours. This type of support would be used for questions such as, "How can I run a list of patients who had EKG's done in the last year?"

BOX 8–1. **MEDICAL SOFTWARE COMPANIES**

- **Keystone Medical Systems**
  Lemoyne, PA 1-800-800-0763
- **Versyss Corporation Mends II Practice Management System**
  Westwood, MA 1-800-899-6400
- **MD VersaForm**
  Applied Software Technology
  Campbell, CA 1-800-678-1111
- **Med-EZ**
  American Voice Computers
  Milpitas, CA 408-946-5282
- **The Resident**
  Wallaby Software Corporation
  Mahwah, NJ 201-934-9333
- **MEDx**
  ASP Software
  Sunnyvale, CA 1-800-822-7832
- **PAS-3PLUS System II**
  Artificial Intelligence
  Seattle, WA 1-800-533-8902
- **MDX**
  Calyx Corporation
  Brookfield, WI 1-800-558-2208
- **Control-o-fax Corporation**
  Waterloo, IA 1-800-344-7777
- **Medicalis**
  CyCare Software Publishing
  Scottsdale, AZ 1-800-545-2488

- **MBS (Medical Business System)**
  DataGraph Software Techologies
  Austin, TX 1-800-800-6433
- **Elcomp Systems**
  Pittsburgh, PA 1-800-441-8386
- **Excalibur Practice Management Systems**
  Execu-Flow Systems
  Edison, NJ 908-287-9191
- **Script Systems**
  Hackensack, NJ 1-800-724-8500
- **+MEDIC**
  MEDIC Computer Systems
  Raleigh, NC 1-800-334-8534
- **MegaMED**
  MegaWest Systems
  Salt Lake City, UT 1-800-999-0788
- **Physician Partner**
  Physician Micro Systems
  Seattle, WA 206-441-8490
- **Physicians Practice Management**
  Indianapolis, IN 1-800-428-3515
- **Medical Manager**
  Systems Plus
  Mountain View, CA 1-800-222-7701
- **ACCLAIM Medical System**
  Sentient Systems
  Kensington, MD 1-800-966-9419

BOX 8–2. COMPUTER-GENERATED APPOINTMENT SCHEDULE

REPORT DATE: 03/12/92   --DAILY APPOINTMENT SCHEDULE--

APPOINTMENT DATE: 03/13/90 WEDNESDAY

TIME	PATIENT NAME PATIENT ADDRESS	DUR	ACCNT/# PHONE #	APPNT TYPE	#MSSD APPTS	APPNT COMMENT	PRIVATE BALANCE	INSUR BALANCE	LAST SVC DATE	APPNT DATE	DOCTOR	LOCATION	ROOM/TP
100P	ADAMS MATTHEW	15	4001	EST PT	0	ANNUAL PHYSICAL	.00	40.00	03/30/91	03/13/92	ADAMS	BOSTON	
115P	ANDERSON MARY	15	2006 329-6141	EST PT	0	POST OP VISIT	30.00	15.00	03/06/91	03/13/92	ADAMS	BOSTON	
130P	SMITH JANE	15	2011 (617) 444-2836	EST PT	2	HEADACHES	.00	15.00	11/04/91	03/13/92	ADAMS	BOSTON	
145P	CARRIER JAMES	15	4021 (603) 669-0846	EST PT	0	BACK PAIN	225.00	493.00	09/20/91	03/13/92	ADAMS	BOSTON	
200P	MULLEN JOHN A	15	3002 (603) 497-5623	EST PT	1	HIGH BP	70.00	460.00	02/01/91	03/13/92	BROWN	BOSTON	
215P	CASEY WILLIAM	30	NEW ACCNT	NEW PT	0	238-7744	.00	.00		03/13/92	BROWN	BOSTON	
245P	BROWN GILBERT	60	1003 472- 1254	EST PT	1	BRINGING INS INFO	.00	87.00	12/01/91	03/13/92	BROWN	BOSTON	TREADMILL

DAILY APPOINTMENT SCHEDULE

REPORT DATE 03/12/91 TUESDAY

TIME	PATIENT NAME	ACCOUNT #	DOB	PHONE #	NSA	APPT/PATIENT COMMENT	PHY
100P	MATTHEW ADAMS	4001	01/05/28	327-7611	1	ANNUAL PHYSICAL PROCARDIA	1
115P	MARY ANDERSON	2006	12/21/20	426-2900	0	POST OP VISIT	1
130P	JANE SMITH	2011	12/06/51	488-2670	2	HEADACHES	1
145P	JAMES CARRIER	4021	06/14/56	462-2244	0	BACK PAIN	1
200P	JOHN A. MULLEN	3002	08/18/19	327-9192	1		1
215P	WILLIAM CASEY	N	06/04/20	462-3441	0	238-7744	1

The daily appointment schedule provides a professional and concise report of daily appointments. This report may also be generated alphabetically to easily pull patient charts for the next day's activity.

(Courtesy of VERSYSS, Inc.)

PURCHASING HARDWARE

Hardware Options

When shopping for hardware, buy a system that is more system than you need at that time. If your office is new to computerization, the office will see more and more ways to become more efficient with the use of the computer. Buying a larger system allows for practice growth, faster speed, and less hassle. The average medical office should be considering a 486 machine

Hardware Support

Hardware support is just as important as software support. It is important to know how much "downtime" the computer system has. Call the references and ask, "Have you had much down time with your XYZ computer system?" This is important, especially if the printer jams and you are in the middle of running your monthly statements. Some vendors may give you a false sense of security, so it is important to ask other medical offices who are using the same equipment. Some hardware problems can be corrected easily by following instructions given over the telephone by a hardware technician. Get to know your hardware technician; someday you might need help in a hurry, and being friends will help get her or him to your office sooner! Most individuals working as hardware and software technicians are knowledgeable and quick to respond (Figure 8–4).

Training and Orientation

It is critically important to have the staff properly trained in the use of the new computer system. Purchas-

---

BOX 8–3. COMPUTER PRINTOUT OF MISSED APPOINTMENTS

03/12/92   --MISSED APPOINTMENT LIST--   DOCTOR: DR ADAMS

DATE	TIME	DR	ACCT#	PATIENT	AGE	D-O-B	MISS APT	TYPE OF VISIT/ COMMENTS	LAST SVC DT	PRIVATE BAL/ INS/OTHER
03/04/92	1:30	1	1007	RUSSELL JONES 111 ELM STREET WEYMOUTH MA 02190	28	07/02/61 (617) 329-7330	4	STRESS TEST PROCARDIA	07/16/90	65.20 13.73
03/05/92	9:30	1	1003	KEVIN JOHNSON 44 EAST STREET PLYMOUTH MA 11111	47	05/13/42 (617) 746-6666	0	SURGICAL FOLLOW-UP	01/02/92	220.00 .00
03/07/92	3:30	1	1035	LISA MORTON ONE SOUTH STREET NATICK MA 01760	31	12/04/58 (617) 365-2569	1	NEW PATIENT VISIT GASTRIC DISTURBANCES		.00 .00
03/08/92	9:00	1	1030	MARY PIKOSKY 763 E. LARK DRIVE MIAMI FL 32958	30	1/25/60 (305) 629-8475	3	HOLTER MONITOR LONITEN/VISKEN	07/08/89	45.00 25.00
03/08/92	4:30	1	1032	DAVID COOK 12 EATON ROAD BARRINGTON RI 02806	37	05/04/52 (401) 245-7909	4	NEW PATIENT VISIT HEADACHES		.00 .00

The Missed Appointment List helps office personnel keep track of those patients who have missed previously scheduled appointments. This may be helpful in rescheduling appointments or in determining whether or not a charge should be applied to the account.

(Courtesy of VERSYSS, Inc.)

BOX 8–4. **COMPUTER PRINTOUT SPECIFYING INFORMATION MISSING FROM INSURANCE FORMS**

03/12/92		MISSING BILLING INFORMATION ON BLUE SHIELD FORMS	
FILE	KEY	ELEMENT	HELD/DOCUMENT ACCOUNTS
PROCEDURE	93521	NEEDS SPECIAL DOCUMENTATION	6788
PATIENT	3780	D.O.B.	3780

03/12/92		MISSING BILLING INFORMATION ON WELFARE FORMS	
FILE	KEY	ELEMENT	HELD/DOCUMENT ACCOUNTS
PATIENT	5429	CERT # VERIFICATION	5429
PATIENT	8541	STREET	8541

03/12/92		MISSING BILLING INFORMATION ON MEDICARE FORMS	
FILE	KEY	ELEMENT	HELD/DOCUMENT ACCOUNTS

NO ERRORS

> *Unbilled services are checked for complete information required for claims to be reimbursed. If inadequate information is recognized, the system will automatically print the account and charge and then put the account on hold for review. The system also notes any procedures that may require special handling such as "individual consideration" procedures.*

(Courtesy of VERSYSS, Inc.)

---

ing a new computer system, or even just changing an existing one, can be a source of severe stress for the employees. Have them become involved in the quest for the new system from the beginning, so that they feel comfortable with the decision and are mentally prepared for the change. Several on-site training sessions and even a few off-site training sessions should be part of the package once the computer has been selected (Figure 8–5). That old phrase "Use it or lose it" is highly pertinent at a time like this. The more the staff use the new computer, the more comfortable with it they will be.

Parallel Processing . . . Used as a Crutch?

Parallel processing consists of running the old computer system or the manual system simultaneously with the new computer system. Running a parallel system can provide the office with benefits and problems. It can be helpful in identifying problems when they arise as a result of the addition or changing of systems. However, because the operations are bound to be different, it is almost impossible to compare any results from tasks that have been performed, and the chances of making errors is much greater. In addition, it places extra stress on the staff because of the extra work involved in performing the same tasks twice. Parallel running of systems should not exceed more than 4 months. Once 4 months have gone by, any bugs that might have been in the new system will have been worked out.

The Old System to the New

If the office already has a computer in place and is in need of an upgrade, there are few options to consider. There are two main ways to accomplish this awesome task: run parallel systems or balance-forward all information into the new system.

BOX 8–5. COMPUTER-GENERATED PATIENT PAYMENT JOURNAL

03/13/92   --PAYMENT JOURNAL--

                              ALL DATES   PREVIOUS A/R: 703,774.72

ACCT#	PATIENT/INSURED NAME	TICKET#	CODE	T	DATE	REFERENCE	PAYMENT	ADJ/REF
1002	GREG SMITH	10014	TPPH	P	03/13/92		110.00	
1002	GREG SMITH	10014	TAPH	A	03/13/92			20.00
1002	GREG SMITH	10014	TOPH	O	03/13/92			25.00
1002	GREG SMITH	10014	TIBR	I	03/13/92			-25.00
1006	RUSSELL JONES	10013	TPM	P	03/13/92	CK 1234	124.00	
1006	RUSSELL JONES	10013	TAM	A	03/13/92	CK 1234		35.00
1006	RUSSELL JONES	10013	TOM	O	03/13/92			26.00
1006	RUSSELL JONES	10013	TIP	I	03/13/92			-26.00
			BATCH BD TOTALS:				6034.00	325.00
								****5709.00
1001	JOHN ANDERSON	10001	TPM	P	03/13/92	EOB #5755	920.00	
1001	JOHN ANDERSON	10001	TAM	A	03/13/92	EOB #5755		110.00
1001	JOHN ANDERSON	10001	TOM	O	03/13/92			310.00
1001	JOHN ANDERSON	10001	TIP	I	03/13/92			-310.00
1001	JOHN ANDERSON	10002	TPM	P	03/13/92	EOB #5755	1120.00	
1001	JOHN ANDERSON	10002	TAM	A	03/13/92	EOB #5755		106.00
1001	JOHN ANDERSON	10002	TOM	O	03/13/92			405.00
1001	JOHN ANDERSON	10002	TIP	I	03/13/92			-405.00
			BATCH KK TOTALS:				2040.00	216.00
								****1824.00
1003	KEVIN JOHNSON	10005	TPP	P	03/13/92	CH 444	630.00	
1004	SALLY SMYTH	10006	TPP	P	03/13/92	CH 123	403.00	
1010	KAREN WINSLOW	10012	TRF	R	03/13/92			-30.00
			BATCH OC TOTALS:				1033.00	-30.00
								****1003.00
			GRAND TOTALS:				10137.00	129.00
								****11266.00
			PREVIOUS A/R PAYMENTS					692,478.72

> *All payments have a clear audit trail. Daily payment activity can be monitored paying particular attention to professional courtesies and adustments in detail. Totals are summarized by provider, location, department and operator.*

(Courtesy of VERSYSS, Inc.)

BOX 8–6. COMPUTER-GENERATED ANALYSIS OF PROCEDURES BY PROVIDER AND LOCATION

03/12/92   --PROCEDURE STATISTICS ANALYSIS--

PRIMARY SORT OPTION: PROCEDURE CODE   SECONDARY SORT OPTION: PROVIDER   TERTIARY SORT OPTION: LOCATION

CODE	STANDARD DESCRIPTION	DEPT	PROVIDER	LOC	M-T-D UNITS	M-T-D SERVICES	Y-T-D UNITS	Y-T-D SERVICES
93000	EKG WITH INTERPRETATION	4	1 DR ADAMS	1	28	2940.00	90	9544.00
		PROVIDER 1	LOCATION 1 TOTAL		18	1890.00	30	3150.00
			PROVIDER 1 TOTAL		28	2940.00	90	9544.00
		4	2 DR. BROWN	1	39	4134.00	125	12890.00
		PROVIDER 2	LOCATION 1 TOTAL		24	2546.00	78	8750.00
			PROVIDER 2 TOTAL		39	4134.00	125	12890.00
			PROCEDURE 93000 TOTAL		67	7074.00	215	22434.00
93015	STRESS TEST	2	1 DR. ADAMS	1	35	2840.00	123	9963.00
		PROVIDER 1	LOCATION 1 TOTAL		28	2268.00	103	8343.00
			PROVIDER 1 TOTAL		35	2840.00	123	9963.00
		2	2 DR. BROWN	1	41	3321.00	140	11340.00
		PROVIDER 2	LOCATION 1 TOTAL		34	2835.00	119	9639.00
			PROVIDER 2 TOTAL		41	3321.00	140	11340.00
			PROCEDURE 93015 TOTAL		76	6161.00	263	2805.00
94010	PULMONARY FUNCION	2	1 DR. ADAMS	1	27	3510.00	57	7420.00
		PROVIDER 1	LOCATION 1 TOTAL		22	2860.00	47	6370.00
						3510.00	57	7420.00
						3806.00	94	12240.00
						3642.00	88	11440.00
						3806.00	94	12240.00
			PROCEDURE 94010 TOTAL		57	7316.00	151	19660.00

Procedure statistics can be analyzed in detail to gain a deeper understanding of the consistency of each procedure performed. Charges can be checked across the board, providers can be compared, locations can be rated on profitability, and departments can be closely monitored for inventory needs. Flexibilities of this report allow just monthly totals to print or procedure totals without the supporting details.

(Courtesy of VERSYSS, Inc.)

As mentioned in the preceding section, running parallel systems means that you run both the new and the old systems simultaneously. You simply pick a date at which time you will enter any new charges into the new system only. The only data entry done on the old system would be the application of charges to existing bills.

If you choose to use the balance-forward method, any unpaid balance in the old system would be converted to the new system by a one-line entry stating "balance forward." There would be no details of the services rendered on the new system except for the new services entered. All the details from the old system can be purged out onto sheets and kept in folders until the time you no longer need them. For a fee, computer companies

BOX 8–7. COMPUTER-GENERATED ANALYSIS OF PAYMENT TRANSACTIONS

03/12/92   --TRANSACTION ANALYSIS--

CODE	DESCRIPTION	TYPE	ALT. SORT	M-T-D DOLLARS	Y-T-D DOLLARS
PCO	COLLECTION PAYMENT	PAYMENT	0	1388.45	8011.67
PPM	PATIENT PAYMENT MAIL	PAYMENT	0	27132.72	86315.07
PP	PATIENT PAYMENT TOS	PAYMENT	0	14254.00	39713.50
PB	B/S PAYMENT	PAYMENT	0	25161.09	129615.00
PM	MEDICARE PAYMENT	PAYMENT	0	69854.34	208208.93
PW	WELFARE PAYMENT	PAYMENT	0	5681.75	26644.27
PC	COMMERCIAL PAYMENT	PAYMENT	0	12093.83	43342.22
AW	WELFARE ADJUSTMENT	ADJUSTMENT	0	2122.64	7647.22
AC	COMMERCIAL ADJUST	ADJUSTMENT	0	3427.00	11641.01
ACO	COLLECTION ADJUST	ADJUSTMENT	0	1388.45	9116.77
AP	PATIENT ADJUSTMENT	ADJUSTMENT	0	991.01	5007.01
AB	B/S ADJUSTMENT	ADJUSTMENT	0	4277.64	13264.33
APC	PROF COURT ADJUST	ADJUSTMENT	0	2188.32	7005.44
AM	MEDICARE ADJUSTMENT	ADJUSTMENT	0	51171.86	145074.03
RP	REFUND PATIENT	REFUND	0	-2544.50	-4768.80
RI	REFUND INSURANCE	REFUND	0	-3665.57	-10114.62
RB	REBILL	OTHER	0	12647.20	31261.10
IC	TRANSFER TO COMM	OTHER	0	-32367.50	-88675.29
OB	TRANSFER FROM B/S	OTHER	0	12452.90	31419.11
OM	TRANS FROM MEDICARE	OTHER	0	26349.80	80146.97
IP	TRANSFER TO PATIENT	OTHER	0	-30365.51	-87746.48
OW	TRANSFER FROM WELFARE	OTHER	0	4360.00	11397.84
OC	TRANSFER FROM COMM	OTHER	0	10647.78	28891.38
IB	TRANSFER TO B/S	OTHER	0	-10327.20	-38364.27
ICO	TRANS TO COLLECTION	OTHER	0	.00	-6473.28
OCO	TRANS FROM COLLECTION	OTHER	0	.00	.00
IM	TRANSFER TO MEDICARE	OTHER	0	-30115.60	-84673.21
OP	TRANSFER FROM PATIENT	OTHER	0	4365.00	11499.50
IW	TRANSFER TO WELFARE	OTHER	0	-142.00	-237.00

Any payment patterns that may have developed can be tracked easily, especially paying close attention to adjustment figures and professional courtesies. Analyzing the profitability of participating with an HMO or calculating the collection rate at the time of service are just two of many analyses drawn from data contained in this report.

(Courtesy of VERSYSS, Inc.)

will electronically convert your patient demographics from your old system to your new one. If the medical practice is quite extensive, this might be an option to consider.

If the practice is changing from a manual system to a computerized system, the staff can spend extra time entering patient demographics before the system goes live (the day you start using only the computer system).

What You Can Do When You Go Electronic

FILING INSURANCE CLAIMS ELECTRONICALLY

Electronic insurance claims are submitted via the telephone lines and take only a *short time to transmit*. The software of the computer translates, edits, and for-

---

BOX 8–8. COMPUTER-GENERATED RECALL LETTER

Medical Associates
123 Main Street
Springfield, ST 55320

March 12, 1992

Jane Smith
200 Taylor Road
Springfield, ST 55320

Dear Jane,

Our records show that you are due for your yearly physical in April. Please call our office (555-9000) at your earliest convenience to set up an appointment.

It is very important that you understand the necessity for a yearly examination. Your vital statistics will be monitored and yearly tests allow us to keep your current condition in a very controlled state. Please do not neglect this notice.

Sincerely,

Janet Roe, M.D.

> *Letters can automatically be generated to patients with recall dates. These personal reminders are effective in practicing preventative healthcare and maintaining a steady patient flow. The system will also track any patient who fails to make an appointment. The doctor can review this list to determine who needs to be contacted.*

(Courtesy of VERSYSS, Inc.)

BOX 8–9. **COMPUTER-GENERATED PATIENT LETTER FOR**
         PAST-DUE ACCOUNT

Medical Associates
100 Main Street
Springfield, ST 55320

March 12, 1992

Scott Ford   Patient: Peter Ford
25 Bell Street   Total Balance: $48.00
Springfield, ST 55320   Overdue Balance: $24.00

Dear Mr. Ford:

To date, several statements have been sent regarding the overdue balance shown above. As of the above date, we have not received a response from you. If you have insurance information that would help in paying this balance, you need to forward us this information in order to process a claim. If no insurance is available, you need to make payment today.

Please contact the billing office immediately so that we may resolve this problem.

Sincerely,

J.B. Dunn
Credit manager

> *Custom letters can be printed to remind patients of past due balances. These letters integrate with data from the patient's record to give accurate balances and proper aging of the account. Keeping collection activity in your office results in more money coming into your practice without sacrificing a percentage to the collection agency.*

(Courtesy of VERSYSS, Inc.)

mats the data according to the requirements of each specific insurance carrier.

Before purchasing electronic claims submission software for the office, there are a few things you might want to consider:

- Ask neighboring practices if they have any experience filing claims electronically. Ask if you can come to see their system in operation.

- Contact the insurance carriers with whom you would be filing claims electronically and ask them for recommendations of qualified vendors.

- Consider attending the next professional meeting to speak with vendors and look at their displays.

- Ask the office's health care consultant, if the office has one, for recommendations on a qualified vendor.

- Ask the vendor how long it has been involved with electronic claims submissions.
- Ask the vendor for the names of offices for which it has installed electronic claims systems.

- Call these offices and ask them about the vendor's service and support.
- Ask about charges associated with these electronic claims packages.

BOX 8–10. COMPUTER-GENERATED COLLECTION REPORT

03/12/92   --COLLECTION REPORT--

----------------GUARANTOR INFORMATION---GUARANTOR #:   1034
                                                                                                                  PATIENT #:   1034

MITCHELL, TODD B.   EMPLOYER: THOMPSON CO.
10 MAIN STREET   3333 ELM STREET
APT #3   BOSTON, MA 02026
WESTWOOD, MA 02090   329-4141
(617) 329-4444

                                           REMARKS: WIFE WORKS AT HOSP

---------------PATIENT INFORMATION --
MITCHELL, TODD B.   RELATIONSHIP TO THE ABOVE: S
10 MAIN STREET   DATE OF BIRTH: 01/06/64
APT #3   PATIENT'S SEX: M
WESTWOOD, MA 02090   MARITAL STATUS: M
(617) 329-4444
---------------INSURANCE INFORMATION--
CODE   NAME   POLICY HOLDER   REL   CERTIFICATE #   GROUP #   MBR #

B   BLUE SHIELD   TODD B. MITCHELL   S   2587251
---------------BALANCE INFORMATION-- DIAGNOSIS INFORMATION -------------------
PATIENT BALANCE: 645.00   DATE LAST SERVICE: 08/07/91   CODE   DESCRIPTION   NOTES
INSURANCE BALANCE: 110.00   DATE LAST STATEMENT: 02/22/92   750.6   HIATAL HERNIA   RECURRING
OTHER BALANCE: 5.00   DATE LAST PAYMENT   06/20/91
UNAPPLIED CREDITS: .00   PATIENT PMTS Y-T-D   25.00
---------------SERVICE DETAIL INFORMATION---

TICKET #	SERV DATE	BILL DATE	PD ST	LOCA TION	PROV IDER	RE SP	INSUR- ANCE1	INSUR- ANCE2	INSUR- ANCE3	TOTAL CHARGES	TOTAL PAYMENT	TOTAL ADJUSTS	TKT BALANCE
10054	05/20/91	05/22/91	B	1	1	P	PATIENT			50.00	25.00	.00	25.00

DIAG 1	DIAG 2	PROCEDURE	PROCEDURE DESCRIPTION	T.O.S.	PROC FEE	UTS	EXTETION
750.6		90050	EST PATIENT LIMITED OFFICE VISIT	6	50.00	1	50.00
		CODE	TRANSACTION DESCRIPTION	DATE	TYPE		AMOUNT
		TPP	PATIENT PAYMENT	05/20/91	P		25.00

TICKET #	SERV DATE	BILL DATE	PD ST	LOCA TION	PROV IDER	RE SP	INSUR- ANCE1	INSUR- ANCE2	INSUR- ANCE3	TOTAL CHARGES	TOTAL PAYMENTS	TOTAL ADJUSTS	TKT BALANCE
10053	07/01/91	07/03/91	B	1	1	P	PATIENT			40.00	.00	.00	40.00

DIAG 1	DIAG 2	PROCEDURE	PROCEDURE DESCRIPTION	T.O.S.	PROC FEE	UTS	EXTENSION
750.06		90020	COMPREHENSIVE EXAM	6	40.00	1	40.00

> *By selecting from a variety of criteria, accounts requiring collection work may be readily identified and sorted by highest balance first. A clear detailed summary of each patient permits complete follow-up work to be done with minimal effort.*

(Courtesy of VERSYSS, Inc.)

BOX 8–11. COMPUTER-GENERATED YEAR-END STATEMENT

PROFILE ANALYSIS FOR 1992

	SERVICES	PAYMENTS	ADJ/REF	NET	YTD	---M-T-D--- PROFILE	COLL	---Y-T-D--- PROFILE	COLL
****LOCATION 1: OFFICE			ATB CATEGORY 20: BLUE SHIELD***						
JAN	59242.50	26803.10	5256.10	27183.30	27183.30	83.61%	54.11%	83.61%	54.11%
FEB	54083.00	17644.00	3044.60	33394.40	60577.70	85.28%	38.25%	84.26%	46.55%
MAR	20547.50	.00	.00	20547.50	81125.20	00.00%	00.00%	84.26%	39.40%
APR	.00	.00	.00	.00	81125.20	00.00%	00.00%	84.26%	39.40%
MAY	.00	.00	.00	.00	81125.20	00.00%	00.00%	84.26%	39.40%
JUN	.00	.00	.00	.00	81125.20	00.00%	00.00%	84.26%	39.40%
JUL	.00	.00	.00	.00	81125.20	00.00%	00.00%	84.26%	39.40%
AUG	.00	.00	.00	.00	81125.20	00.00%	00.00%	84.26%	39.40%
SEP	.00	.00	.00	.00	81125.20	00.00%	00.00%	84.26%	39.40%
OCT	.00	.00	.00	.00	81125.20	00.00%	00.00%	84.26%	39.40%
NOV	.00	.00	.00	.00	81125.20	00.00%	00.00%	84.26%	39.40%
DEC	.00	.00	.00	.00	81125.20	00.00%	00.00%	84.26%	39.40%
TOT	133873.00	44447.10	8300.70	81125.20	81125.20				
**** LOCATION 1: OFFICE			ATB CATEGORY 21: BLUE SHIELD REVIEW						
JAN	14712.36	4267.85	2045.52	8398.99	8398.99	67.60%	42.91%	67.60%	42.91%
FEB	13364.92	1334.26	672.56	11358.10	19757.09	66.48%	15.01%	67.33%	29.63%
MAR	1469.51	.00	.00	1469.51	21226.60	00.00%	00.00%	67.33%	28.16%
APR									28.16%
MAY									28.16%
JUN									28.16%
JUL									28.16%
AUG									28.16%
SEP									28.16%
OCT	.00	.00	.00	.00	21226.60	00.00%	00.00%	67.33%	28.16%
NOV	.00	.00	.00	.00	21226.60	00.00%	00.00%	67.33%	28.16%
DEC	.00	.00	.00	.00	21226.60	00.00%	00.00%	67.33%	28.16%
TOT	29546.79	5602.79	2718.08	21226.60	21226.60				
****LOCATION 1: OFFICE			ATB CATEGORY 30: MEDICARE						
JAN	49488.50	26675.92	10214.40	12598.18	12598.18	72.31%	74.54%	72.31%	74.54%
FEB	52244.98	10214.58	2944.13	39086.27	51684.45	77.63%	25.19%	77.63%	49.20%
MAR	19947.70	.00	.00	19947.70	71632.15	00.00%	00.00%	77.63%	68.34%
APR	.00	.00	.00	.00	71632.15	00.00%	00.00%	77.63%	68.34%
MAY	.00	.00	.00	.00	71632.15	00.00%	00.00%	77.63%	68.34%
JUN	.00	.00	.00	.00	71632.15	00.00%	00.00%	77.63%	68.34%
JUL	.00	.00	.00	.00	71632.15	00.00%	00.00%	77.63%	68.34%
AUG	.00	.00	.00	.00	71632.15	00.00%	00.00%	77.63%	68.34%
SEP	.00	.00	.00	.00	71632.15	00.00%	00.00%	77.63%	68.34%
OCT	.00	.00	.00	.00	71632.15	00.00%	00.00%	77.63%	68.34%
NOV	.00	.00	.00	.00	71632.15	00.00%	00.00%	77.63%	68.34%
DEC	.00	.00	.00	.00	71632.15	00.00%	00.00%	77.63%	68.34%
TOT	121681.18	36890.50	13158.53	71632.15	71632.15				

This report provides an extensive analysis of payment profiles and collection ratios for any given month or on a year-to-date cumulative basis. Profiles and collection ratios are displayed for provider/insurance responsible combinations. The percentages allow the practice to readily recognize trends and are a strong indicator of future collections.

(Courtes y of VERSYSS, Inc.)

- Ask about the cost of service contracts.
- Ask about updates on the software.
- Ask whether training is available for the staff and physician.

HANDLING THE TICKLER SYSTEM

The tickler system is a method that the practice uses to recall patients to the office for various reasons—an annual physical, an annual Pap Smear, a follow-up exam after the removal of a polyp, etc.

Manual tickler systems take the form of 3 × 5 cards filed by the months of the year. However, they can be much more efficiently done on a computer. For example, the computer can be programmed to pull the names of all patients who had a physical in June of last year and print a reminder that can be mailed in May of this year. It can send collection notices to all patients with a balance overdue 60 days or longer.

GENERATING LETTERS

Just as it does with the tickler system, the computer will automatically print correspondence that is preprogrammed into the system upon the request of the user. For instance, if a patient passes away, the user can print

---

BOX 8–12. COMPUTER-GENERATED MEDICAL RECORD

03/26/92   --ACTIVITY LISTING--

PATIENT		SEQUENCE	DATE	TYPE	DESCRIPTION	CATEGORY DESCRIPTION
1302	THOMPSON JOHN	51	01/04/92	CLINIC	HYPERTENSION	1

HEIGHT: 72   WEIGHT: 235   TEMPERATURE: 98.5   BLOOD PRESSURE: 140/98   PULSE RATE: 98   SODIUM LEVEL: 50
CURRENT MEDICATIONS: PROCARDIA - 25MG 2X A DAY

NOTES: DISCUSSED HIGH SODIUM LEVEL WITH PATIENT AND THE IMPORTANCE OF BEING
COMPLIANT WITH DIET. HE AGREED TO SET UP AN APPOINTMENT WITH THE DIETICIAN.

1302	THOMPSON JOHN	52	02/01/92	CLINIC	HYPERTENSION	1

HEIGHT: 72   WEIGHT: 229   TEMPERATURE: 98.4   BLOOD PRESSURE: 135/90   PULSE RATE: 96   SODIUM LEVEL: 41
CURRENT MEDICATIONS: PROCARDIA 25MG 2X A DAY

NOTES: PATIENT IS APPARENTLY BEING MORE COMPLIANT WITH DIET. EVIDENT IN
DECREASING SODIUM LEVEL AND WEIGHT LOSS.

1302	THOMPSON JOHN	53	03/26/92	CLINIC	HYPERTENSION	1

HEIGHT: 72   WEIGHT: 226   TEMPERATURE: 98.5   BLOOD PRESSURE: 132/90   PULSE RATE: 95   SODIUM LEVEL: 35
CURRENT MEDICATIONS: PROCARDIA 25MG 2X A DAY

NOTES: PATIENT COMPLAINS OF "FEELING FLUSH" FOR 1/2 HOUR TO AN HOUR AFTER TAKING MEDICATION.
FACE, NECK AND SCALP ARE PINK AND HOT. WILL MONITOR AND IF STILL A COMPLAINT AT NEXT
MONTH'S VISIT WE WILL DISCUSS ADJUSTING MEDICATION.

> *The following patient medical record can be reviewed on the operator terminal or printed as shown. Cross indexing of various type visits, tests or drugs is also easily obtained.*

(Courtesy of VERSYSS, Inc.)

BOX 8–13. **COMPUTER-GENERATED HEALTH EXAMINATION FORM**

PHYSICIANS HEALTH EXAMINATION

NAME: Melissa Brimmer   DOB: 06/08/71   SEX: F
ADDRESS: 140 Cresent Street, Springfield, ST 02169   PHONE: 770-3406
PARENT/GUARDIAN: Peter J. Brimmer

IMMUNIZATIONS		DATES			
DPT	09/28/71	01/06/72	02/18/72	05/05/72	01/30/74
DT	01/14/88				
TUBERCULIN	03/14/89				
POLIO	01/06/72	02/18/72	05/05/72	01/30/74	10/07/77
MMR	04/12/89				
HIB-CONJUGATE					

HISTORY - INCLUDING MAJO
CHICKEN POX - Y/N?N

> Forms can also be created using Letterwriter. This camp physical form integrates information stored in the patient's medical records regarding lab tests, immunizations and physical history.

LABORATORY TESTS

	DATE	RESULT
URINALYSIS		
LEAD TEST		
HEMATOCRIT	03/14/91	41%
CHOLESTEROL	06/23/91	211
OTHER		
OTHER		

NO ENTRY ON A DATE MEANS A NEGATIVE OR NORMAL RESULT.

PHYSICAL EXAMINATIONS-MOST RECENT AND CURRENT MEDICATIONS
PHYSICAL DATE: 03/14/91   HEIGHT: 60   WEIGHT: 131   BP: 106/85   PULSE:
EXAMINATION WAS NORMAL UNLESS ABNORMALITIES ARE LISTED BELOW:

THIS PATIENT IS FIT FOR COMPETITIVE SPORTS AND PHYSICAL EDUCATION UNLESS NOTED OTHERWISE BELOW:

PEDIATRIC ASSOCIATES   DOCTOR'S SIGNATURE:_____
ONE BROOKSTONE PLACE   DOCTOR'S NAME:_____
SUITE 327   DATE: 03/12/92
SPRINGFIELD, ST 22146   PHONE: (708) 555-8585

(Courtesy of VERSYSS, Inc.)

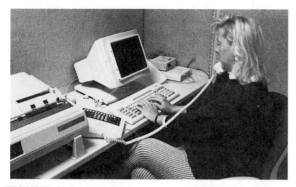

FIGURE 8–3. A software company's hotline operator is always friendly and eager to help customers.

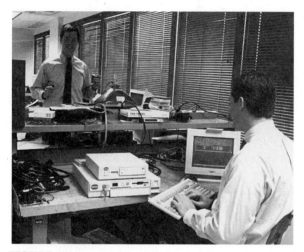

FIGURE 8–4. Hardware technicians are knowledgeable, friendly, and quick to respond.

out a preprogrammed letter of condolence to the family with just the push of a few buttons. By accessing a patient referral letter, the user can generate and print out a thank-you letter to the physician or patient who provided the referral. As you and your staff begin to use the computer's letter-generating capability, you will begin to think of more and more uses for it.

PRINTING DATA MAILERS

As discussed in Chapter 6, there is a difference between data mailers and patient statements. The data mailer is either a four-part or six-part one-piece bill that is generated from the computer. The mailer prints the patient's bill and the address on the envelope at the same time. A front sheet is attached so that the medical biller can see what was actually printed on the bill on the

inside of the mailer. This front sheet can be easily removed and thrown away after review of the bill. All that is needed to mail the bill to the patient is a stamp! If you are thinking of using data mailers, make sure the printer you have is a workhorse and is able to handle the thickness of the data mailer. The amount of space on a data mailer is limited, so if you wish to print a lot of information regarding services and payments, it might be better to consider a patient statement.

PERFORMING END-OF-DAY BACKUP

Every computer trainer will emphasize to the office the importance of the end-of-day backup. If files are not backed up onto a disc or tape at the end of every day, there is a possibility of losing all the work that was entered for that day. If you have a backup and something happens to the computer overnight, it is easy to reeducate your computer by simply installing the backup tape or disc and restoring the computer to the end of the day before. No matter how little work is entered into the computer on a single day, never shut it down without first backing up (Figure 8–6)!

DESIGNING THE PATIENT ENCOUNTER FORM

Once you have chosen your hardware and software vendors, you need to give some thought to the type of forms that you want to use with the new system. Many vendors supply the forms necessary for your use. If not, they will give you the names of suppliers of forms.

One of the most important forms you might want to

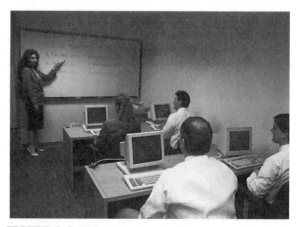

FIGURE 8–5. Training on the use of the computer system is important.

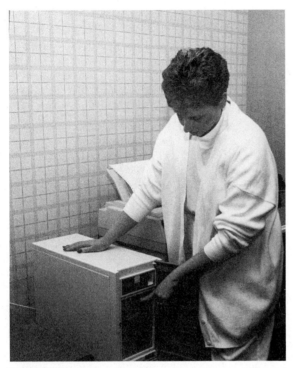

FIGURE 8–6. A receptionist inserts a backup tape for end-of-day procedures.

- secondary
- Patient's insurance numbers

Account Balance

This area of the fee slip/Patient Encounter Form should include the balance due on the patient's account. It is advisable to show this balance in the following areas:

- Due by patient
- Due by insurance
- Previous balance
- Today's charges

This area can be extremely helpful when outstanding balances are due. The area shows the amount the patient owes, so that it can be collected at the time of the patient's appointment.

FROM THE AUTHOR'S NOTEBOOK

The area that shows the patient balance can be highlighted so that it gets the patient's attention.

design is the fee slip, or Patient Encounter Form. It needs to include areas for the following information:

- Patient demographics
- Account balance
- Evaluation and management codes
- Procedure codes
- Laboratory and x-ray codes, if applicable
- Diagnosis codes
- Date for return appointment

Some offices like to include an area for procedures that need to be scheduled. Other offices like to include an area for the physician's signature.

Patient Demographics

This area of the fee slip/Patient Encounter Form should include the following information:

- Patient's name
- Patient's address
- Patient's phone number
  - at work
  - at home
- Patient's date of birth
- Patient's insurance company
  - primary

Evaluation and Management Codes

This area should include all levels of service of evaluation and management codes. The physician's choices will be much easier when she or he is able to see the various levels from which to choose. These levels should include the following:

- New-patient codes
- Established-patient codes
- Consultations (referred by another physician)
- Confirmatory consultations
- Preventive medicine codes

Procedure Codes

This area should include the procedures most commonly provided done in the office, for example, the electrocardiogram or fiberoptic sigmoidoscopy.

Laboratory and X-Ray Codes

This area should include any laboratory or x-ray studies that would be performed in the medical office, such as a complete blood count, urinalysis, or x-ray of a right foot for an x-ray study.

Diagnosis Codes

This area should include the diagnoses most commonly used in the office. There should also be ample room left for additional diagnoses to be written in. This should include V codes and E codes when applicable.

Date of Next Appointment

This is the area of the form where the physician communicates to the front-desk personnel when the patient is to return for a follow-up appointment. The physician might want to see the patient for follow-up in 6 weeks or maybe not for 3 months. This can be written by the physician in this area.

DESIGNING THE HOSPITAL TRACKING FORM

A form similar to the fee slip/Patient Encounter Form can be designed for use with hospital patients. The areas that should be included on the Hospital Tracking Form are

- Patient's name
- Patient's date of birth
- Admission date
- Discharge date
- Authorization/precertification number
- Insurance company
  - Primary
  - Secondary
- Insurance numbers
- Diagnosis code area
- Procedure code area
- Total charge area
- Physician's signature area

Patient's Name/Date of Birth

This area should include the patient's name with a middle initial and the patient's date of birth. The date of birth is especially important, because there might be two patients with the same name in the hospital at the same time.

Authorization/Precertification Number

This number is required by some insurance companies for payment of the hospital stay. It is important to include this number on the billing sheet so that the billing department can access it.

Diagnosis Codes

Space for diagnosis codes can be provided on the Hospital Tracking Form in two ways. One way is to designate an area where diagnoses can be written in by the physician or biller. They MUST be in order of priority. It is sometimes helpful to set up the diagnosis code area as follows:

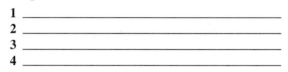

Diagnosis:

1 _____
2 _____
3 _____
4 _____

It is important to remind the physician that diagnosis coding is her or his responsibility. It is unfair to expect billing personnel, or even clinical personnel, to be able to specify patients' diagnoses.

Another way to provide space on the Hospital Tracking Form for diagnosis codes is to provide a list of common diagnoses with blanks in front to prioritize them. Additional open space must be left for diagnoses that are not listed. This is not always the best way to set up the diagnosis section of the Hospital Tracking Form. Hospital diagnoses can be too numerous to mention, and, depending on the specialty, it may be too difficult to set it up in this manner. An example would be:

_____ 530.11 Reflux Esophagitis
_____ 682.9 Cellulitis, Non-Spec
_____ 786.59 Chest Discomfort
_____ 724.5 Backache, Unsp
_____ 244.9 Hypothyroidism
_____ 451.2 Deep Vein Phlebitis

Remember . . . Be Wise . . . Prioritize!

GENERATING REPORTS

Many financial reports and other types of reports can be generated by the computer system. These reports can be used to assess the practice's financial status, to track the number of procedures performed, or to track the number of new patients seen. The computer also can produce many statistics that can be helpful for forecasting the future of the practice. The following is a partial list of reports that can be produced:

- Accounts receivable aging analysis
- Patient master file
- Analysis of patient demographics

- Listings of charges, payments, and adjustments by month to date (MTD) and year to date (YTD)
- Location masterfile
- Analysis of referring physicians
- Audit trails
- Billing reports
- Master insurance file
- Analysis of procedures
- Analysis of diagnoses

Some computer systems are designed to provide payroll and tax services. They keep track of all business transactions and their effects on the assets and liabilities of the practice. They maintain daily records of deposits and withdrawals, print balance statements, and print the checks for both payroll and payables. These functions would be assigned passwords so that only specific individuals could access them.

MANAGING RX's

If you have the right software, you can use the computer to manage the office prescriptions. You can print out prescriptions and track the medications, saving the physician valuable time and improving the quality of medicine. Patients' allergies can be clearly displayed on the computer screen to avoid the improper prescribing of medication. Medication conflicts and medication-mandated laboratory work can also be flagged in the computer system. Prescription renewal alerts can be established for every patient, and a complete list of the patient's medication, with directions and precautions, can be given at each visit.

With this type of software, physicians can easily choose a medication from a list of medications in the database and tailor it to the parameters necessary for that individual patient. The capabilities of checking and double-checking are phenomenal, and the percentage of errors is decreased. Medication interactions are promptly pointed out if the physician prescribes a medication that interacts with another.

This software not only prints out the appropriate prescription, but also enters an entry of the medication prescribed into the patient's record. These programs can be passworded should a physician feel a need to do so.

KEEPING MEDICAL RECORDS ON-LINE

The computerized medical record is a fantasy that's about to become a reality for the medical office. Some feel that computerization of medical records provides

high-quality and cost-effective medical care for the patients. Computerized medical records

- Increase the availability of the patient's medical history and preserve accuracy.
- Facilitate clinical research by providing comprehensive views of health care delivery.
- Provide diagnostic and therapeutic problem-solving support.
- Increase efficiency of the staff by reducing time spent retrieving information.
- Eliminate overhead and administrative costs associated with paper transfer and storage.
- Maintain a comprehensive legal record of patient care.
- Ensure confidentiality of patient data through the use of passwords.

What the future holds in terms of computerized medical records can dazzle even the most high-tech of physicians. As computer systems become linked together in a network throughout the country, the patient's lifetime medical records can be made available wherever the patient seeks service. Redundant tests will not have to be ordered, therefore saving money on unnecessary testing. Physicians will not have to worry about relying on patients' memory regarding historical medical events such as prior illnesses, drug allergies, etc. All the medical information available on that particular patient will be accessible to them.

Computerized medical record systems can contain the following information:

- Laboratory results
- Radiology results
- Pharmacy
- Respiratory therapy
- Cardiology
- Physical therapy
- Physician's orders
- Record text consisting of
  - History and physicals
  - Progress notes
  - Operative reports
  - Pathology reports
  - Discharge summaries

These records can also contain nursing care information such as

- Nursing assessments
- Progress notes
- Care plans
- Vital signs
- Counseling (dietary, cardiac, etc.)

- Patient acuity levels
- Charting and clinical documentation

Health care providers, even physicians, are realizing that computers can make their lives easier, helping them to manage the many changes that occur in health care on a daily basis.

The Tie That Binds the Medical Office and the Hospital

Information systems must accommodate the infrastructure of the health care entity of the future. They must address the daily functions of both the hospital and the office and must play a major role in patient care. Each entity must have the support of the other in an effort to increase quality care and decrease costs. Medical offices will find themselves more efficient when a computer system linked to the hospital's computer system is situated in their office for their own personal use. This system can be used to find lab and x-ray reports that never seemed to make it to the office, saving office staff time in calling to obtain the report, while the patient is waiting in the office. Billing and insurance information can also be easily shared by both the hospital and the office. This can eliminate claims denials or delays due to incorrect insurance information provided by either the hospital or the office. The office hospital biller will no longer have to go to the hospital medical records department or the billing department for insurance and billing information. It will be as simple as turning on the computer and pulling up the information. On the other hand, the patient might provide the office with more information then they provided to the hospital. No matter how you look at it, shared information makes everyone a winner.

References

Farber, L. *Encyclopedia of Practice and Financial Management.* Oradell, NJ: Medical Economics Books, 1988.

Simkin, M. G. *Discovering Computers.* Dubuque, IA: William C. Brown Publishers, 1990.

Tappert, E. "Improve Practice Productivity." *Group Practice Journal,* May/June 1992, pp. 25–26.

Whinnery, S. "Electronic Claims Submission Helps Group Practice Cut Costs." *Group Practice Journal,* July/August 1989, pp. 26–58.

9

Employee Benefits

Employee Benefits

An employee benefit is any benefit or service other than wages for time worked that is provided to an employee in whole or in part by her or his employer (Figure 9–1). Employee benefits became an important issue during World War II and the Korean War, when wage freezes were in effect. Today, many offices offer a variety of employee benefits in lieu of higher salaries, and benefits for employees can usually be secured at a lower cost through group arrangements rather than on an individual basis. The employer reaps tax benefits for offering certain types of employee benefits.

Most office managers believe that a job's benefits package is just as important as its salary. In our fast-paced and competitive society, we are always looking for more benefits. We require child care and tuition reimbursement. We need flexible schedules to balance our family life with our professional life. Although it is not easy, medical offices should recognize the needs of their staff and meet them when possible. This recognition makes for happy employees, which makes for a happy office. According to a survey done by the U.S. government, the costs of employee benefits amount to approximately 39.2% of payroll, and this percentage is expected to rise approximately 2% annually. The major employee benefits offered are medical and retirement plans. The costs of medical and retirement benefits have risen consistently every year by about 1%. Vacation costs have shrunk slightly each year since 1989 and are expected to continue to decline. The cost of health care benefits for an employee in a medical office ranges from $1,400 to $9,398 per year, depending on the size and type of the medical practice. Because of this increase in costs, more and more employers are raising the deductibles of their medical plans. This same government survey also showed that there is a definite trend toward flexible benefit plans, or *cafeteria benefits.* Cafeteria benefits allow the employee to choose from a variety of benefit options to fit her or his specific needs.

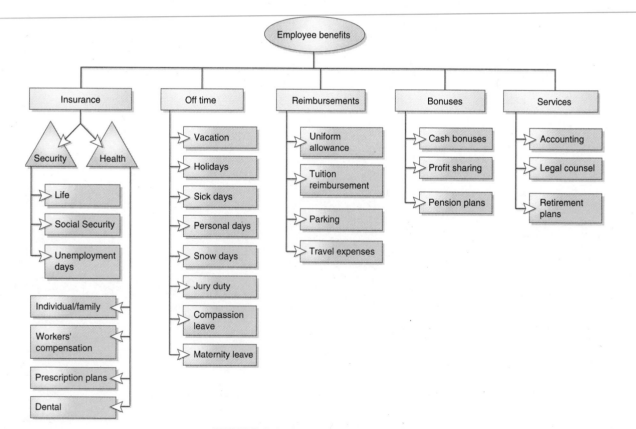

FIGURE 9–1. Types of employee benefits.

CATEGORIES OF BENEFITS

There are five categories in which an employer pays a benefit to an employee. They are

- Private insurance plans
- Bonus cash payments
- Social insurance plans
- Services
- Payments for time off

Private insurance plans consist of premiums or payments made to cover life insurance, disability insurance, health insurance, and retirement plans. *Bonus cash payments* consist of payments made in addition to salary or wages, such as tuition reimbursement, Christmas bonuses, profit-sharing plans, and savings plans. *Social insurance plans* consist of Social Security contributions, Workers' Compensation payments, and unemployment compensation. *Services* include van pools, free parking, day care, clothing or uniform allowances, and wellness and fitness programs. *Payments for time off* include sick time, compassion time, maternity leave, vacation time, holidays, and jury duty.

PRIVATE INSURANCE PLANS

Life Insurance

The oldest and most common of the life insurance plans is "term" insurance. This type of life insurance benefit provides death benefits only and does not build up any cash value. Most group life insurance plans are designed to provide coverage during the employee's years at work and are usually canceled upon termination of the employee. Section 162 of the Internal Revenue Code allows employers to deduct payments made to group term insurance companies. This is considered an ordinary business expense for the employer, and therefore it is rewarded with favorable tax treatment. The employee cannot deduct any contribution she or makes as an individual. Any payroll deductions for group term insurance are included in the employee's taxable income.

Disability Insurance

Group disability insurance supplies employees with partial or total replacement of income while they are out of work as a result of sickness or accident. In the medical office, disability insurance is one of the benefits that are least likely to be offered, yet it is probably the most important to the employee. During a recent survey, it was found that only two-thirds of American businesses offered short-term disability benefits. Only one-third offered long-term disability benefits.

Health Insurance

Health insurance is the most significant type of group insurance in terms of the number of employees covered and the dollar amount paid to cover them. With the exception of very small medical practices (generally solo practices), most physician offices offer some type of medical insurance coverage to their employees. At one time, group medical insurance was provided at no cost to the employee. However, with the skyrocketing cost of health care today, many offices have changed coverage plans to those that require employee contributions. Today's employers are providing more extensive health insurance coverage for employees than the employers of the past provided. The three basic coverages provided are

- Hospital expense benefits
- Surgical expense benefits
- Physician expense benefits

The newer coverages that are currently being included are

- Home health care
- Ambulatory care
- Extended care
- Hospice care
- Birthing center care
- Vision care
- Prescription drug benefits
- Preventive care

Retirement Plans

Along with medical insurance, retirement plans are the most commonly offered employee benefit and account for the largest portion of expenditures for each employee. Retirement income can come from employment earnings after retirement, from individual savings accounts, from Social Security, or from employer-sponsored retirement plans. The federal government offers incentives in the way of tax benefits to physicians who sponsor retirement plans for their employees.

BONUS CASH PAYMENTS

Some compensation plans include plans for cash bonuses to be paid to employees immediately after achievement of a goal or to be deferred until employees' employment anniversary date or birthday or until they have been employed a certain amount of time. Many of these bonus payment plans are based on merit or on the growth of the practice. They are sometimes set up to reward an employee for attaining a certain goal or objective within the practice. For instance, a billing manager who has achieved an objective of decreasing aged account balances of over 90 days by $20,000 might be rewarded with a $500 bonus. Bonuses have been found to increase not only revenues, but also productivity and morale.

SOCIAL INSURANCE PLANS

A large portion of the money employers spend on benefits for their employees is used to make legally required payments to social insurance programs. For medical offices with small benefits programs, this contribution may account for the majority of the total benefit package for each employee. The term "Social Security" refers not only to the payments people get when they retire, but also to survivors' benefits, disability benefits, unemployment benefits, and Medicare hospitalization and supplementary medical insurance benefits provided by the federal government insurance program.

Workers' Compensation

Workers' Compensation laws were enacted to require employers to provide benefits to employees for losses resulting from a work-related injury or illness. These laws are based on liability without fault. These benefits are all subject to statutory maximums. These plans are state run and regulated. Office managers should be aware of their state's regulations regarding employee injury or illness. Offices must purchase coverage for their employees through an insurance company that handles Workers' Compensation insurance. All employers must pay the full cost of this insurance for their employees. Workers' Compensation laws provide benefits for medical care, disability income, death benefits, and rehabilitative services.

Unemployment

Before the Social Security Act of 1935, few employees had any protection for lost wages during a period of unemployment. The Social Security Act provided for a payroll tax to cover employees during this time. This act has two objectives: to provide the individual with income during unemployment and to aid in the employment search. To be eligible for unemployment benefits, employees must meet the following requirements:

1 They must have a previous working record within a certain base period. In most states, this period is either 52 weeks or four quarters before the time of employment.
2 They must be physically and mentally able to work and must be available for work.
3 They must be actively seeking work. Most states require that an individual make an honest effort to obtain a job.
4 They must comply with a 1-week waiting period before benefits start.
5 They must be free of any disqualifications that would result in cancellation, postponement, or reduction of benefits. These disqualifications include
   • Voluntarily leaving a position.
   • Being discharged for misconduct.
   • Refusing to accept a suitable job.
   • Being involved in a labor dispute.

You may find it quite helpful to purchase an employment regulations book from the state. This book explains all state rules and regulations regarding employment. It will contain more information than you will actually need, but it is a valuable resource for any office manager.

SERVICES

Benefits can be offered to employees in the way of services. Such services could be

• Accounting services
• Legal services
• Medical services
• Pharmaceutical services

The practice accountant's services can be offered to employees at tax time. The fees for such services could be absorbed by the office. The same can be done with the practice attorney. Employees can consult the attorney regarding such matters as wills and housing settlements, and the bill for the consultation can be changed to the office. Medical services should be provided to employees and their families. If an employee requires the services of a specialist, perhaps the physician could ask the specialist for a professional discount for the employee. Some offices will pay for their employees' medications. These are generally small offices whose medical insurance coverage does not include a prescription plan.

PAYMENTS FOR TIME OFF

Being paid for days not worked is a pleasant benefit for any employee. Paid days off may include holidays, sick days, personal days, snow days, etc. Some physicians' offices give the Friday after Thanksgiving as a paid holiday. Others pay for time off for immediate family medical emergencies. This translates into instant goodwill between the employee and the employer.

√Cafeteria Plans

HOW CAFETERIA PLANS WORK

Employers are now offering their employees a choice of benefits. An increasing number of physician's offices are adopting the cafeteria plan for their employee benefits program. In this plan, each employee is presented with a list of available benefits from which to choose and a specific total dollar amount to spend on their chosen benefits. The advantage of this plan to the business side of the medical practice is that the benefits that the employees choose are deducted from their salary and are not an added expense for the business. The advantages for the employees are that they are allowed to convert part of their taxable income into nontaxable dollars and can choose only the benefits they need. In a typical cafeteria plan, an office manager might choose a disability plan as part of her or his benefits package, whereas a computer operator may choose child care benefits. Employees are also given the option of additional salary equal to the cost of the benefit package. If they take this option, employees are responsible for paying taxes on these dollars. It is important for the office manager to understand that certain employee benefits such as Workers' Compensation, are the financial responsibility of the employer and are not to be included in the financial part of the cafeteria benefits package.

In the last 10 years, the number of cafeteria plans has grown to the extent that it has been predicted that by 2000, most employers in the United States will provide employees with cafeteria plans. Some feel that employees may choose their benefits unwisely, and there is concern about employers' moral and legal obligation to prevent financial injury to employees. This concern has been incorporated into the design of the plan, which specifies that certain basic benefits must be offered, providing a certain degree of security for each employee. A selection of optional benefits is then presented, from which employees can add to their plan. The basic benefits provided in a cafeteria plan are generally

- Medical insurance
- Disability income insurance
- Term life insurance
- Travel accident insurance (when an employee is on a business trip)
- Pension and profit-sharing plans

The optional benefits are generally equal to 3% to 6% of the employee's salary. They can include

- Additional life insurance
- Accidental death insurance (when basic travel insurance does not apply)
- Term life insurance on dependents
- Dental insurance
- Annual physical examinations for the employee
- Vacation time
- Cash
- Tuition reimbursement
- Wellness and fitness program
- Child care program
- Adult day care program
- Personal days
- Free parking
- Transportation
- Moving expense reimbursement
- Paid jury days
- Financial planning
- Legal services
- Accounting services

If the employee does not have enough credits to purchase optional benefits, additional monies can be deducted from her or his pay to cover the costs of the desired benefits.

> **MANAGER'S ALERT**
>
> When establishing a cafeteria plan, the office must do it on a strictly nondiscriminatory basis. All of the full-time employees must be included!

RATIONALE FOR A CAFETERIA PLAN

Many employers think that employees are unaware of the dollar value of the fringe benefits they receive.

A cafeteria plan makes employees more aware of the costs of benefits. Often, once employees are educated to the costs of such benefits, they are more appreciative of the benefits being offered to them.

The inflexibility of conventional benefit plans usually causes them to fall short of the needs of each employee. For example, an employee with no children cannot get excited about a fringe benefit of child care. This can cause employee dissatisfaction and contribute to constant employee turnover. With a cafeteria plan, there is increased employee satisfaction, which results in better employee retention and an increased ability to attract qualified employees for positions in the office. There is a lot to be said for promoting goodwill between the employer and employee. Everyone wins in this situation.

Many employers use cafeteria plans as a way to contain costs of escalating benefit programs. Between the federal and state regulations, and the inflation rate, employee benefits can become quite costly. Because a cafeteria plan is a "defined contribution" plan rather than a "defined benefit" plan, it provides many opportunities for controlling increased costs.

DRAWBACKS OF THE CAFETERIA PLAN

The office manager should realize that if the office chooses to adopt a cafeteria plan, it faces a complex and time-consuming project in putting it in place.

Another drawback of the cafeteria plan is that the incurred costs of designing and adopting such a plan are slightly higher than those of a conventional plan. Most incurred costs come from the development and administration of the plan. The continuing costs of the plan depend on such factors as what benefits are involved, the number of options presented, the frequency with which the employees are allowed to change benefits, and whether all employees are covered by the plan.

The 10 Most Common Employee Fringe Benefits

The following are the 10 employee fringe benefits most commonly offered by medical practices today:

1 Paid vacations
2 Paid holidays
3 Paid sick days
4 Medical insurance
5 Prescription plans
6 Dental insurance
7 Personal days
8 Snow days
9 Pension plans
10 Profit-sharing plans

PAID VACATIONS

Vacations can be granted in a variety of ways. Vacation options should be described completely in the *Office Procedure and Policy Manual.* The following are models in which the office might grant vacations.

Model 1

1st year: no vacation
2nd year: 1 week of vacation
3rd year: 2 weeks of vacation
4th year: 3 weeks of vacation
5th year and beyond: 4 weeks of vacation

Model 2

1st year: no vacation
2nd–4th year: 2 weeks of vacation
5th–9th year: 3 weeks of vacation
10th year and beyond: 4 weeks of vacation

Model 3

After 6 months: 3 days of vacation
After 12 months: 1 week of vacation
After 3 years: 2 weeks of vacation
After 5 years: 3 weeks of vacation
Vacation caps at 3 weeks

Model 4

1 vacation day for every 60 days worked
Vacation caps at 18 days

These models are for full-time employees only. Part-time employees follow a rated schedule commensurate with the number of days they work per week. For instance, if an employee was part-time (working 2 days a week) and the office followed Model 1 for its full-time employees, the part-time employee would receive no vacation pay the first year. The second year, the part-time employee would receive 2 days of vacation pay; the third year, 4 days of vacation pay; the fourth year, 6 days of vacation pay; the fifth year, 8 days of vacation pay; and so on.

PAID HOLIDAYS

The six paid holidays most frequently observed in the medical office are New Year's Day, Memorial Day, Fourth of July, Labor Day, Thanksgiving Day, and

Christmas Day. Some additional holidays that may be given to employees include Martin Luther King Jr. Day, President's Day, Good Friday, Easter Monday, the day after Thanksgiving, Christmas Eve, and New Year's Eve. Some offices may also elect to give employees their birthday off as a paid holiday. Offices with Jewish, Muslim, and other religious persuasions will wish to observe their religious holidays in addition to the six most common holidays.

PAID SICK DAYS

The number of paid sick days given to employees must be decided between the office manager and the physician. The minimum number of sick days given as a benefit in a medical office is 5. The maximum number is generally 12. Any number in between can be chosen as the sick day benefit for the office. Some offices give a minimum number of sick days but also give personal days.

MEDICAL INSURANCE

Medical insurance is the most important fringe benefit that a medical office can offer today. This insurance can be a Blue Cross/Blue Shield plan, a managed care plan, or a commercial insurance plan. When thinking about employee medical insurance, the office manager should investigate many different plans to compare their benefits and costs. A few offices still offer coverage for family members.

PRESCRIPTION PLANS

Prescription plans are becoming more popular as a medical office benefit. Many managed care plans provide a reasonable rate for the additional prescription plan for the employees. With prescription prices continuing to soar, employees are most appreciative of this benefit.

DENTAL INSURANCE

Dental insurance is not as commonly offered by employers as medical insurance is, but it is still among the top 10 benefits. Dental insurance can become quite costly, and most employers are attempting to keep costs down. As is done with medical insurance companies, the office manager should investigate various companies that provide dental insurance and compare the benefits of the plan and the costs. An office might provide employees a managed care plan for their medical

insurance and Blue Shield for their dental insurance. It is important to shop around to get the most for the office's money!

PERSONAL DAYS

The number of personal days given as a benefit in a medical office ranges widely—from none to 10. This benefit should be decided in conjunction with the other benefits offered. A few offices today still do not provide personal days to their employees. However, these offices are the exception, not the rule. Most offices recognize employees' need for personal days to tend to medical or dental appointments, child illness, parent illness, car repair, financial business, etc. Personal days are found to be a much needed and much appreciated benefit. Many office employees work full-time, which does not leave time for much else. By providing these days as a benefit, the physician and office manager will promote much goodwill.

SNOW DAYS

If the office is located in a geographical area where snow and ice can be a problem, it is best to have a snow day policy in place. Some offices grant a set number of days per year for which they will pay employees' wages when snow keeps them home. Other offices never close in bad weather and feel that their employees should be able to get to work. They deduct any days lost from employees' pay. Other practices pay the employee if the office is closed because of snow but do not pay the employee if the office is open but the employee cannot make it to work. In this case, the office must have a policy as to whether the employee will be docked for this time or whether the employee will be allowed to make up the time at a later date. In any case, it is best to have a snow policy in place before you need it. It should be included in the *Office Procedure and Policy Manual* so that employees are aware of it ahead of time. An example of a fair snow day policy is shown in Box 9-1.

PENSION PLANS

In an effort to recognize the hard work and good efforts of her or his employees, an employer may wish to establish a money purchase pension plan for the exclusive benefit of all eligible employees and their beneficiaries. In this plan, the employer makes a contribution to the employee's pension every year. This retirement benefit is provided totally at the employer's expense and does not consist of any monies from the employee.

> **BOX 9–1. SAMPLE SNOW POLICY**
>
> If the office is officially closed due to bad weather, employees will be paid for these days. If the office is open on a day of bad weather and the employee either cannot make it to work or chooses not to come to work, the employee will be paid but will be expected to make up this time at a later date.

When the employee retires or leaves the practice, she or he receives the value of this account. These plans are developed to the specifications of the Employment Retirement Income Security Act of 1974. A sample plan is shown in the Appendix.

PROFIT-SHARING PLANS

A profit-sharing plan is designed to allow a relatively short-term deferral of income and is a somewhat more speculative benefit to the employee, because the employer's contribution is based on profits. This plan is in contrast to the pension plan, which is designed to provide income at retirement. A profit-sharing plan can provide for a totally discretionary employer contribution. This means that even if the office makes a profit in a certain year, the employer does not necessarily have to make a contribution to the plan that year. There is no minimum-funding rule; however, there must be a substantial and recurring contribution, or the plan will be looked upon as terminated. A profit-sharing plan is considered more of an incentive than a predictable source of income. Employees may be permitted to withdraw from their profit-sharing plan before retirement; however, these early withdrawals may be subject to a penalty.

A sample employee benefits booklet is included in the Appendix.

Additional Benefits That Some Offices Offer Their Employees

LIFE INSURANCE

An employee benefit that is not as commonly offered as others is life insurance. Some medical insurance plans come with a piggyback life insurance policy. This policy can range from $10,000 to $50,000 in life insurance benefits.

TUITION REIMBURSEMENT

Many offices pay for or reimburse employees for their educational expenses. Most offices are delighted that their employees are interested in improving their skills. Employees can deduct their educational expenses if the education maintains or improves a skill related to their position or is directly related to maintaining this position. If the office reimburses employees for this education, the deduction can be made as a tax-free form of compensation.

UNIFORM ALLOWANCE

Occasionally, one will find a small medical office that offers its employees uniform allowances. This is generally not found in larger practices, where it becomes too costly. Employees can deduct from their taxes the cost of any uniform required for the position. Some offices require a specific uniform and provide an allowance toward the purchase of this uniform. For instance, a physician might want her or his office staff to dress in blue scrubs with white jackets. Colored scrub outfits are very popular today and have become more reasonable in price than many white uniforms. Employees generally prefer wearing colors, as opposed to the traditional whites.

References

Beam, B. T., Jr., & McFadden, J. J. *Employee Benefits.* Homewood, IL: Irwin, 1988.

Holley, W. H., & Jennings, K. M. *The Labor Relations Process.* Hinsdale, IL: Dryden Press, 1991.

10

Health and Safety Regulations

What Is OSHA?

The Occupational Safety and Health Act of 1970 was enacted by Congress to establish protocols and standards for occupational health and safety. The Occupational Safety and Health Administration (OSHA), part of the Department of Labor, issues standards that must be followed by all employers and employees and makes site visits to ensure compliance. These regulations are critically important to all medical offices, clinics, ambulances, and hospitals. It is necessary for medical office managers to know these regulations and to follow them strictly. Under federal law, OSHA has the right to inspect all private health care facilities and hospitals in all 50 states, the District of Columbia, Puerto Rico, and U.S. territories. Federal agencies, including military bases and veterans hospitals, may also be inspected.

History of OSHA's Development of Blood-Borne Pathogen Standards

OSHA's involvement with medical practices began in 1983, when it issued a set of voluntary regulations intended to decrease the risk of occupational exposure to the hepatitis B virus (HBV). Since then, the regulation of medical workplaces has increased slowly but steadily. In 1986, the American Federation of State, County, and Municipal Employees petitioned OSHA for emergency temporary standards to reduce workers' risk of contracting certain infectious diseases. That petition was probably the origin of the blood-borne pathogen regulations that were put into effect officially in 1992.

In 1987, the U.S. Department of Labor and the U.S. Department of Health and Human Services issued a joint advisory notice urging employers to institute universal precautions set forth by OSHA wherever workers might have contact with blood or other potentially infected fluids. They also published an advance notice of their intention to initiate a rule-making process on reducing occupational exposure to HBV. In 1988, OSHA started sending selected advisors on fact-finding inspections of medical offices, and in May 1989 OSHA published a blood-borne disease proposal. Receiving increasing pressure from the public to "do something" about acquired immune deficiency syndrome (AIDS), in 1989 Congress began holding hearings on the proposed new OSHA rules. In March 1991, Congress increased the financial penalties for noncompliance with these rules in the workplace, and in October of that year it

directed OSHA to issue the blood-borne disease regulations by December 1, 1991. Finally, on December 6, OSHA published its blood-borne pathogen standards in the *Federal Register,* and the rest is history!

OSHA's Blood-Borne Pathogen Standards

The final OSHA standards regarding exposure to blood-borne pathogens are important to all medical facilities where there is a risk of exposure to infectious materials and blood-borne pathogens. Settings that are found to be noncompliant are subject to penalties of up to $70,000 per incident. Since the implementation of OSHA's final ruling on the blood-borne pathogen standards in January 1992, federal OSHA agents have visited 293 medical surgical hospitals in the United States and found 1,453 violations of these standards. These regulations include:

- A Hazard Communication Plan
- An Exposure Plan
- A Medical Waste Management Plan
- Housekeeping Policies
- Personal Protective Measures
- General Safety Precautions
- A Fire Safety Plan
- A Staff Development/In-Service Training Program

Guidelines of the Occupational Safety and Health Administration (OSHA)

THE HAZARD COMMUNICATION PLAN

The purpose of the Hazard Communication Plan is to help employers understand the policies and procedures governing OSHA's Hazard Communication Standard of 1987. This standard is also known as the "Right to Know law." Employees must be informed of hazardous chemicals in their place of employment, and they must be made aware of the health risks associated with these chemicals. There should be a labeling system in place that identifies all hazardous chemicals, their purpose, and their location. One staff member should be appointed to be in charge of OSHA compliance. This employee should make a list of all hazardous materials in the office setting and post it. Some items that might be forgotten are

- Printer or copy machine ink

- Typing correction fluid
- Glass and surface cleaner
- Antibacterial soaps
- Chemicals used for instrument cleaning
- Furniture polish

As you can see, even ordinary household items are hazardous and should be treated as such.

There must be a material safety data sheet for each hazardous chemical in the office. This can be obtained from the manufacturer. Most companies have these sheets on file and can easily put one in the mail to you. These sheets should be kept together in a binder labeled "MSDS—Material Safety Data Sheets." The potential risks of all hazardous chemicals in the office should be discussed in a meeting with all personnel.

The OSHA Hazard Communication Plan also requires that medical offices

- Report accidents and incidents.
- Post notices of new and revised MSDS for 10 days on employee bulletin board.
- Inform contractors of hazardous chemicals.

THE EXPOSURE CONTROL PLAN

The Exposure Control Plan is one of the most important plans of the Occupational Safety and Health Administration and was adopted in 1991. The purpose of this plan is to prevent or control employee exposure to blood, body fluids, and other potentially infectious materials. The office's Exposure Control Plan must be written and available to all employees and must be annually reviewed and updated. The purchase of any new equipment or the addition of a new procedure requires an update of the plan. The Exposure Control Plan consists of several components, any of which can be inspected by OSHA at any time during the course of the year. The components of the Exposure Control Plan are

- Exposure determination
- Compliance regulations
- HBV vaccination
- Postexposure evaluation
- Hazards communication to employees
- Record-keeping requirements

The determination of which jobs include potential exposure to infectious materials is a part of the exposure determination. The office manager must list any position, and its function in the office, that would pose potential risk of exposure to infectious materials. The use of protective equipment should come into play when compiling this list.

To comply with the OSHA Exposure Control Plan regulations, the office must make sure the *Office Procedures and Policy Manual* contains sections on

- Biohazard labeling
- Classification of exposure categories
- Engineering controls
- Exposure determination
  - Needlesticks and cuts
  - Injury on the job
  - Exposure incidents to blood/body fluids
  - HBV immunizations
- Protective equipment

Biohazard Labeling

Biohazard labeling is done with a biohazard symbol or by the use of red bags or red containers, and is done in an effort to warn employees of potential hazards (Figure 10–1). **Any contaminated waste, containers of regulated waste,** and refrigerators and freezers or other containers used to store, transport, or ship blood or other potentially infectious materials must be labeled. The standard warning labels that can be purchased include the universal biohazard symbol followed by the word "Biohazard." The label must be fluorescent orange or orangish red, with lettering or symbols in a contrasting

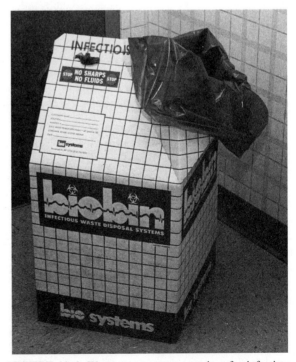

FIGURE 10–1. Waste management container for infectious material. (Courtesy of BioSystems.)

color. The label must be affixed to the container. Red bags or containers may be substituted for specific labeling.

Labeling is not required for the following:

- Containers of blood, blood components, and blood products that have been labeled as to their contents and released for transfusion or other clinical use because they have been screened for HBV and the human immunodeficiency virus (HIV) prior to their release
- Individual containers of blood or other potentially infectious materials that are placed in secondary labeled containers during storage, transport, shipment, or disposal
- Specimen containers in a facility that uses universal precautions when handling all specimens
- Laundry bags or containers in a facility that uses universal precautions for handling all laundry
- Regulated waste that has been decontaminated

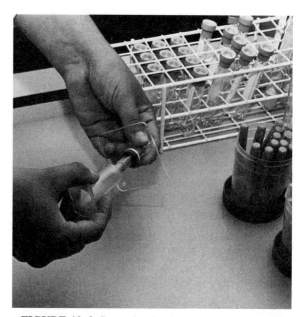

FIGURE 10–2. Protective barrier capping mechanism.

Classification of Exposure Categories

The Classification of Exposure Categories is a written list of job categories that expose employees to bloodborne pathogens. To create this list, the office manager first defines all duties, tasks, and procedures of each and every position in the office that puts an employee at risk of exposure. From this list, the manager then develops a classification of related jobs. If all employees within a specific job classification perform the same pathogen-exposing duties, a list of the specific tasks and procedures for each position is NOT required. For instance, if the office employs three nurses, it is only necessary to develop one nurse job classification that encompasses all three positions.

Engineering Controls

Engineering controls are used to eliminate or minimize employee exposure. These controls include isolation of the employee from such hazards as sharps containers and self-sheathing needles. Because needlestick injuries occur from a variety of devices, there is not a single device or policy that can be used to prevent all needlestick injuries. Contaminated needles CANNOT be recapped by hand, or removed from disposable syringes by hand, unless there is no feasible alternative or recapping is required during a specific medical procedure. This would include the drawing of blood gases (which is never done in an office setting) and the

administration of incremental doses of medications to the same patient (which DOES sometimes occur in a medical office). Mechanical devices and plastic shields that are available for such purposes (Figure 10–2). Bending, shearing, or breaking of contaminated needles is prohibited.

ALL needles MUST be placed in a sharps container for proper disposal (Figure 10–3). Some sharps containers are reusable; however, in an office setting, it is advised to use the disposable ones. These containers must be accessible to employees. For example, they must be located next to the phlebotomy chair, not across the room. In exam rooms, they should be located near the exam table area, where they would be most frequently used.

Exposure Determination

Exposure determination involves many components. Administration of the HBV vaccine is one component of this category and is discussed in detail later in this chapter. Should an exposure occur, a confidential medical examination and documentation are immediately required. The employee must identify the patient source, and that patient's blood must be tested as soon as possible after consent is obtained to determine HIV or HBV infectivity. Any information on the patient's HIV or HBV test must be provided to the evaluating physician. A copy of the OSHA guidelines must be obtained and followed explicitly.

Protective Equipment

The use of protective equipment is an important factor to remember if a lab is located in the medical office. The technician MUST wear gloves during the phlebotomy process. (The only exception to this rule is phlebotomy performed in volunteer blood donation centers.) If an employee is found to be allergic to the gloves, the employer must provide an alternative, such as the use of hypoallergenic gloves, glove liners, powderless gloves, or simply a different brand of glove. Whatever it takes, the office is required to solve the problem!

Face and eye protection is required when there is a potential for splashing, spraying, or spattering of blood or other potentially infectious materials. Prescription glasses may be used as protective eyewear as long as they are equipped with solid shields. If protective eyewear is chosen over the use of a face shield, the eyewear must be worn in combination with a mask to protect the nose and mouth.

MEDICAL WASTE MANAGEMENT PLAN

The purpose of the Medical Waste Management Plan is to protect the public and environment from becoming endangered by infectious medical waste that has been improperly handled, stored, or disposed. Policies must be written to cover

- Categories of waste
- Disposal of sharps
- In-service training
- Medical waste containers
- Preparation of medical waste for pickup
- Storage of medical waste
- Tracking of medical waste
- Weighing of medical waste

HOUSEKEEPING POLICIES

The OSHA housekeeping policy requires employers to maintain clean and sanitary conditions in the workplace. Schedules should be implemented for appropriate cleaning of rooms where body fluids are present. Housekeeping employees must wear appropriate personal protective equipment during all cleaning of blood, body fluids, or other potentially infectious materials and during decontaminating procedures. Disinfecting must be done with a chemical germicide. The office manager should have a workable housekeeping procedure in place at all times. This means that the office should be clean and sanitary at all times. There should be a written schedule for any method of decontamination. Provisions should be made for the disposal of contaminated material in such a way that the materials necessary to perform the disposal are easily accessible. This includes contaminated laundry. OSHA has outlined specific regulations for the treatment of contaminated laundry, and they must be followed to the letter.

FROM THE AUTHOR'S NOTEBOOK

Regular household bleach in a 1:10 dilution can be used for disinfecting. This has been approved by OSHA and is less expensive than commercially purchased solutions.

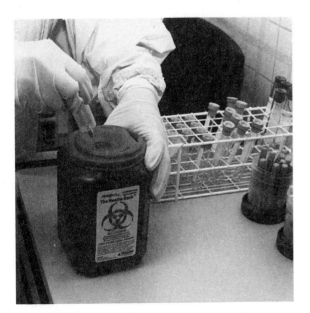

FIGURE 10–3. Disposable-sharps container.

PERSONAL PROTECTIVE MEASURES

The purpose of the Personal Protective Measures plan is to minimize occupational exposure to blood-borne pathogens through the use of personal protective equipment and procedures.

Equipment

What is personal protective equipment? It is clothing and equipment designed specifically to protect health care workers from direct exposure to blood, body fluids, or other potentially infectious materials. Physicians and office managers should be aware that OSHA mandates the use of personal protective equipment by all employees directly involved with patient care. The staff must be provided, at no cost to themselves, the equipment that OSHA specifies as necessary. This equipment includes

- Gloves
- Eye protection
- Resuscitation bags
- Masks or face shields
- Mouthpieces
- Splash guards
- Gowns and laboratory coats
- Protective jumpsuits
- Eye wash stations
- Surgical caps or hoods
- Shoe coverings when appropriate

Any personal protective equipment is appropriate if it prevents blood or other liquids from passing through to the staff's clothing or body. All employees are required to use personal protective equipment, unless they refuse to use the equipment because, in their personal and professional judgment, it would prevent the delivery of quality health care or public safety or would pose an increased hazard to their safety or the safety of a co-worker. Should these situations arise, they must be carefully documented.

It is the physician's or office manager's responsibility to ensure that all protective gear is in the proper sizes and is clean and laundered has been disposed of if it has been used and is disposable. The physician or office manager is also responsible for the repair and replacement of any equipment that is no longer effective. It is the office manager's responsibility to see that all employees are using the various protective devices available in an effort to eliminate the risk of exposure to infectious materials that they can come in contact with during the course of their duties.

Procedures

OSHA requires procedures for

- Handling and or disposing of used needles
- Classification of exposure categories
- Employee health programs

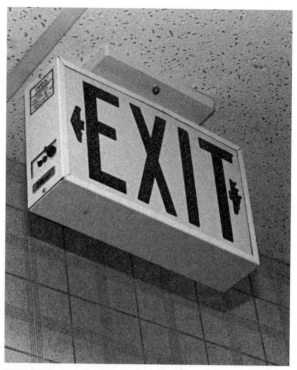

FIGURE 10–4. Illuminated emergency exit sign. (Courtesy of Gastrointestinal Specialists, Inc.)

- Handwashing
- The use of gloves and gowns
- The use of masks
- Capillary blood sampling

GENERAL SAFETY PRECAUTIONS

The General Safety Precautions plan requires the employer to provide a safe working environment for all employees. Each office should have safety policies and procedures regarding employee health, exposure categories, first-aid kits, hazardous and toxic substances, protective equipment, and smoking.

FIRE SAFETY PLAN

Each office must develop a fire safety plan that contains written policies and procedures regarding

- Exits (Figure 10–4)
- Fire alarm pull stations (Figure 10–5)
- The sound of the fire alarm
- Fire drills and classes on how to use a fire extinguisher
- Fire extinguishers (Figure 10–6)
- Fire prevention

- Floor plans
- Hazardous areas
- Inspection of heat/air conditioning systems
- Testing of fire alarms
- Testing of sprinkler systems

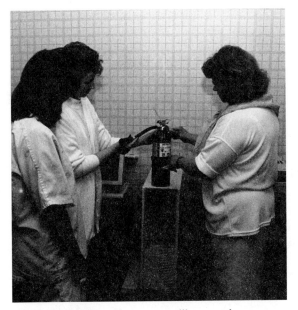

FIGURE 10–6. The office manager illustrates the proper use of the fire extinguisher.

- Treatment of the injured
- Methods of evacuation
- Missing persons
- Discovering a fire
- Emergency telephone numbers
- Emergency lighting (Figure 10–7)

STAFF DEVELOPMENT/IN-SERVICE TRAINING PROGRAMS

One of OSHA's most important functions is developing standards for the education and training of employees. Providing employee training is a vitally important part of complying with OSHA policies and procedures. Training must be provided to employees at the beginning of their employment and annually thereafter. Every employee who is at risk of exposure to blood or other infectious materials must participate in these training sessions. No one may be excused! These training sessions must be provided during working hours and before a new employee starts a position. Training must consist of the following elements:

- Explanations of the epidemiology and symptoms of HBV and HIV infection
- Explanations of the modes of transmission of HBV and HIV
- Explanations of the Exposure Control Plan
- Explanations of the use of personal protective equipment

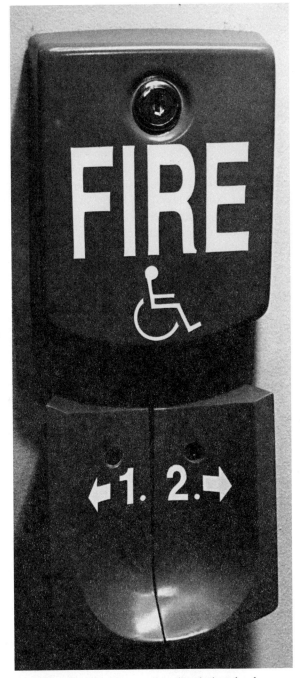

FIGURE 10–5. Fire alarm pull station designed to be accessible to persons with disabilities. (Courtesy of KevCor, Ltd.)

- Explanation of universal precautions
- Information on the HBV vaccine
- Procedures to follow should exposure occur
- Explanation of signs, label, tags, and color coding denoting biohazards

Compliance

All medical offices must follow OSHA's universal precautions, and they must be enforced at all facilities. Therefore, all employees should assume that all materials are infectious and are to be dealt with in that manner. These regulations outline the engineering that should be used to reduce the chances of occupational transmission of infectious diseases. These should consist of any forms of technology that would help to decrease the risk of exposure. A venipuncture recapping device is an ex-ample of this type of technology. All types of equipment must be checked regularly to ensure that they continue to be effective in reducing exposure. The regulations mandate that controls be in place to reduce the risk of exposure.

One of the most obvious work practice controls is proper handwashing. Each medical office should have facilities that are easily accessed by the staff. The physician is responsible for ensuring that all employees wash their hands at the appropriate times.

The second most obvious mandated work practice control is the proper disposal of sharps. These regulations now state that syringes should NOT be recapped, bent, or removed. It is strictly prohibited to shear off or break a contaminated needle. The only exception to this rule is to provide information that there was no alternative to recapping available to the employee. All sharps must be placed in appropriately marked containers until they are picked up for processing. Some states have already used a similar regulation for the sharps disposal, according to the Department of Environmental Resources. These sharps containers must be labeled with an orange and black sticker that reads "Biohazard."

Many other commonsense procedures are included in the OSHA rules and regulations. They are:

- Eating or drinking in areas where occupational exposure could occur is prohibited.
- Storage of food and drink in refrigerators, in freezers, on shelves, in cabinets, or in other places where infectious materials might be stored is prohibited.
- Pipetting or suctioning of blood or potentially hazardous material by mouth is prohibited.
- Packaging infectious materials in any container that is not leakproof or labeled is prohibited.
- The use of "Biohazard" labels is mandatory.

Requirements for HBV Immunizations/Evaluations

Physician offices are required to make the HBV vaccine available at no cost to all employees with jobs that carry the risk of occupational exposure. The only exceptions are employees who have already received the vaccination, employees who have demonstrated that they are immune through an antibody test, and employees who for medical reasons cannot accept the vaccine. If an employee refuses the vaccine, the physician or office manager must obtain her or his signature on the

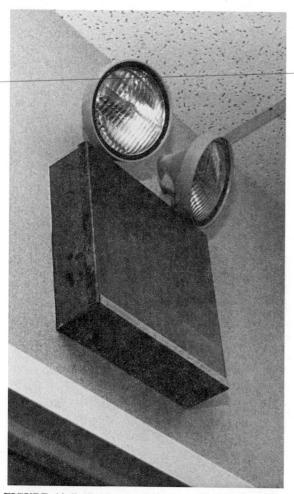

FIGURE 10–7. Emergency lighting. (Courtesy of Gastrointestinal Specialists, Inc.)

appropriate employee consent form. A sample of this form is shown in Box 10–1.

The HBV vaccine should be administered after the employee has received training in the prevention of occupational exposure and within 10 working days of the start of employment. Office managers should be aware of these time constraints and be available to train the new employee within the first week of her or his employment. The regulations do not require that an employee specify a reason for refusing vaccination; however, documentation is always helpful when the OSHA inspectors are at the door. Employees who refuse the vaccine are allowed to change their mind at any time during the course of their employment, and if they do, the physician is obligated to provide this vaccine for them at no cost.

Is Your Office "OSHA Ready"?

The initial panic that you are likely to experience when the OSHA inspector unexpectedly arrives can be fended off by having an understanding of what will take place during the inspection. Once you've undergone your first inspection, you will find the thought of one much more bearable! An OSHA inspection can occur at any time during your office hours. Being prepared for this inspection will help to eliminate chaos and will allow the inspection to proceed smoothly and efficiently.

THE INSPECTION

OSHA inspections are comprised of three parts:

Initial meeting—The inspector interviews the physician.

Walk-through—Office compliance is assessed. Employees are sometimes interviewed privately.

Final meeting—The physician is informed of any apparent violations.

Initial Meeting. During the initial meeting, the inspector asks to see the Exposure Control Plan. This plan must be complete, accessible, and presentable. It must be reviewed and updated annually or whenever changes in job classifications or risk of exposure occur. Keep this in mind: 90% of all violations found in medical offices are due to inadequate Exposure Control Plans.

Walk-Through. The walk-through is the part of the inspection during which the inspector checks office procedure for compliance with the OSHA regulations. Some inspectors go so far as to observe a patient procedure to evaluate the use of personal protective equipment and work practice policies. The inspector also asks to see the procedure for waste disposal and housekeeping policies. If the office contains a laboratory, the inspector will observe the collection, handling, and disposal of blood and its components for compliance with OSHA regulations.

Final Meeting. The final meeting consists of a listing of violations that the inspector believes are present in the office.

VIOLATIONS AND PENALTIES

The inspector reports the violations to OSHA, where a compliance report is compiled and any appropriate citation is prepared. If the medical office receives a citation, it is given 15 days in which to file an appeal. A hearing is then scheduled before an administrative law judge, at which time a determination will be made. A list of OSHA regional offices is provided in Box 10–2.

Penalties for OSHA violations range from $70 to $70,000 for each violation cited. The amount of the fine is based on the severity of the violation and its impact on infection control. There are four categories of violations that can be cited:

1 willful
2 serious
3 repeat
4 other

Each violation is judged by each individual case presented, and good intentions will not keep an office from receiving a citation and fine. The office manager is responsible for monitoring and controlling the compliance of the office and should therefore take a good, hard look at all office policies and procedures to ensure that they comply with OSHA regulations.

THE MOST COMMON VIOLATIONS OF THE BLOOD-BORNE PATHOGEN STANDARDS

The following is a list of the most common violations of the blood-borne pathogen standards found during OSHA inspections in 1 year.

- Improper storage containers were used for non-sharp waste.
- The schedule and method of implementation of a standard were not included in the Exposure Control Plan.
- Work surfaces were inappropriately decontaminated.

BOX 10–1. **HEPATITIS B IMMUNIZATION CONSENT FORM**

I understand that due to the nature of my position, there is a risk of occupational exposure to blood or infectious materials. I understand that I may be at risk of acquiring hepatitis B virus (HBV) infection. I have been given the opportunity to be vaccinated with the HBV vaccine at no cost to myself and have received information regarding HBV. The following information has been explained to me:

1 I may request HBV antibody testing prior to deciding whether or not to receive the HBV vaccine;
2 If I am found to be immune to HBV by antibody testing, then my employer is not required to offer to me the HBV vaccine;
3 If I refuse the HBV vaccine and at a later date decide to accept the vaccine, I may do so at that time in accordance with the policies governing HBV immunizations and at no cost to myself.

I have been informed that the side effects of this vaccine might include:

1 soreness at injection site
2 local reaction
3 rash
4 fatigue
5 joint pain
6 headache
7 dizziness
8 fever

I hereby
    [   ] accept
    [   ] refuse
the HBV vaccine.

_____

Employee Signature

_____

Date

Prescreening date: _____

Results: _____

Dates of vaccination

1st: _____

2nd: _____

3rd: _____

I certify that the above-named individual received a copy of the HBV information sheet and has been fully explained the contents. I certify that I reviewed with the above-named individual our established HBV immunization policy and procedures.

_____   _____

Date   Signature—Title

- Signed refusal of the HBV vaccine was not available.
- Employees did not comply with personal protective equipment.
- HBV vaccine was not available.
- Improper warning labels and signs were on containers of regulated waste.
- A written Exposure Control Plan was not available.
- A listing of job classifications for all employees exposed was not available.

- A listing of tasks when some employees were exposed was not available.
- Handwashing was not performed properly.
- Face protection was used improperly.
- A written schedule for cleaning and decontamination of an area was not available.
- Documentation that employees were trained within 90 days of standard was not available.
- Name of person who trained staff on OSHA regulations was not documented.

BOX 10–2. OSHA REGIONAL OFFICE LOCATIONS

REGION I
(CT, MA, ME, NH, RI, VT)
1st Floor
133 Portland Street
Boston, MA 02114
(617) 565-7164

REGION II
(NJ, NY, Puerto Rico, Virgin Islands)
Room 670
201 Varick Street
New York, NY 10014
(212) 337-2378

REGION III
(DC, DE, MD, PA, VA, WV)
Gateway Bldg, Suite 2100
3535 Market Street
Philadelphia, PA 19104
(215) 596-1201

REGION IV
(AL, FL, GA, KY, MS, NC)
Suite 587
1375 Peachtree Street
Atlanta, GA 30367
(404) 347-3573

REGION V
(IL, IN, MI, MN, OH, WI)
Room 3244
230 South Dearborn Street
Chicago, IL 60604
(312) 353-2220

REGION VI
(AR, LA, NM, OK, TX)
Room 602
525 Griffen Street
Dallas, TX 75202
(214) 764-4731

REGION VII
(IA, KS, MO, NE)
Room 406
911 Walnut Street
Kansas City, MO 64106
(816) 426-5861

REGION VIII
(CO, MT, ND, SD, UT, WY)
Federal Bldg, Room 1576
1961 Stout Street
Denver, CO 80294
(303) 844-3061

REGION IX
(American Samoa, AZ, CA,
Guam, HI, NV, Trust
Territories of the Pacific)
Room 415
71 Stevenson Street,
San Francisco, CA 94105
(415) 744-6670

REGION X
(AK, ID, OR, WA)
Room 715
1111 Third Avenue
Seattle, WA 98101-3212
(206) 442-5930

The Clinical Laboratory Improvement Amendments of 1988

The Clinical Laboratory Improvement Amendments of 1988 set forth performance requirements for laboratories. These rules and regulations were amended in 1993, with the final version of the performance requirements. In-office laboratories are now subject not only to state regulations, but also to federal regulations. Each physician-owned laboratory (POL) and hospital or independent laboratory is responsible for payment of a compliance fee. This fee varies from state to state and is based on an hourly rate determined by each state government, as opposed to the average amount for each of the 11 compliance fee schedules. Hourly inspection rates range from $19.52 in Puerto Rico to $84.54 in Michigan. More than 80,000 POLs have applied for certification for their laboratories.

The CLIA inspection process is focused on the quality of lab services provided. CLIA inspections are intended to provide on-site education regarding accepted lab procedures. They are also intended to determine whether a lab is complying with CLIA standards and will aid in the decision to issue certificates. During this inspection, lab personnel may be asked to perform procedures, show the inspector all areas of the lab, and provide requested documentation. These inspections are conducted by Health Care Financing Administration (HCFA) regional surveyors and state agency personnel. HCFA will provide written guidelines to assist regional surveyors and state agency personnel with federal inspections. These guidelines are available from the National Technical Information Service at (703) 487-4650 (regular orders) or 1-800-553-6847 (rush orders). Request "Appendix C," document #PB-92-146-174. The price is approximately $38.00.

References

Cavalli, K. "Is Your Office Ready for an OSHA Compliance Inspection?" *Physician's Management,* July 1993, pp. 94-95.

Federal Register, December 1991, pp. 64175-64181.

Universal Precautions. Garden Grove, CA: Medcom, 1992.

Valiant, C., & Roberts, R. "OSHA's Rules on Bloodborne Pathogens Affect Physicians and Their Employees." *Group Practice Journal,* May/June 1992, pp. 48-50.

Watson, L. "Handling Medical Waste." *Advance Laboratory,* March/April 1993, pp. 14-18.

Wold, C. "New OSHA Regs Will Target Physicians' Offices." *Physician's Management,* July 1992, pp. 165-176.

11

Responsibilities of the Medical Office Manager

A Hard Act to Follow

The Bad Manager
- *The Manager Who's Had No Management Training*
- *The Wimp*
- *The Task Master*
- *The Phantom*
- *The Intimidator*

The Three Goals of a Medical Office Manager

The Competent Office Manager's Areas of Expertise

Management Principles to Live By

Leadership and the Medical Office Manager
- *Management Styles*
- *Characteristics of the Creative Manager*

The Office Manager and the Physician—A Happy Duo?

Policy and Procedure Manuals That Work

The Health Care Consultant

A Project List That Can Keep You on Target

The Physician Demographics Sheet

Condolences

Memo Writing Made Easy
- *Step 1: Know Your Purpose*
- *Step 2: Keep It Short and Get to the Point*
- *Step 3: Avoid Catchy Phrases*
- *Step 4: Maintain a Backlog of Successful Memos*
- *Step 6: Personalize the Memo*
- *Step 7: Make It Easy for the Recipients to Give Feedback*

Managing Desk Clutter

Staff Meetings
- *Meeting Planning Checklist*
- *Getting Them There on Time*
- *The Making of Effective Staff Meetings*

The Patient's Bill of Rights

Practice Mergers
- *Finances*
- *Employees*
- *Fee Schedules*
- *Time for the Attorney*

Snap Decisions: Harmful or Helpful?

The National Practitioner Data Bank

The Physician's CV—That First Impression

The Beeper: Friend or Foe?

Lost in Translation

Purchasing Power: Buying Equipment, Furniture, and Office Supplies
- *Control of Costs*
- *Bargain Shopping for Equipment and Supplies*
- *Leasing Versus Buying*
- *Copiers*
- *The Fax Phenomenon*
- *The Security of a Paper Shredder*
- *The Security System—A Must!*
- *Desk Accessories*
- *The Supply Order Log*

Employee Theft

"Other" Office Insurance
- *Injury Liability*
- *Personal Property Insurance*

The Facility
- *Office Leases*
- *Moving the Office*
- *Building a New Facility*
- *Don't Move . . . Spruce Up!*
- *Revamping of Present Space*

Be Humble . . . Apologize

Professional Societies
- *Medical Group Management Association*
- *Professional Association of Health Care Office Managers*

A Hard Act to Follow

"Whenever you hear that everything is going as planned, somebody is either a fool or a liar."
—Management Guru Ted Levitt

It is not easy to step into someone else's shoes. Facts are, the staff probably liked the last office manager and are not easily swayed into liking a replacement. The manager who held this job previously is a hard act to follow. It is difficult to overcome self-doubts and prove yourself under adverse conditions. Staff members will be resistant to changes, saying, "But we always did it this way!"

When you are trying to fill these big shoes, the worst battle is within yourself. There is generally a buildup of anxiety that far exceeds the resistance from staff members. Remind yourself of all the positive things that you are doing, counsel yourself, and downplay the fears. You know you would not be there if you couldn't do the job! Avoid justifying your decisions and actions. When you are told that the other way was better, simply tell the staff that you appreciate their suggestions and will consider them. Tell them that your way of doing things may be a little different, and say it firmly. The staff members will eventually come around. Make sure that the wide range of emotions that you feel every day are not shown. Your success is tied directly to your self-discipline. Failing to keep your emotions under control can cause failure. Look secure and confident, and the staff members will soon look at you that way!

The Bad Manager

In many articles and books regarding managers, supervisors, and bosses, the unspoken implication is that bad ones are few and far between. Not so, says psychologist Mardy Grothe, co-author of *Problem Bosses: Who They Are and How to Deal With Them*— There are more bad ones than good ones! In a study conducted by the University of Southern California, 75 out of 100 people polled said they had experienced difficulties with a boss or manager. Let's face it, the medical office manager will usually not win a popularity contest; however, an environment of mutual respect and friendliness will work. Such an environment can be stymied by employee behaviors that can make an office manager cranky. The following is a partial list of types of employees you can expect to put you in a cranky mood:

- Employees who insist on talking to you even though you are actively involved in a telephone conversation
- Employees who insist on asking questions at the same time
- Employees who constantly whine
- Employees who stampede for the front door at the end of the day
- Employees who give matter-of-fact answers when really they are unsure
- Employees who take forever to say something
- Employees who insist on standing at the office door when you return from vacation, wanting all the details of the trip . . . meanwhile there are mounds of paperwork on the desk waiting for attention
- Employees who don't produce a requested piece of information until you ask them for it a second time
- Employees who have an excuse for everything
- Employees who are chronically late
- Employees who always have an emergency
- Employees who are always "sick"

THE MANAGER WHO'S HAD NO MANAGEMENT TRAINING

Of all the problem managers today, the most common seems to be the office managers who have been promoted into their management position without proper training and education. This office manager is often found in the office talking on the telephone for the better part of the day. To avoid being this type of manager, it is important to develop a list of areas, such as creating the budget or interviewing job applicants, where inadequacies seem to be prevalent. Then sign up for workshops and seminars (at the office's expense) to gain skills in these areas. Once you have attended these courses, you will have more confidence and feel generally better about the position. It is also important to not stay in your office; get up and walk around all areas of the office. Stop and ask individual employees how they are doing. Ask them about their work.

> **FROM THE AUTHOR'S NOTEBOOK**
>
> A good office manager is a "working" office manager. An individual who knows what staff are doing is a successful office manager.

THE WIMP

The wimpy office manager has a difficult time dealing with conflict and making a firm decision. This office manager is afraid to ask an employee to perform a certain task and often performs the task her- or himself. This manager cannot handle employee conflicts and would rather have the employees slug it out before getting involved! To avoid being this type of manager, again consider taking a seminar or workshop on personnel management. Weekly or monthly staff meetings will also help you feel more comfortable with facing the staff. To get some of the confidence you need, ask the physician for feedback on your work.

THE TASK MASTER

Some office managers think the more hours worked, the more work done. This is not always the case. Employees will fill time with paper shuffling if they are made to stay and work long hours. Look for ways for each employee to be more productive and efficient during the time allotted for her or him. Perhaps a reassessment of job descriptions would be helpful. In addition, do not expect all workers to work at the same speed, and understand that employees have responsibilities outside the office that also require their attention. Very few people feel that their job is their life!

THE PHANTOM

The phantom manager makes an appearance at the office, does one or two things, and then leaves. This forces employees to address their questions and suggestions for alternatives to an empty chair, usually by sticking Post-It notes on it. To manage, you must be there! It is unfair to expect employees to make judgments and decisions they might not be equipped to make but have to make because of an absent "leader." You know the old saying: "The band cannot play without the bandleader. How would the trumpets know when to come in?!"

THE INTIMIDATOR

Intimidators attempt to make themselves feel better about their own inadequacies by controlling and bullying the employees. They correct an employee in front of others, causing an embarrassing situation for the employee. The old saying "You can catch more flies with honey than you can with vinegar" seems to fit here. It doesn't help any situation to be nasty. Any reprimanding should be done in your office with the door closed; it should never be done in public. Behavior like this will cause a chronic staff turnaround problem.

The Three Goals of a Medical Office Manager

1 Quality of Care
2 Happy Employees
3 Achievement of Goals

Quality is important in any product or any service. If the product or service a business provides is not of high quality, the business loses customers, and a medical office is no different. Providing a happy environment for employees to work in is a key to successful office management. Happy employees are more productive employees and take pride in their accomplishments. The achievement of goals is another key to successful medical office management. In Box 11–1, you will find a blueprint for achievement.

The Competent Office Manager's Areas of Expertise

The competent office manager possesses expertise in three areas: clinical, financial, and psychological.
Clinical Knowledge. Knowledge of the clinical

BOX 11–1. **BLUEPRINT FOR ACHIEVEMENT**

BELIEVE while others are doubting
PLAN while others are playing
STUDY while others are sleeping
DECIDE while others are delaying
PREPARE while others are daydreaming
BEGIN while others are procrastinating
WORK while others are wishing
SAVE while others are wasting
LISTEN while others are talking
SMILE while others are pouting
COMMEND while others are criticizing
PERSIST while others are quitting
—William Arthur Ward

aspects of a medical practice can be most helpful to an office manager. It can be helpful in understanding the triage of patients to be seen by the physician and in determining the correct code for the service provided. Having some type of clinical background can be as important as having a business background, depending on the type of medical practice.

Financial Knowledge. Knowledge of finances is another major aspect of the office manager's competence. Physicians are concerned about revenues and expenses, as well as about patient care. To many physicians, an important responsibility of the medical office is to keep an eye on the bottom line. It is necessary for physicians to know the overhead costs, the turn-around time of billing, and other financial ratios to be able to budget for the coming year, and it is the office manager who gives them these pieces of financial information.

Psychological Knowledge. Personnel management is the most difficult part of the medical office manager's job. Many managers say it would be easy to manage a medical office, were it not for personnel problems. These, unfortunately, are a reality. The medical office manager should be a counselor and advisor to the staff. She or he should be able to make decisions that do what's good for the office and yet address some of the needs of the employees. This is discussed in detail in Chapter 2. Psychological knowledge can also come in handy when dealing with physicians and other contacts, such as hospital employees, salespersons, etc. As Priscilla Gross of the American Medical Association once said, "A personnel manager should possess a sensitive ear, a caring heart, and the skin of a rhinoceros."

Management Principles to Live By

Many people have had ideas about management. Some of these ideas have endured, and some haven't. The following are eight management ideas that have stood the test of time:

Mile's Law: Where you stand depends on where you sit. Mile's Law forces the manager to focus on the big picture, negotiating and building strengths. According to Mile's Law, the manager builds a sense of teamwork by walking around. Don't just sit at your desk; walk around, talk to employees, get updates.

Parkinson's Law: An activity expands to fill the time allotted to it. In 1957, An English historian found that the more people who were hired, the more work they created, without necessarily increasing the office's output. A corollary to this law is that activity speeds up as a deadline approaches.

GIGO: Garbage in, garbage out. An anonymous, frustrated computer operator coined this phrase to account for the fact that a computer's output is totally dependent on what's put into it. Likewise, the output of any project is totally dependent on the quality of input (the people, materials, budgets, and information).

The Law of Effect: Behaviors immediately rewarded increase in frequency, and behaviors immediately punished decrease in frequency. The educational psychologist E. L. Thorndyke believed that timely feedback is one of the manager's most powerful motivators. The Law of Effect is a particularly suitable tool for a proactive manager. Catch employees in the act of victory and thank them on the spot. Just as quickly point out mistakes when you find them.

The Peter Principle: People tend to be promoted until they reach a level beyond their competence. A bestseller entitled *The Peter Principle* proposed this simple explanation as to why competent performers become less effective when promoted.

Pareto's Law (the 80–20 Rule): The significant elements in any group usually constitute only a small portion of that group. Pareto, an Italian engineer, developed the law of the "trivial many" and the "significant few." Eighty percent your productivity comes from 20% of your effort.

The Pygmalion Effect: Our expectations for others condition our behavior toward them, which in turn affects how they behave. According to this law, if you believe your employees are lazy and apathetic, you will respond with minimal delegation and trust. They, in turn, will fail to improve, and you will end up with a group of employees who are lazy and apathetic.

Murphy's Law: If anything can go wrong, it will. Murphy's Law warns us to always have a contingency plan. This law is most evident when you attempt to implement change in the office. Try to anticipate your employees' objections to an innovation and defuse them before they arise.

All of these laws contain a common thread: the admonition to treat people well, also known as the Golden Rule.

Leadership and the Medical Office Manager

"Leaders are like eagles. They don't flock. You find them one at a time."

—Anonymous

In a medical practice, leadership skill is crucial not only because patients, physicians, and staff members expect it, but because quality improvement demands it. Who is a leader? A leader is a person who is assertive, resilient, proactive, charismatic, innovative, focused on the big picture, and quality oriented and who puts these traits into the service of inspiring and guiding employees through day-to-day operations. Employees' success in performing their duties relies on four factors:

1 What the manager says
2 How the manager says it
3 Whether the manager believes it
4 How the manager acts

You will accomplish creative leadership by directing the efforts of others in an effective, innovative way to accomplish the goals of the practice. Results are one way to measure the success of your method. Truly successful leaders also look for changes in attitude and commitment on the part of the employees. If you are an effective leader, your employees will perform at the same level regardless of whether or not you are there to supervise them.

MANAGEMENT STYLES

Ohio State University conducted research on different management styles and the effectiveness of each. It identified four management styles (Box 11–2) that office managers should recognize and try out before attempting to establish when to use each type of style.

Directing. Style 1 is Directing. Directing managers give their employees a lot of direction and little support. They

- Set goals and expectations.
- Set plans for action.
- Control the decision process.

BOX 11–2. **LEADERSHIP STYLES**

Style 1: Directing
High Directive
Low Supportive

Style 2: Coaching
High Directive
High Supportive

Style 3: Supporting
High Supportive
Low Directive

Style 4: Delegating
Low Supportive
Low Directive

- Determine evaluation methods.
- Provide specific directions.

This style is appropriate in a crisis or emergency situation, where there is little or no time for consultation or evaluation of the problem. It is not so good for day-to-day personnel management.

Coaching. Style 2 is Coaching. The office manager, when using this style, obtains more feedback from the employee than is obtained in the Directing style and encourages motivation. The amount of direction the manager gives remains high because the employee is still learning the job. Coaching managers

- Set goals and action plans but still consult with employees.
- Encourage two-way communication between them and the staff.
- Explain the big picture—why things are done a certain way.
- Give lots of feedback, both positive and negative.
- Make final decisions and evaluate performance.
- Continue to teach, train, and provide direction.

The Coaching style is most effective with employees who are still learning their jobs and need encouragement to maintain their motivation. This management style involves a lot of hands-on training.

Supporting. Style 3 is Supporting. When they adopt this style of management, office managers

- Share responsibility for problem solving with staff.

- Delegate some goal-setting and decision-making tasks.
- Involve employees in performance evaluations.
- Listen and provide feedback.
- Encourage self-evaluation and independence.

This style allows seasoned employees to solve their own problems. The amount of direction given is reduced, because employees know their jobs. The manager wants to encourage more independence.

Delegating. Style 4 is Delegating. When managers are using this type of style, they reduce both their support and direction. Delegating managers

- Collaborate with employees to set individual goals.
- Encourage employees to monitor and evaluate their own work.
- Do not provide feedback or much direction.
- Demonstrate trust and confidence in employees by encouraging independent thought and action.
- Allow employees to take responsibility and give them full credit.

As stated previously, by training staff and then motivating them, the medical office manager frees up time to do other necessary tasks, such as planning the overall goals of the practice and the budget for the practice. A good leader provides stimulation, encouragement, support, and inspiration to all employees, allowing them to grow and achieve. Some feel that at this point, the manager gives up supervision in favor of consultation. It is good to encourage employees to solve their own problems in their own ways and to come to you only when these ways have failed. This approach to management can be risky, but it is beneficial in that you reap the benefits of energized employees.

CHARACTERISTICS OF THE CREATIVE MANAGER

"Leaders should spend no more than four hours a day in their offices. The rest of the time, they should be out with their people. They should be talking with employees and getting feedback on problem areas. They should be patting people on the back!"
—Lecturer Perry M. Smith

Caring for Employees' Psychological Health

Part of being a creative manager is realizing that all employee efforts and accomplishments must be recognized. Always thank employees for a job well done. It's a good idea even to say "Goodbye and thank you" at the end of the day. This is called caring for employees' psychological health. Don't indulge in careless and picky criticism. It is destructive to your employees and to the general office environment.

Removing Employees Who Are Roadblocks to Efficiency

By the same token, incompetence is not to be tolerated. You have the responsibility to run an efficient office, and employees who ultimately stand in the way of your meeting this responsibility must be removed. This can be a difficult task, but it can be done with grace.

Seeing the Big Picture

It's good to see the "small picture," the details, but a progressive office manager is also constantly concerned about the big picture. An office manager with long-term vision is a valuable asset to the medical office.

Dealing with Employees' Inflexibility

When a medical office has just opened, employees' roles are generally loose and flexible. In addition, communication is usually good, because the office is small. When the office starts becoming experienced, roles start to become more defined, and when the office starts growing, rules and procedures are developed to ensure consistency and quality. As the office manager, you may begin to think in terms of positions, rather than in terms of the people in them. Keep in mind that once employees have been doing a task a certain way for a long time, they are likely to fight change. Simply giving them a new telephone will send some employees into a frenzy. It may be difficult for these employees to adapt to changes that you, as a creative leader, wish to make. When implementing changes, be aware of this inflexibility and proceed with caution. Changes can be made—maybe not quickly, but they can be made.

Balancing the Need for Employees To Trust You with the Need To Serve the Office's Best Interests

Trust is vital to good leadership. However, fulfilling this trust cannot overrule the need to do whatever's necessary for the good of the office. Some decisions may be very difficult to make. As an example, you might agree to change the position of an employee to a recently opened different position. After interviewing new candidates, you feel the office would run smoother if the new employee would take the open position because of her/his qualifications, and the established employee would stay in the position she/he is currently in. This can be disappointing for the employee but is in the office's best interests.

Teaching Your Staff

Good leadership in a medical office depends greatly on teaching. Leaders must be teachers, willing to share insights, skills, and experiences with their staff, helping them to grow as employees.

Managing the Demands on Your Time

Time management and organization are integral components of effective management. You will find that your travel plans, telephone calls, mail, and schedules can get out of hand. Staying busy and working longer hours do not always solve the problem. Control over your schedule and discipline are what's needed.

Keeping Up Your Physical Stamina

Without stamina, you cannot be a good leader. It is wise to build some type of exercise program (jogging, swimming, racquetball, etc.) into your schedule, so that you can get some relief from stress. The demands of a medical practice can take their toll on an office manager in a short period of time.

Knowing How to Run a Meeting

Another sign of creative management is knowing how to run a meeting. This is discussed later in this chapter, but the following are a few basics to remember: Good leaders are actively involved in the meeting, express their views and concerns, know how to draw conclusions and wrap up the meeting, and set the date and agenda for the next meeting.

Being Able to Laugh

Humor can be a great reliever of tension. You should let your employees know that work is not so important that you can't sit back and laugh a little. Don't confuse humor and laughter with making fun of someone, however. Humor delivered with a sharp tongue and off-color humor are unacceptable!

Balancing the Need to Take Risks with the Need to Be Reliable

Risk taking is sometimes an essential part of decision making. However, it is important to always listen to all sides before making any decisions. Most decisions cannot wait, and many times office managers must implement these decisions rather quickly. The office manager should understand what would be the best and the worst possible outcomes of the decision, weigh them carefully, and then, with the consistency of the past, make a good, quick decision. It is important to realize that there is an element of risk involved every time an office manager needs to make a snap decision. However, the office staff are aware that the office manager makes all decisions with a certain amount of consistency and begin to rely on that element of the office manager's persona. Office managers should be careful when making commitments to these decisions and should realize that a nondecision is also a decision in itself. Reliability is a component of a good office manager and must be present to provide strength and stability to the office.

Managing with Flexibility and Integrity

Flexibility and integrity are also essential to the medical office manager. The best office managers are those with open minds and a willingness to deal with new ideas. Even more important than flexibility is integrity. In fact, of all the qualities a good office manager should have, integrity is probably the most important. Good leaders do not talk about integrity— they just operate at its highest level. Integrity must be ingrained in all staff members and must be supported by you and the physician.

There are several leadership qualities a good manager should have. They are listed in Box 11–3. After reading this list, try to evaluate what qualities you possess that are strong or weak. Try to work on the weak qualities to improve your leadership capabilities and to secure your position as a competent medical office manager.

BOX 11–3. LEADERSHIP QUALITIES FOR MEDICAL OFFICE MANAGERS

- Is honest and sincere.
- Uses delegation effectively.
- Has respect for employees and elicits respect from them.
- Is empathetic.
- Is fair.
- Is committed to the goals of the practice.
- Realizes the importance of patient satisfaction.
- Has good communication skills and is an active listener.
- Encourages and rewards good work by staff members.
- Is straightforward and consistent in behavior.
- Is able to admit mistakes and use them as learning experiences.
- Has good counseling skills.

---

to help make the day better. Recognize when the physician is having a bad day and ask if there is anything you can do. This will be greatly appreciated, and the physician with insight will be pleased that you can recognize a bad day and are willing to help to make it better.

After the solid relationship has been established, carefully choose a time to present your new idea. Timing is a critical factor in whether your new idea is accepted. Don't present the physician with a new idea as she or he is racing down the hall toward the hospital! There is no formula for determining when the window of opportunity is open. After working with a physician for a while, you will be able to sense when the time is right to spring a new idea on her or him. In addition, have documentation available to back up your idea, and present it in such a manner that it evokes a positive response from the physician (Figure 11–1). If your presentation requires handwritten material, keep it clear and short. Nobody has the time to read a large amount of material, so your success will depend in part on whether you can present your information completely yet briefly. Practice the presentation before attempting it on the physician; this will help you identify any flaws or glitches in it. Good Luck!!

The Office Manager and the Physician—A Happy Duo?

It is most important to have a good working relationship with the physician. It is not a relationship that is built easily; it requires hard work on the part of both parties. It is important to understand clearly what the physician expects. Find out from the physician what the goals of the practice are, what the goals of the office manager's position are, what the responsibilities of the position are, and whether there are any obstacles that may prevent you from doing a good job. It is only after you have obtained full and clear answers to these questions that you will be able to be effective and productive.

Getting a new idea across to the physician requires excellent timing and the right content. If you have a strong, open relationship with the physician, it is easier for the development of new ideas for the practice. If the strong relationship does not exist, you might first want to work on that aspect before attempting to go further. Show the physician that you are a capable, dependable, and responsible manager with the best interests of the practice in mind at all times. Help the physician to make the best and effective use of her or his time and keep the lines of communication open at all times. Ask the physician on a regular basis if there is anything you can do

Policy and Procedure Manuals That Work

The *Office Procedure and Policy Manual* can be an important tool for the manager of a medical office. Any

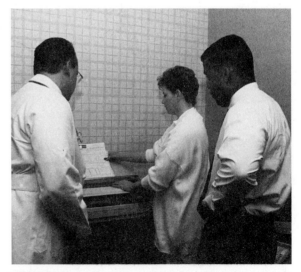

FIGURE 11–1. The office manager brings the computer transmission dilemma to the physician's attention.

medical practice consultant will tell you that a manual should be in place in every medical office. This manual explains the policies of the office and tells employees what is expected of them. The office will run more smoothly and misunderstandings between employees and management will be kept to a minimum. Every manual should cover certain key areas. These areas are

An introduction
A mission statement (the vision of the practice)
The office's address and phone number
The name and address of the hospital where the physician is on staff
Office hours
Gossip
Confidentiality
Orientation and training period
Employee evaluations
Employee benefits
Sick time
Maternity leave
Compassion leave
Vacation policy
Continuing education
Discipline, resignation, and termination
Breaks
Lunch periods
Smoking policy
Jury duty
Part-time employment
Parking
Employee grievances
Snow days/inclement weather
Personal phone calls
Conduct and appearance
Workstation appearance
Public relations
Job descriptions
Holidays
Pay schedule
General questions

The Health Care Consultant

More and more physicians' offices are calling on the expertise of the health care consultant. This consultant is asked to observe the day-to-day workings of the office, the personnel, and, yes, even the physician, with the purpose of identifying areas that need to be more productive and efficient. To work successfully with a health care consultant, the office staff, the office manager, and the physician must be committed to the overall good of the office. Health care consultants are brought on board for advice on

- Starting a practice
- Closing a practice
- Expanding a practice
- Staff attrition
- Problems caused by decreased in patient loads
- Problems caused by recession and government changes that affect the office bottom line
- The problem of personnel turnover
- Investments and taxes

It is important to remember that the health care consultant is not the enemy, but rather a partner who is attempting to solve the practice's problems. A qualified consultant can tell the physician whether the office needs an insurance agent, a billing service, an investment advisor, or a lawyer. There are more than 500 medical practice management consulting firms in the United States. The best place to get a reference on a consultant is an office that used that consultant.

A number of consultants should be interviewed by both the office manager and the physician, so that the person who best fits the needs and vision of the practice is selected. When you are interviewing the consultant, note whether the consultant asks the appropriate questions and whether the consultant listens to answers that are given. Does the consultant act anxious to help or distracted? Ask about backup resources and about individual experience. Ask the consultant about her or his approach to the problems presented. Not all consultants take the same approach.

Most consultants will not charge you for the initial interview (which can take more than an hour), but be sure that fees are discussed before signing any contract. Beware of a consultant who comes in with a lower fee. You get what you pay for! Pick a consultant whose fee is in the same ballpark as the others. Make sure that the terms of the contract are clear to avoid problems later. By the end of the interview, a good consultant not only will have helped the physician and manager understand their objectives, but also will have a tentative plan for meeting them.

Consultants bill for their services in one of two ways: either by the hour or by the project. Once the practice's objectives have been identified, the consultant who bills by the hour states a time frame in which the objectives can be accomplished and quotes a fee for that time. Health care consultant fees range from $100 an hour to

$300 an hour. This rate includes time spent in the office, time spent in travel, time spent doing research, and time spent preparing reports for the practice. A 3-month project for a consultant to come into an office and evaluate it could cost as much as $10,000, depending on the types of services the consultant performs. Consultations regarding practice location and office layouts can be even higher in cost.

Consultants will try to disrupt the practice as little as possible, while continuing to become knowledgeable about all aspects of the practice. The office should be open to the suggestions for improvements that the consultant makes. You hired the consultant for her or his expertise, so use it! Smart consultants know their limitations; when they are faced with questions that require an expertise they don't have, they contact the appropriate person and obtain the answer. Generally, good consultants have a broad base of specialists in different areas of health care and business on whom they can call for information. Most consultants say that unless a practice is in very bad shape, they will increase practice income only by about 10% and will reduce costs by about 5%. Once the consultant's work is done, the practice must assess whether the goals decided on in the initial interview were met. Remember, by bringing on a practice consultant, the office is reflecting a innovative, progressive philosophy for strengthening the practice.

A Project List That Can Keep You on Target

On a normal day, office managers can find themselves working on as many as 10 different projects. What with the constant interruptions from both staff members and the physician, managers may find it difficult to keep track of the various projects on which they are working. A project list can help office managers stay on target in each project. This simple list specifies the project name, the starting date, the finishing date, and an area for comments regarding that project.

A sample of a blank project list is shown in Box 11–4. It can be photocopied and used as is, or it can be customized to fit the individual needs of any office. A sample of a project list in use is shown in Box 11–5. It shows that on August 1, 1993, the office manager began evaluating a way to reduce petty cash expenditures (Box 11–5). After a few days of working off and on to cut costs, the Reduction in Petty Cash Expenditures project

was completed on August 14, 1993. Some projects are more detailed and require a longer amount of time. The purpose of this list is simply to remind the office manager that certain projects are still on the table and must get some type of closure soon. Projects such as developing or revising the policy and procedure manual can take a long period of time. An office manager should not have open projects on this list for more than 3 months. Another reason for keeping an accurate project list is that it is useful at performance review time. You can present this list to the physician as an accurate account of your work for the year.

The Physician Demographics Sheet

The Physician Demographics Sheet comes in handy for many tasks. This sheet can be prepared by you or by any one of your staff who has access to the appropriate information. The Physician Demographic Sheet contains information necessary for recredentialing of the physician for either insurance companies or hospitals. A completed Physician Demographic Sheet contains the following items:

- Physician's name
- Physician's date of birth
- Physician's place of birth
- Physician's social security number
- Physician's medical license number
- Physician's Drug Enforcement Agency (DEA) registration number
- Physician's Continuing Medical Education information
- Name of the malpractice insurance company
- Office's address
- Office's hospital affiliations
- Physician's education
- Positions held by the physician
- Physician's tax ID number

The above items are the items generally requested on recredentialing forms. If a sheet containing this information is already in the office manager's file, an employee can simply copy the sheet and attach it to the form. Office managers and office staff not in the know have spent many hours completing recredentialing forms. By using this method, a recredentialing form can be completed in just minutes. The staff will still have to copy medical licenses, DEA registration, and malpractice face sheets to attach and mail along with form, however.

BOX 11–4. **BLANK OFFICE MANAGER'S PROJECT LIST**			
Project	Started	Finished	Comments

BOX 11–5. **OFFICE MANAGER'S PROJECT LIST**

Project	Started Finished	Comments
PETTY CASH	8/1/95 * * * * * * * * * 8/14/95	EXPLORING WAYS OF REDUCING PETTY CASH
TYPIST	8/4/95 * * * * * * * * * * *	INTERVIEWING FOR ADDITIONAL TYPIST
POLICY AND PROCEDURE MANUAL	8/10/95 * * * * * * * * * * *	REVISING CURRENT MANUAL
PHYSICIAN'S WEEKEND SCHEDULE	8/10/95 * * * * * * * * 8/10/95	REVISION OF SCHEDULE FOR MONTH OF SEPT.

Condolences

The office should have a policy as to how to handle the death of a patient. Condolences might be handled differently, depending on how long the patient was with the practice and how often the patient was seen. Some offices send flowers or cards. A few offices even attend the viewing and funeral. The most common way to express condolences is to send a condolence letter to the surviving spouse or family. This letter should be short but should offer support, sympathy, and caring at this difficult time. Families of the deceased appreciate that the office took the time to send a note of sympathy. This can be done by the office manager or by the typist at the direction of the office manager. Before typing the letter, check with the physician to see if there is a special note that she or he would like to include. If not, type the letter and place it on the physician's desk for a signature. Make sure that the letter offers the staff's condolences too!

Memo Writing Made Easy

It takes about an hour for most people to write a memo successfully. Many office managers do not have that kind of time. There are a few short steps that can ease the pain of memo writing forever. If you follow these steps, your memos will be polished and will produce results.

STEP 1: KNOW YOUR PURPOSE

The first step in memo writing is to determine what it is you want to accomplish. Decide what it is you want to say, and say it! Start by writing, "I'm writing to tell you that" and then continue with your thought. After you have finished, go back and delete the first six words. This should make an excellent start for your memo.

STEP 2: KEEP IT SHORT AND GET TO THE POINT

The second step in memo writing is to keep it short. Mystery novels may hold someone's attention, but a long memo won't. No one has the time or the desire to read long, rambling memos. State what you want to say as clearly and simply as possible. Don't belabor the point you are trying to make; ask for the action at the beginning of the memo. One way to make sure that you

are keeping it short is to imagine that you are sending a telegram and have to pay for every word! After finishing a part, go back and reread it; you might be able to delete even more. As Blaise Pascal said, *"I have only made this memo long because I have not had time to make it shorter!"*

STEP 3: AVOID CATCHY PHRASES

A memo is not the place to be flip or cute. Often, what comes across as witty wordplay to you while you're writing will just be bothersome to the people reading your message. Write the memo as if you were speaking in person to the persons receiving the memo. Your memo is a reflection of you, so be professional.

STEP 4: MAINTAIN A BACKLOG OF SUCCESSFUL MEMOS

Keep copies of other memos so that you can refer to them if necessary. You can often find the style you need by reading other people's memos. Also, keep any memos that you write that you think are excellent pieces of work. You can turn to them should you ever have a sudden case of writer's block.

STEP 6: PERSONALIZE THE MEMO

Everyone likes attention, and everyone likes to be remembered. If you are sending the same memo to more than one person, take a minute to jot a quick note on each one to personalize it for each recipient. The flattered person is the person who will be disposed to help you in the future if you need a favor.

STEP 7: MAKE IT EASY FOR THE RECIPIENTS TO GIVE FEEDBACK

Make it easy for everyone who receives your memo to respond to it by inviting the recipients to simply write their answer on your memo and send it back. This will save time and result in quicker responses.

Managing Desk Clutter

As discussed in Chapter 2, everyone has her or his own work style. Some say that desk clutter is a sign of a highly creative process going on. Others say that desk clutter does nothing but promote missed meetings, late reports, etc. and that "A neat desk is an organized mind." Organization is very important to a medical office manager. The lack of it can defeat even the best managerial skills. A good office manager makes it a practice to have on the desk only what is being worked on at the time. Once that project is finished, the file should be closed and put away. It is then time to move on to the next task. Edwin Bliss, author of *Getting Things Done: The ABC's of Time Management* states, "No matter how important all your projects may be, you can only concentrate on one at a time. Everything else is a distraction." A good habit to get into is to clear your desk before leaving the office at the end of the day. Delegate, dump, or do each project that was sitting there for the entire day. Having a cluttered desk constantly reenforces the fact that there are projects to be done but no time now to do them. The manager ends up playing mental shuffleboard, moving files around from spot to spot, always thinking about them. This is distracting from the current project.

Desk clutter can result in the following problems if not addressed immediately:

- Lost files and disks
- Errors and incomplete information
- Low morale
- Delays in completing work
- Confusion

The office manager is sometimes to blame for clutter in the office. Perhaps there is a need for additional closet space or shelving. This is not the fault of the employee. The office manager should be continually evaluating the needs of the office and should be addressing any storage needs that may arise. An office manager cannot expect an employee to keep an area neat if there is no room to store supplies and equipment.

Staff Meetings

"Diplomacy is the art of letting somebody else have your way."

—David Frost

The main objective of the medical office staff meeting is to instill a team spirit so that staff members will work together to create a more efficiently run office. Monthly meetings should be worked into the schedule and should not be cancelled for any reason. These meetings may or may not include the physician. Some medical offices have found that they get more accomplished when the physician is not present. Others say the opposite. It is

best to hold meetings both ways to see which works best for your office. Employees will not freely give up their own time for these meetings, so they must be scheduled during their working hours. It is best to block off an hour or so during a workday and have the answering service answer the telephone. Some offices hold meetings over lunch periods.

Problems with individual staff members should not be addressed in staff meetings; these should be discussed privately. If a meeting is held to discuss a change in policy, do not ask the staff for their approval; instead, explain the change firmly and ask staff members for input on how to make the new policy successful. Successful meetings mean exchanges of ideas. Be careful not to let go of control of the meeting, however, by being too open-minded. Always be positive about some aspect of the staff's work. Too many negatives cause low morale and reticent behavior.

MEETING PLANNING CHECKLIST

1 Before the meeting, decide the general purpose of the meeting and then the specific objectives of the meeting. Figure out clear, reasonable due dates for each task that will be assigned at the meeting.

2 Determine the degree of decision sharing and group autonomy. Is this a recommendation group or decision-making group?

3 Choose the type of meeting format: roundtable discussion, brainstorming, consultative, directive, non-directive, etc.

4 Choose who will participate.

5 Select those who might perform a task during the meeting, such as taking notes, chairing the meeting, etc.

6 Schedule the time, place, and duration of the meeting as appropriate to the task and purpose.

7 Determine how and when participants will be briefed as to their individual meeting responsibilities—by telephone, written notice, etc.

8 Determine any audiovisual aids that might be needed and make arrangements for them to be at the meeting place.

9 Develop an agenda and distribute it before the meeting if possible.

Keep this list available for all meetings and use it as a reference. A meeting action plan should be completed during every meeting, so that the office manager will know which task is to be completed by whom and when. A sample meeting action plan is shown in Box 11–6.

BOX 11–6. **MEETING ACTION PLAN**

Date: _____

Action to Be Taken	Person Responsible	Deadline
_____	_____	_____
_____	_____	_____
_____	_____	_____
_____	_____	_____
_____	_____	_____
_____	_____	_____

Key Issues

_____

_____

_____

_____

_____

_____

Recorder: _____

GETTING THEM THERE ON TIME

No one likes meetings that go on forever. This can be partially eliminated if everyone arrives on time. It is not fair to others if repeat offenders constantly breeze in 15 minutes after the meeting started. Be sure to post the date, time, and place of the office meeting to give everyone proper notice. Then there can be no excuses. You may find that sometimes scheduling a meeting at an odd time will help people remember it. In other words, a meeting that would normally be scheduled for 9:00 AM could be scheduled for 9:45 AM.

Another way to cure latecomers is to discuss important items first. Latecomers can also be motivated to be on time if items of their interest are scheduled for the beginning of the meeting. If you issue an agenda a few days before the meeting, staff members can see what is to be discussed and when. It can also be helpful to involve staff members in the meeting. Perhaps they can report on new coding ideas or new ideas for appointment scheduling. This does wonders for office morale, can be a pleasant learning experience for everyone, and creates the desire to be on time where once there was none.

If none of the above ideas seem to work on chronic latecomers, take them aside and discuss the problem privately. Emphasize that it is not only that they are habitually late, but that their input is important to the group and very much needed.

THE MAKING OF EFFECTIVE STAFF MEETINGS

It is important to start the meeting at the designated time, even if all members of the staff are not present. Starting the meeting on time conveys the seriousness and formality of the meeting. Always close the door when starting the meeting. This reenforces the meeting's importance and indicates that any intrusion after this point is disruptive. As mentioned, use a format whereby the most important information is covered first.

After a while, regularly scheduled office staff meetings can become unproductive, because they are routine to the staff. At this point, meetings should not discuss work in progress. Instead, have each staff member hand in a written update of the project or task on which she or he is currently working, and focus the meeting on issues such as marketing, patient satisfaction, and teamwork.

An effective manager holds staff meetings at odd times, as already mentioned, and just before lunch (Figure 11–2). Holding the meeting just before lunch ensures that staff will stick to the matters at hand. In addition, think about your office's appointment schedule before scheduling a meeting. At US Healthcare, the president issued a policy that no staff meetings of three or more could be held between 9:00 AM and 4:00 PM, because this was their busiest time. It made no sense to have staff meetings to discuss better customer relations when the customers needed the staff at that time.

Keep the topics confined, because broad topics can cause the group to lose focus. If the office is large enough to have department heads, meetings with department heads should be scheduled before meetings with the rest of staff. When writing the agenda, be sure to be specific. For instance,

The wrong type of agenda listing:

III) Marketing Strategies

The right type of agenda listing:

III) New Marketing Strategy: Patient Information Booklets

A specific agenda helps the meeting stay on course and keeps the staff members focused. As mentioned, give the staff members the agenda before the meeting, so that they might prepare statements and opinions. In addition, always issue follow-up notes after the meeting that outline what was discussed, what was decided, and how it is to be handled. This way, all staff members are clear as to the role they play in completing this task. When something is written in black and white, it is less easy for employees to say they misunderstood.

An effective meeting leader is like a talk show host. Try to get each member's input without jeopardizing the focus. To do this, simply word questions specifically instead of generally. In other words, ask, "Ann, how does this change in data entry affect your position?" instead of "Ann, what do you think?" A specific question requires a specific answer, and the meeting is kept under control. When people get off track, gently but firmly pull them back on track by stating "That's very interesting, but how does that relate to our issue?" They will see that they were a bit off the subject and will apologize, allowing the meeting to move on.

It is a good idea to allow time at the end of the meeting for "Potpourri." This is generally a 15-minute session in which any staff member can bring up a topic for discussion, with the understanding that it must be brief. If the topic is too long, discussion of it can be finished in the office manager's office after the meeting.

Visual aids always help get a point across. The office manager can use a variety of items: flip charts, slides, or handouts. Slides should be used for large groups, and flip charts and handouts for smaller groups. The important thing to remember is if they see it, they retain it.

The Patient's Bill of Rights

The American Hospital Association (AHA) published the "Patient's Bill of Rights" in 1973. This AHA wrote the Patient's Bill of Rights to provide more effective care and greater satisfaction for the patient, physician,

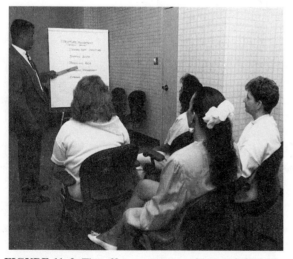

FIGURE 11–2. The office manager conducts an informative staff meeting.

and hospital. The office manager might want to copy this document and place it in the waiting room for patients to either read in the office or pick up and take home. At the hospital, the Patient's Bill of Rights is generally given to the patient at admission. The physician–patient relationship takes on new dimensions when the patient is in the hospital setting. Not only is the physician responsible for the patient, but the hospital as an institution also accepts responsibility for the patient. The patient's rights should be supported by both the hospital and the physician; they are an integral part of the patient's recovery. Because this document has been prepared by professionals rather than consumers, it would probably be admissible as evidence in a case where the rights of the patient are concerned. Box 11–7 presents the AHA's Patient's Bill of Rights. The office manager might want to develop a particular Patient's Bill of Rights for the medical office. This can be included in the *Patient Information Handbook* or can be made into a pamphlet and placed in the waiting room for patients to pick up. A sample Patient Bill of Rights for a medical office is shown in Box 11–8.

Practice Mergers

Many have predicted that there will be a merging of medical practices across the United States in response to the current climate in the health care field of government regulation and decreased reimbursement. Some believe that the market will force all physicians to join some type of group practice and the days of the solo practitioner will be gone. Regardless of the external forces being applied to the medical practice, there are some definite advantages to practice mergers:

- Centralized billing
- More efficient bill collection
- Group purchase discounts
- Overhead economies of scale
- Better quality total management
- Practice transition

To get to these advantages, however, some storms must be weathered. One of the major problems that occurs when two practices merge is that the wrong practices merge. It is best to determine compatibility before taking this big step. It is like a marriage; the only difference is that it involves more personalities, which makes it even worse! There are three major areas to assess before a merger should take place: finances, employees, and fee schedules.

FINANCES

The finances of the two practices should be assessed and compared. Each practice's history of collections, accounts receivable, adjustments, and productivity should be included in this assessment. Information should be obtained from the accountant regarding liabilities. The office managers can share information such as overhead and billing turnaround times. Discussion of issues such as Medicare participation and managed care participation is essential. Retirement plans, employee medical insurance plans, and profit sharing also need to be addressed. The office manager should work closely with the physician, the accountant, the lawyer, and the other practice's counterparts. It is in the office manager's best interests to cooperate completely during this discovery period.

EMPLOYEES

Employees and their salaries must be considered. If the merger takes place, there will be duplication of many positions among the practices. The salary structures should be analyzed along with the benefits package that each office offers. Developing new policies and salaries can be difficult, but consensus must be worked out before any merger takes place. Consideration should be given to valuable staff and staff who have been employed for many years. Of course, each practice wants to keep its employees, so this can be a very difficult aspect of the merger. Often, the employees who are retained are those who are the most cost-effective to retain. As an office manager, the best position to take is to be pleasant and as helpful as possible and have a positive outlook about the merger process. This will be of great benefit.

FEE SCHEDULES

The fee schedules and coding, both procedural and diagnostic, of both practices should be considered and compared. The newly formed practice will need a uniform fee schedule. The office manager might want to suggest to the physicians that a management consultant be brought in to review both offices' fee schedules and advise. Existing computer systems and billing systems need to be evaluated by either the office manager or a management consultant. The two offices' coding practices should be studied and a single list of codes created.

BOX 11–7. THE AMERICAN HOSPITAL ASSOCIATION'S PATIENT'S BILL OF RIGHTS

1 The patient has the right to considerate and respectful care.

2 The patient has the right to obtain from his [sic] physician complete current information concerning his diagnosis, treatment, and prognosis in terms the patient can be reasonably expected to understand. When it is not medically advisable to give such information to the patient, the information should be made available to an appropriate person in his behalf. He has the right to know, by name, the physician responsible for coordinating his care.

3 The patient has the right to receive from his physician information necessary to give informed consent prior to the start of any procedure and/or treatment. Except in emergencies, such information for informed consent should include but not necessarily be limited to the specific procedure and/or treatment, the medically significant risks involved, and the probable duration of incapacitation. Where medically significant alternatives for care or treatment exist, or when the patient requests information concerning medical alternatives, the patient has the right to such information. The patient also has the right to know the name of the person responsible for the procedures and/or treatment.

4 The patient has the right to refuse treatment to the extent permitted by law, and to be informed of the medical consequences of his action.

5 The patient has the right to every consideration of his privacy concerning his own medical care program. Case discussion, consultation, examination, and treatment are confidential and should be conducted discreetly. Those not directly involved in his care must have the permission of the patient to be present.

6 The patient has the right to expect that all communications and records pertaining to his care should be treated as confidential.

7 The patient has the right to expect that within its capacity a hospital must make reasonable response to the request of a patient for services. The hospital must provide evaluation, service, and/or referral as indicated by the urgency of the case. When medically permissible, a patient may be transferred to another facility only after he has received complete information and explanation concerning the needs for, and alternatives to, such a transfer. The institution to which the patient is to be transferred must first have accepted the patient for transfer.

8 The patient has the right to obtain information as to any relationship of his hospital to other health care and educational institutions insofar as his care is concerned. The patient has the right to obtain information as to the existence of any professional relationships among individuals, by name, who are treating him.

9 The patient has the right to be advised if the hospital proposes to engage in or perform human experimentation affecting his care or treatment. The patient has the right to refuse to participate in such research projects.

10 The patient has the right to expect reasonable continuity of care. He has the right to know in advance what appointment times and physicians are available and where. The patient has the right to expect that the hospital will provide a mechanism whereby he is informed by his physician or a delegate of the physician of the patient's continuing healthcare requirements following discharge.

11 The patient has the right to examine and receive an explanation of his bill regardless of source of payment.

12 The patient has the right to know what hospital rules and regulations apply to his conduct as patient.

(Courtesy of the American Hospital Association.)

TIME FOR THE ATTORNEY

Once fee schedules, employees, and finances have been carefully examined and decisions have been made, it is time to contact an attorney to handle other issues: corporate structure, assets, management, compensation, and buyouts. These are not a part of the office manager's duties and can be quickly passed off to the practice attorney. There are no easy mergers, but the most important factor is the compatibility of the physicians. If they are not happy, no one else will be!

Snap Decisions: Harmful or Helpful?

A good manager is a good decision maker. Decisiveness inspires support, intimidates the opposition, and gives you control. Sometimes a not so great decision made quickly is better than a good decision made slowly. Movement in any direction brings a new perspective to any situation, making the right decision more apparent. There's something to be said for people who care enough to always do their best; however, nine times out of ten, an adequate decision made in a timely fashion is worth a lot more than an agonized but late perfect choice. The following decision-making guidelines can help you be more decisive:

- Know that you might blow it.
- Calculate the risks.
- Know that you can change your mind.
- Refuse to decide.
- Don't get hung up on fact finding.
- Know when to proceed with caution.

- Break out of your usual thought patterns.
- Search for a solution.
- Respect hunches and gut feelings.
- Ask an expert.

The National Practitioner Data Bank

The National Practitioner Data Bank was started in 1990 by the Health Resources and Services Administration. The purpose of this data bank is to store adverse information regarding physicians. Malpractice insurers, hospitals, and state licensing boards began sending information about physicians and dentists, mostly reports of malpractice insurance payouts, adverse information that was uncovered during credentialing, and licensure decisions. The organizations allowed to query the data bank are hospitals, medical societies, licensing boards, and certain health maintenance organizations.

There is some concern regarding the confidentiality of the information stored in the National Practitioner Data Bank. Most feel that this bank comes with many problems, such as erroneous accusations and mix-ups with records. It is best to advise the physician to check

---

BOX 11–8. ONE PRACTICE'S PATIENT'S BILL OF RIGHTS

In our years of practice, we have often heard patients complain about doctors. We have tried to live by certain principles. We have decided to write them down for you.

A patient has the right to know what his or her illness is and what trouble it is likely to cause.

A patient has the right to have the illness explained in ordinary English, not medical terms.

A patient has the right to know the treatment options, the advantages and disadvantages of each, and what each will cost.

A patient has the right to know the doctor's qualifications and experience.

A patient has the right to consult other doctors without me being insulted or angry that the patient wants another opinion.

A patient has the right to understand my fees.

I have also tried to live by these standards:

I will spend a patient's money as wisely as if I were spending my own. I will look for and recommend the least expensive way of solving my patient's problems.

I will not recommend surgery unless the patient needs help that only surgery can provide.

If a patient feels I have not provided him or her with my best efforts, I will refund the money he or she paid me—no questions asked. I can't guarantee results of treatment, but I can guarantee you my best efforts to treat you honestly and fairly.

periodically on the status of her or his record. The physician is supposed to be notified if someone deposits data on her or him, but the physician is not notified of withdrawals of information. To find out who has been looking at the physician's file, the office must fill out a form available from the bank. Photocopies are not accepted. The address of this bank is

National Practitioner Data Bank
P.O. Box 6048
Camarillo, CA 93011-6048

Hospitals often tap the bank when credentialing new physicians for admittance to the staff of their hospital. This practice is beneficial to the hospital and its staff members. This bank was designed because of the public's concern about physicians who were guilty of poor medical practice and were relocating to another state to continue these same poor medical practices. The following is the information that goes into the bank on each physician:

- Name and address
- Work address
- Social security number
- Date of birth
- Name of each professional school attended
- Each professional license number and state
- DEA number
- Names and addresses of hospitals of affiliation

In reference to malpractice cases, the following additional information is stored:

- Site where claim has been filed and the case number
- Date and description of the acts or omissions that gave rise to the claim
- Date and description of the case and the amount of the judgment

In reference to sanctions by licensing boards and peer review bodies, this additional information is stored:

- Description of the acts, omissions, and other reasons for the board's actions or limitation of clinical privileges
- Description of the sanction, the date it was imposed, and the date it went into effect

The Physician's CV— That First Impression

Many physicians don't realize the importance of the professional look of a CV. CV, of course, standing for *curriculum vitae,* which is Latin for "a short account of one's career and qualifications prepared typically by an applicant for a position." Obviously, physicians use their CV when they are on a job search, but a physician's CV is also used for other purposes:

- When the physician has been invited to lecture (for example, by a drug company), the sponsoring party will circulate her or his CV as a form of advertisement.
- Hospital medical staff offices make the physician's CV a part of her or his file.
- Law firms using the physician as an expert witness request a copy of the physician's CV.

The physician should be made to realize the importance of this document; after all, it is her or his autobiography. You can help the physician prepare her or his CV. Be sure that the heading is clear and specifies the physician's name, address, and phone number. The CV should be outlined in both logical and chronological order. The standard form for the CV is as follows:

- Heading
- Education
- Postgraduate education
- Certification
- License
- Experience
- Honors
- Publications

Remind the physician not to leave gaps in the CV. If she or he spent a year traveling around Europe, this trip should be listed. Such gaps can also be listed as "sabbatical" or "personal leave."

Print the CV on a laser printer or ink-jet printer, as opposed to a dot matrix printer. The quality produced by a dot matrix printer is unacceptable for a CV. Try to avoid a typewriter also. If the office does not have a laser or ink-jet printer, have the CV printed at a local print shop; it isn't very expensive, and the finished product is excellent. Remember, this is the first impression of the physician—make it good!

The Beeper: Friend or Foe?

Most physicians think their beeper is more a nuisance than an asset. To make the physician's life more bearable, consider some of the following factors before purchasing a beeper:

- Always get the smallest beeper possible. Believe it or not, beepers can get heavy and tug on clothing.

The physician will appreciate your thoughtfulness.

- Purchase a beeper that not only beeps, but vibrates. This is especially helpful to physicians when they are attending or giving a lecture, reading a bedtime story to their youngest, or intently listening to an irregular heartbeat.
- Purchase a beeper that stores messages. This is especially helpful when the physician is in surgery or in transit between the office and the hospital. Although most physicians now have car phones, many prefer to answer routine messages when they arrive at their destination.
- Don't give the beeper number to anyone unless the physician instructs you to.
- It's a good idea to be nice to the answering service. This is very important, because they will happily hold messages and will learn how to triage your calls.
- Advise the physician to obtain a cellular phone. This can save a hassle if indeed the physician is beeped for an emergency. The cellular phone eliminates the necessity of finding a pay phone while in transit.
- Education of the patient is most important when attempting to make a beeper system work for you. This can be done through the *Patient Information Handbook*. In the handbook, you should explain the office's policy regarding patients' routine questions about their conditions and their medications.

Lost in Translation

The United States has long been a melting pot for people of Hispanic, Slavic, Asian, Indian, Anglo-Saxon, and many other lineages. Medicine is currently grappling with a surge of patients who don't speak English. Many barriers inhibit communication between patients and physicians, but none is more serious than the inability to speak English. Health care workers often find themselves in the waiting room asking for the friends or family of a patient to serve as an interpreter. Many hospitals have hired telephone interpreters or bilingual staff members in an effort to provide the best quality of care for all patients, even those who do not speak English. Having a translator who is not well versed in the language of medicine comes with its own set of problems. One must worry about explanations getting lost in translation. The best solution, of course, is to use trained medical interpreters. These, however, are few and far between. They can be borrowed from hospitals and clinics as the need arises.

AT&T has a Language Line service covering more than 140 languages. They can also be called on in an emergency. The number for this service is 1-800-628-8486, and the cost of a call is approximately $3.50/minute. This 24-hour line can be charged on a credit card and partially covered by both Medicare and Medicaid, when the amount is reasonable and the care is necessary. Bell Telephone has special telephone services for people with either a hearing or speech disability. The customer service guide at the beginning of the telephone book explains all the details necessary for offices in need of these services.

Even with the help of a good interpreter, treatment of non-English-speaking patients can be tricky. Always speak directly to the patient, as if there were no interpreter in the room. This will help to establish a bond with the patient. Allow the interpreter to get the patient's whole story and *then* relate it to office personnel and the physician. Sentence-to-sentence translation becomes difficult in a medical setting. After the physician and the office personnel have given instructions to the patient, have the translator ask the patient to repeat them. This will help to avoid any misunderstandings. Any time information is conveyed through another, there is a greater chance the information will be distorted, diluted, or completely erroneous. Remember the childhood game "Whisper Down The Lane"? The first child whispered a phrase to another child, who whispered it to another, and so on down the line. By the time the last child heard the phrase, it had become distorted. What started out as "I'm going to the movies after school" had become "I'm quitting school to be a movie star!"

The translator can also help the medical office understand a patient's culture. For example, a patient who stares at the floor during the entire conversation with the physician might give the physician the impression that she or he is depressed or disinterested, when actually the person is showing respect. Some cultures don't believe in germ-based illnesses; they believe that illness is caused by evil spirits, so an immunization shot that may cause a healthy child to become sick for a day doesn't make sense to them. Patience and understanding are the best tools to work with at times like this. No one said it would be easy meshing American-style medicine with various cultures, but it is rewarding.

Many agencies are available to help the office communicate with deaf patients also, who are legally entitled to a certified interpreter through the Americans with

Disabilities Act of 1990. Schools for the deaf and agencies for the deaf can be of assistance in this situation.

Purchasing Power: Buying Equipment, Furniture, and Office Supplies

CONTROL OF COSTS

"You do not need an MBA from Harvard to figure out how to lose money."

—Robert Little, Chair, Textron

Medical office managers should realize that one very important function on their list of many is to control costs in the office. Some practices are charged for the amounts of electricity and water they use in their particular office space. Even if the office does not pay separately for these utilities, unwise use can increase these bills for the owner of the building, which will eventually be passed on to the office in the form of an increase in rent. Regardless of how the bills are divided, the office should be frugal about utilities.

Everyone should cut costs, because "costs" cost money! The office manager can cut costs by not spending large amounts of money on office decor and on equipment containing "bells and whistles" that might not be necessary. The medical office manager should make employees aware of the costs associated with the running of a medical practice and ask for their help in being as cost conscious as possible. The office manager can institute a few policies that will immediately save on office expense:

- Purchase less expensive supplies by either buying off brands or shopping around for a better price.
- Purchase stock when it is on sale. For instance, if computer paper is on sale this week at a very good price, purchase a few boxes and store for future consumption.
- Assess the staff to evaluate the need for the number of employees working there. Perhaps two tasks could be combined into one, which would reduce the payroll by one employee. However, NEVER stress the employees to the point of breakdown in order to save money on payroll.
- Turn off utilities when not in use. When you are not using an exam room, keep the lights and equipment in there off and close the door to that room.
- Check expiration dates on vaccines and injectables.

Many companies will give you credit upon return and reorder.

- Maintain proper maintenance and cleaning of equipment—it will last longer.
- Cross-train employees so that you have flexibility when needed.
- Monitor inventory to prevent the need to pay for rushed delivery, shipments sent through Federal Express, or supplies that can be purchased quickly through local suppliers but at higher costs.
- Consider installing a computer as an alternative to increasing staff.
- Use part-time employees whenever possible to decrease payroll taxes and the costs of employee benefits.
- Know the cost of seeing a patient in the office and then do not participate in managed care programs that pay less than your costs.
- Look into employee benefits that are tax free.
- Terminate mediocre employees—the cost of nonproductive employees outweighs the cost of hiring and training a new employee.
- Decrease state unemployment taxes by reducing employee turnover.
- Pay income tax estimates on time.
- Avoid paying penalties for errors by knowing the Occupational Safety and Health Administration regulations, the *Current Procedural Terminology* and *International Classification of Diseases, Ninth Revision* codes, and the requirements of the Clinical Laboratory Improvements Amendments of 1988.
- Evaluate the necessity of having service contracts on equipment.
- Evaluate leasing versus purchasing equipment.
- Minimize the need for a collection agency by planning and implementing a collection system at the time of service.
- If the help of a collection agency is needed, shop around for one whose rates are acceptable.
- Submit insurance claims electronically to eliminate the cost of postage and employee time spent on billing.
- Computerize patient appointment scheduling to save staff's and the physician's time.
- Hire a competent accountant to help with budgeting, forecasting, and tax planning strategies.
- Choose a bank with competitive rates and good business packages.
- Hire an attorney for the practice to read over all contracts and agreements.

BOX 11–9. **COST OF SUPPLIES BY MEDICAL SPECIALTY (COURTESY OF MEDICAL ECONOMICS.)**

Specialty	Percentage of gross spent for:		
	Clinical Supplies	Business Supplies	Total
Allergy	5.3%	2.8%	8.1%
Cardiology	0.9%	1.1%	2.0%
Cardiovascular surgery	0.7%	0.2%	0.9%
Dermatology	3.6%	2.3%	5.9%
Emergency medicine	0.5%	0.3%	0.8%
Family practice	5.7%	2.3%	8.0%
Gastroenterology	1.5%	1.6%	3.1%
General surgery	1.4%	1.3%	2.7%
Internal medicine	3.2%	1.9%	5.1%
Neurology	1.1%	1.7%	2.8%
Neurosurgery	0.6%	1.5%	2.1%
Obstetrics/gynecology	2.4%	1.6%	4.0%
Oncology/hematology	10.6%	1.5%	12.1%
Ophthalmology (dispensing)	9.3%	1.7%	11.0%
Ophthalmology (nondispensing)	5.7%	2.4%	8.1%
Orthopedic surgery	2.9%	1.6%	4.5%
Otolaryngology	2.3%	1.9%	4.2%
Pediatrics	8.5%	2.6%	11.1%
Plastic surgery	3.2%	1.9%	5.1%
Psychiatry	0.1%	1.7%	1.8%
Radiology	0.7%	1.0%	1.7%
Urology	6.7%	1.6%	8.3%

As Box 11–9 shows, the percentage of its gross income a practice spends for medical supplies varies widely depending on specialty. The mean percentage for office supplies is 1.65%, a figure that varies only slightly from specialty to specialty.

BARGAIN SHOPPING FOR EQUIPMENT AND SUPPLIES

Medical offices spend an average of 6% of their gross income on medical and office supplies. Depending on the type of specialty, it could be higher. The office manager should be bargain shopping whenever possible for best prices and discounts. There is much competition now, and many companies will negotiate prices with medical offices in order to be promised the account. Even desks and filing cabinets can be purchased inexpensively if they have a small dent or scratch. It is possible to negotiate deals in which the office can get as much as 50% off by buying equipment that is slightly dented or scratched.

You can also check with local medical suppliers to see if they have any used equipment for sale. If the practice is new, you and the physician might want to consider purchasing used equipment until the practice becomes profitable. The used equipment can then slowly be replaced with new equipment. Many young, new physicians today want to open an office with all new equipment. Try to dissuade them of this, explaining that it would be easier to start out with used equipment and replace it as the practice becomes secure. Most new physicians are paying off multiple student loans and will appreciate the advice of a competent, seasoned office manager.

When you are looking for used equipment, it might be advantageous to check the county medical journals or local medical papers. Check journals for classified ads placed by physicians who are retiring or redecorating their offices and wish to sell their office furniture. In the yellow pages in the telephone book, under Used Business Furniture, you might be able to find office equipment that you need. Avoid purchasing used furniture for the waiting room, however; this gives patients one of their earliest impressions of the medical office, and it should be clean, neat, and pleasant looking.

LEASING VERSUS BUYING

Most businesses today have the choice of either leasing or purchasing equipment. Each option has distinct advantages and disadvantages. Leasing helps keep expenses down and can be used as a tax benefit also. Leasing is popular with oncologists, ophthalmologists, and radiologists, because their technology changes so rapidly and is so expensive. The photocopier is always a popular item for leasing, because it gets so much use that the office will want to replace it every few years, rather than have costly repair bills and down time.

FROM THE AUTHOR'S NOTEBOOK

If you plan on using a piece of equipment until it falls apart, buy it. Buying is cheaper than leasing because you can deduct the depreciation.

If the office is preparing to purchase rather than lease, keep in mind the tax consequences of paying cash for the item. Leasing conserves office cash, and the interest paid on the lease offsets the taxable earnings. Medical equipment purchases are 100% depreciable over 5 years; office furniture can be fully written off over 7 years. The office is unable to depreciate equipment that is leased.

Leasing can be the most convenient way to obtain equipment, but it is not the cheapest way. If the office is having cash flow problems, leasing may be the only choice for obtaining the equipment needed.

MANAGER'S ALERT

Watch out for leases that state you have the option to buy. The IRS may take the position that you're buying the equipment, not leasing it.

It is always a good idea to have the practice lawyer read over all leases before signing them. Most physicians don't realize that personal liability is written into some leasing contracts. This is something that should be avoided if at all possible. The office manager must look for certain aspects of the lease to prevent problems with the IRS. There is a gray area between a lease and a purchase loan. To prevent any problems along this line, look for the following aspects:

1 The leasing company must own at least 20% of the equity of the property during the term of the lease. If that is not the case, the IRS could consider the deal a purchase.
2 The leasing company must show that it is making a profit, independent of its own tax benefits.
3 At the end of the lease, the office cannot purchase the equipment at less than fair market value (bargain purchase option).
4 It must be commercially feasible for someone else to use the equipment at the end of the lease.

COPIERS

Choosing the Correct Copier

When you are shopping for a copier, you are shopping for more than just the copier itself. The service and actual down time are very important factors to consider. For instance, if it is going to take the service technician 24 hours to get to the office to do a repair, you might want to consider a different brand of copier or a different dealership. An average time period for a technician to get to the office for a service call is 4 hours. Many dealers offer an even shorter time frame. The copier purchased should also have a generous warranty with it. Many companies are now offering generous warranties, enhanced service, and performance promises with every copier.

The competition is great, so shop around and have an understanding of how the copier works before purchasing. Make a list of the features that your office will need. The following are features available:

- Collator
- Sheet feeder
- Enlarge/reduce
- Automatic contrast
- Multiple paper trays
- Two-sided copying
- Sorter
- Zoom
- Shifting

- Dual-page copying
- Edge erase
- Single-color copying

The following are well-known companies who produce office copiers:

Canon
Fuji Photo Film USA
Lanier Worldwide, Inc.
Mita Copystar America
Panasonic Communications
Ricoh Corporation
Xerox Corporation
Toshiba America
Eastman Kodak
Konica Business Machines
Minolta Corporation
Monroe Systems for Business
Pitney Bowes Company
Sanyo Business Systems
Standard Duplicating Machines
Sharp Electronics Corporation

Guidelines to Help You Get the Most from Your Copier

There are some basic rules to follow to ensure that you get the most from the copier you choose.

- Avoid placing the copier in direct sunlight or by a heating vent.
- Keep the copier out of drafts and make sure there is adequate circulation around it.
- Be careful when trying to save money by buying off brand toners, copy cartridges, drum cartridges, etc. These off brands may damage the copier, and the repairs will cost more than you saved by buying an off brand. One recommendation is that the generic toner from Quill Office Products is generally cheaper than other toners and works well in most machines.
- Use high-quality paper and 20-pound bond.
- Make sure that paper remains dust free. Any paper dust can clog sensors and foul the mechanical parts.
- Keep the glass of the copier clean. This can be done easily with a glass cleaner or alcohol. This will help keep the quality of your copies high.
- Watch what you have near the copier; it doesn't digest foreign objects well! Many is the time the technician has been called to the office for a "repair," only to extract a paperclip, a leaf from a

plant, a staple, a pencil, a push pin, or a scrap of paper from inside the copier. Never, ever, leave a coffee cup or soda sitting on a copy machine. It can easily be knocked over; when liquid gets into the copier, it can cause major damage.

- Paper will curl in excessive heat. This can cause paper jams.
- Clear the exit tray regularly to avoid copy backups that will eventually cause a jam.
- When the paper is full of electricity and sticking together, spray the entire ream lightly with hairspray or static-removing spray.
- The toner should be stored in a cool, dry place; otherwise, it will harden and form clumps. Gently shake the toner before installing it in the copier to remove clumping and clinging to the inside of the cartridge.

Copy Bandits

The need to control the use of the photocopier is essential in a medical office. It is the second most widely abused equipment in a medical office, the first, of course, being the telephone. It has been estimated that 20% of all copies made in an office are copies for personal use by the staff or physicians. Some of these copies are made just in case they are needed at a later date. This practice costs the medical practice in paper, toner, and wear and tear on the copy machine. Some companies sell copy "controllers" that monitor the number of copies produced, with the goal of controlling costs. The controllers are tied into a computer system that reads from them how many copies were made and by whom. Coin-operated copiers can also be purchased; however, these are the type that are seen in the local libraries and post offices—not very sophisticated. One of the easiest ways to keep copy costs down is to make employees aware of the costs of the copier. If they are aware that management is monitoring the copies, they will tend to make fewer personal copies.

Paper for the Copier

The type of paper used in the copier can enhance the copies made. By buying quality paper, you will ensure that your copies come out clear and clean (Figure 11–3). In addition, keep all copy paper dry. This means not on a concrete floor in a basement. All paper should be stored on a shelf in a dry room.

FROM THE AUTHOR'S NOTEBOOK

Fan a ream of copy paper before inserting it into the copier tray. This will help eliminate jams and misfeeds.

THE FAX PHENOMENON

Fax machines are the latest office technology. Many thought at first that there was no need for a fax machine in a medical office. This soon proved wrong. The fax machine has many uses in today's medical office. If the practice has more than one location, it can be extremely helpful to fax patients' records and test results between offices. Hospitals get into the act by faxing test results and information to the office when the office cannot wait for the regular mail and when the contents of the document are too complicated to explain over the telephone. Fax machines also make communication between the medical office and law offices and accountants' offices more convenient. Once there is a fax machine in place, all of the employees in the office will wonder what they did without it!

A basic fax machine is very affordable now and can provide excellent service. A physician's office does not need a fancy machine; a basic fax is more than sufficient

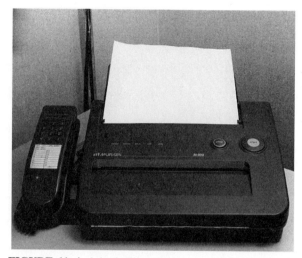

FIGURE 11–4. A basic fax machine is generally all that is necessary for a medical practice.

(Figure 11–4). Some fax machines are more expensive than others because they offer features such as paper cutters, plain-paper usage, auto send/receive functions, programmable keys, and speed dialing. Some fax machines even offer additional memory to allow document storage and mailboxes for certain employees. Within the last few years, plain-paper fax machines have replaced thermal-paper ones in many offices, and color will soon be possible. In 1992, modems with computer links were introduced into the fax market, and these have opened up more new markets and applications.

The fax machine is now definitely a must for a medical office. It has become as important as the photo-copier! It is good practice to use a cover sheet when faxing to ensure that the fax is routed to the proper individual. A sample fax cover sheet is illustrated in Box 11–10.

THE SECURITY OF A PAPER SHREDDER

The Environmental Protection Agency has estimated that the typical employee throws away a staggering 1/2 pound of paper every day. This has created a new industry—the manufacturing of paper shredders. The paper shredder in a medical office cannot save the amount of paper waste, but for many office managers, it's a good place to start. Every business has records that shouldn't be seen by others, and a medical office is no different. Old payroll records, old telephone logs, old cancelled checks, and old meeting minutes can be easily disposed of with a paper shredder. With the confidentiality issue so important, a paper shredder could be a

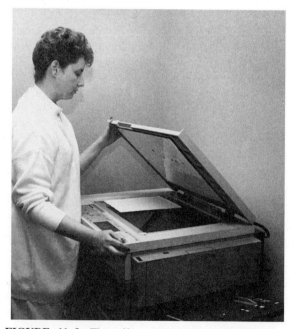

FIGURE 11–3. The office photocopier should be user-friendly and dependable.

valuable asset to a medical office. Shredders come in a wide range of styles, prices, and capacities. There are personal-size shredders and large, centralized shredders. All can do the same job, but some fit the needs of the office more than others. With the paper shredder manufacturing growing at 10% per year, the office manager can find the shredder that is right for the office. When purchasing a paper shredder, be careful to check the warranty. Be sure that it includes the cutters and labor. Check to see what other parts are covered by the warranty.

THE SECURITY SYSTEM—A MUST!

General Considerations

Every medical office needs a security system. It has been proven that burglars break into offices without alarms five times more often than they break into those with alarms.

Many factors must be considered when choosing a security system. One important thing to realize is that no security system is a substitute for a strong door with a deadbolt lock. When you are shopping for a burglar alarm, have the representative come to check over the office. Have her or him check the windows and doors for danger signs such as weak hinges, old wooden frames, etc. Some police departments will do such an inspection at no cost to the office. Some alarm systems are fairly easy to install; however, before getting the physician to do the deed, check on what it would cost to have someone in the business install it for you. Installing a security alarm requires a certain amount of wiring and electronic knowledge.

MANAGER'S ALERT

Remember, although alarm systems deter some burglars, no security company can give you a 100% guarantee that your office will be completely protected against a professional or determined burglar.

BOX 11–10. **FAX COVER SHEET**

DATE: _____

FACSIMILE TRANSMISSION COVER SHEET

TO NAME: _____

LOCATION: _____

PHONE NUMBER: _____

FAX MACHINE NUMBER: _____

FROM NAME: _____

LOCATION: _____

PHONE NUMBER: _____

FAX MACHINE NUMBER: _____

NUMBER OF PAGES: _____ (INCLUDING THIS COVER SHEET)

SPECIAL INSTRUCTIONS: _____

_____

_____

To ensure good security coverage, use both perimeter and area alarms. The area alarm is the backup to the perimeter alarm; it scares the burglar out of the office.

Components of the Alarm System

There are three basic components of the alarm system: sensors and detectors, master controls, and alarm devices.

Sensors and Detectors. Perimeter protection is the first line of defense against a burglar. Perimeter sensors sense the intrusion on the property before the burglar is able to get inside. These can be found in the form of a door sensor, which sounds an alarm if the intruder attempts to open the door, or a window sensor, which sounds an alarm if the intruder attempts to break a window. Area protection is a scanner that scans a specific area, usually with a beam. When the beam is broken, an alarm sounds. This can sometimes be enough to scare away an intended burglar. It is best to install both perimeter and area protection alarms for complete coverage.

One of the most common types of perimeter sensors is a magnetic switch. This is the sensor that is placed on doors, windows, or any other moveable area. This type of sensor will not deter experienced intruders. They simply break the window and put a magnet next to the switch, which simulates that the area is closed. Also, an experienced intruder can cut the glass so as not to trip the switch and climb through the window without disturbing the magnetic switch. To prevent entry of the premises through broken glass, you can use a metal foil or audio sensor.

Area sensors are usually more sophisticated and more commonly chosen as the sensor of choice. Area sensors can be ultrasound, microwave, infrared, floor mat switches, and photoelectric beams. As you can see, protection systems can become elaborate or can be kept simple.

Master Control. The master control is the part of the system that reads the information from the sensors and decides what action to take. This control is programmed by the owner and makes decisions according to what it has been told to do. The master control comes with a variety of features: lockup relay, set switches, automatic shutoff, and delay entry/exit circuits. The individual vendors of systems can explain in detail the features of each type of alarm system.

Alarm Devices. The last part of the alarm system is the actual alarm itself. There are sirens, bells, whistles, and flashing lights. Depending on the vicinity of the office, the physician might want to choose one type over another. The police will most probably suggest that a light be left outside of the office if the office is in a single-structure building. Alarm systems can also be connected to automatic telephone dialers that will call either a switchboard or the local police station. Self-installed alarm systems can be purchased and installed for between $150 and $2,000, depending on the type of system chosen. Professionally installed systems can cost between $500 and $3,000 for full office coverage, both outside and inside. If a system is chosen that involves a security company, be advised that they will charge you an additional $25 per month, on average, for their services. Alarm company decals are also a very popular item today. Many people purchase the decal for the window, without purchasing the actual alarm system. This does deter more inexperienced burglars, who will choose a location without a decal. However, professional burglars are likely to know what kind of system is in place by the name on the decal and are adept at bypassing the alarms. In this case, the decal would definitely be a disadvantage, rather than an advantage. Remember, burglary is a crime of opportunity, so don't make it easy for them!

When choosing the alarm system for the office, you need to consider various external factors (Box 11–11), such as the type of building that the office is located in—whether it is an office building or a single standing structure. If it is an office building, is it a high rise or a condominium style, with all offices on the ground floor? What type of neighborhood is it in? Is it on busy highway with a lot of passer-by coverage? Is the neighborhood well lit, or is the office in a dark area of town? Is the office in a city or a small town? These factors are very important when assessing the needs of the office for a security system.

MANAGER'S ALERT

When buying an alarm system, don't forget to get a battery backup. If the burglars cut the electric line, the office will still be secure.

DESK ACCESSORIES

Containers

Most employees like to work at a desk that has color and personality. The 1990s have seen offices decorated

---

BOX 11–11. HOW TO CHOOSE THE RIGHT SECURITY SYSTEM

Choose a company.

1 Ask your personal property insurance agent for a recommendation of qualified installers.
2 Contact the National Burglar and Fire Alarm Association in Bethesda, Maryland, for a list of their members in the area of your office.
3 Check with the Better Business Bureau for reputable companies.
4 Ask other physician offices about the companies they use.
5 Ask several security companies to survey the prem ises and submit a proposal.

Once you have chosen a company, ask the following questions.

1 What types of alarms do you install?
2 Do you specialize in business or residential systems?
3 Are your employees bonded?
4 How long will it take to install the system?
5 What are the guarantees or warranties of the system?
6 How soon can the system be installed after the decision is made?
7 Does your company operate a monitoring station, or do you use a separate company?
8 What liability will you assume if the office is burglarized because of a system malfunction?
9 Does your system ever experience down time?

---

in burgundy, mauve, navy, slate blue, forest green, and ecru. Many brands of accessories come in these bold colors. Art deco, traditional wood, leather, and marble can still be found, but plastic comes in the widest range of colors. The look that seems to be in demand is plastic with rounded edges and bright colors, although wire has also found its way into the workplace in the form of coiled wire for wastebaskets, pencil holders, etc. Some offices purchase employees' items of choice for them and allow free reign in selection of color and material. Other offices ask employees to purchase their own accessories for their desks and allow them the same openness. Regardless of who buys, allow employees to choose the items they need in the style they want, and the office environment will seem a more content one.

Stacking trays can be helpful on desks where limited space is available. Now, in our age of high technology, almost everyone has a computer on her or his desk. Couple that with an adding machine/calculator, stapler, tape dispenser, pen and pencil holder, desk calendar, Rolodex, and pictures of loved ones, and there is little room left for actual work. Stacking trays can also eliminate desk drawer clutter if they are used as drawer organizers. They can hold a variety of items, such as paper clips, staplers, scissors, rulers, etc. These trays come in letter size and legal size to accommodate all situations.

Writing Instruments

For more than 5,000 years, humans have been recording events by using some type of writing instrument. The Egyptians used hollow reeds, the Chinese used brushes, the Europeans used quills, and the Greeks used a metal stylus very similar to our metal-tipped pens of today. Even though we find ourselves in a high-tech world, we still have the need for the ubiquitous pen and pencil. Each desk in the medical office should be equipped with the appropriate number of pens, pencils, and highlighters.

In 1884, Louis Waterman, from New York, patented the first fountain pen. This pen became very well known and is the pen of choice for most physicians today. The rest of the staff generally use ballpoint pens, which were introduced in 1945. However, there is still a place for the pencil. Pencil lead comes in a variety of colors, which the medical office can use to its advantage. Perhaps the office would like to record the physician's meetings in green pencil, the physician's lectures in red, etc. This can be very helpful in keeping schedules straight. In addition, pencils should always be used when scheduling patient appointments if the office is not using computerized scheduling. *Many* changes take place in the appointment book, so it is easier to use pencil only! Some hospital billers like to use mechanical pencils when doing their billing, because of the constant sharp point. Many bookkeepers also choose to use mechanical pencils. Check with your employees to find out their needs. If they have the equipment that they want, they are happier and more productive.

Pharmaceutical representatives often offer pens and notepads in exchange for seeing the physician. Most office pens can be obtained through these reps, which helps to keep office supply costs down.

THE SUPPLY ORDER LOG

The inventory of supplies should be checked on a weekly basis. This task should be assigned to one person in the clinical area and one person in the clerical area. This person then assumes the responsibility of maintaining and ordering of the supplies needed in each area.

Develop a log in which to track both medical and office supplies that have been ordered (see Box 11–12 for a sample). This can be done very easily by using a three-ring binder. Keep supply order forms in the front and a complete list of vendors' names, addresses, and telephone numbers. It might also be helpful to list the items that are ordered from each vendor, along with their prices. If ordering is done in this organized fashion, it can be done by staff members instead of you. Remember, it is important to delegate as many tasks as possible to give yourself time for more important duties. When items are delivered, it is important for the employee to check the supply order log and verify that the order is complete. Take a special note of items that are back-ordered and check the office stock to ensure that the stock will not be depleted before the new stock arrives.

Employee Theft

Employee theft is a huge and growing problem. The goods and cash lost to theft are estimated to total $120 billion a year. A Massachusettes-based security consultant recently stated that about 30% of American workers plan to exploit their employer by some type of theft. Another 30% are basically good employees, but succumb occasionally. The last 40% are honest. Employee theft comes in a variety of forms. It can be as simple as a pen, notepad, postage stamp, and kleenex or as high level as petty cash and daily cash intakes.

The figures aren't good, and the office manager must take precautions to prevent as much theft as possible. By using personal interviews, credit checks, and reference checks, most office managers can ward off the "rough"

employees. They can also make use of honesty tests. These tests cost approximately $10–$20, which includes the scoring of the test. They predict future behavior based on the test taker's attitudes and past conduct. The biggest providers of these tests are:

London House, Chicago, IL
Reid Psychological Systems, Chicago, IL
Pinkerton Services Group, Charlotte, NC

Although these tests are developed to show "core integrity," they can also forecast absenteeism, accidents, and other problems associated with employees. Use caution in choosing a company to supply such tests, because tests that do not meet the standards of reliability can leave the door open to lawsuits. A set of standards can be obtained from individual test publishers or from the Association of Personnel Test Publishers, 655 15th Street, N.W., Suite 320, Washington, D.C. 20005. Their telephone number is (202) 639-4314. Their publication *Using Integrity Tests To Screen Job Applicants* is free.

One of the best ways to curtail employee theft is to promote positive feelings toward the office and the physician. Employees tend to steal more if they feel that the office has been unfair to them. Studies have shown that there are lower levels of employee theft in offices with low employee turnover and high performance on the job.

Setting up a formal chain of command in cash management can also discourage employee theft. This chain should be set up as follows:

Employee 1 collects money from patients.
Employee 2 processes these payments.
Employee 3 deposits these payments.

If this system is established, it becomes difficult for one person to be able to steal. The report of payments posted for the day should match the daily deposit. Some offices deposit only on a weekly basis; this should be changed to daily if at all possible. If the office cannot change to daily depositing, the daily sheets should be totaled at the end of the week and should then match the weekly deposit.

Payments received through the mail should be tallied on a separate sheet, and a separate deposit should be made for these checks. On the deposit slip, write "mail" somewhere, so that the bookkeeper will know the source of these funds. The employee should also initial each daily sheet and mail sheet, so that it creates a paper trail in case of a problem.

A final way to decrease employee theft is to prosecute employees who steal. This has been proven to be one of the most effective deterrents. Although it costs money

BOX 11–12. **PAGE FROM A SUPPLY LOG**

Supply Log

Date	Vendor	Items Ordered	Date Items Received	Initials

and takes time, the result is that the office gets restitution and doesn't suffer morale problems. Civil restitution is a popular way of recouping losses in a medical office. The physician and the employee work out an arrangement for the repayment of the theft. Many offices prefer to take the easy way out and simply terminate the employee without any type of restitution or prosecution. This sets a bad example for the other employees who are still in the office. Any type of prosecution can send a strong message to others that the office will not tolerate that type of behavior. This can work to the advantage of the office, because any other employees who were stealing or thinking of it will soon stop.

One way to protect the office and the physician is to purchase dishonesty insurance. This insurance can be purchased as part of a package for office liability and personal property. It protects the office from any losses from employee theft. The office manager can also check into purchasing fidelity bonding on the employees who handle cash in the office. Fidelity bonding is a type of insurance that reimburses the practice in the event of employee theft. The employees who handle cash are asked by the insurance company to sign an application for bonding. The employees are then aware that they are being watched, and this tends to keep them honest.

"Other" Office Insurance

Everyone today focuses on malpractice insurance, giving little thought to other types of insurance needs. The office manager should shop around and compare insurance plans before choosing a policy for the office.

INJURY LIABILITY

Injuries from falls and bumps are always occurring in the medical office. All those in business are subject to liability every time an individual steps into their place of business. A medical office has an even greater risk, because many patients are ill and fragile.

> **MANAGER'S ALERT**
>
> Patients can sue you successfully even when their injuries are partly their own fault!

The office manager should carefully walk through the office to evaluate any potential disasters that might

cause a need for this additional insurance. The manager should also check to see exactly where the liability ends. If the office is located in a free-standing dwelling, liability extends to the edge of the property.

PERSONAL PROPERTY INSURANCE

Evaluate and prepare a list of equipment for personal property insurance and make sure the coverage is ample for fire, theft, flood, or any other disaster that may find the office. Planning for these type of events helps to make them less painful if they occur. Check into "continuing business coverage," so that in the event of disaster, the office can rent temporary accommodations and continue to see patients while repairs are being made. This coverage will also handle cleaning of the office. Some physicians will ask a colleague about sharing space in their office in an event of an emergency situation. One of the most important things to remember is that if the office is computerized, copies of the daily, monthly, and yearly backup disks should be kept in a fireproof cabinet so that they are not lost. Finally, don't forget the patients! Someone should be designated to call the patients, explain the situation, and reschedule appointments at a designated time and place.

> **FROM THE AUTHOR'S NOTEBOOK**
>
> One way to safeguard against loss of files in the computer in the event of disaster is to have the computer operator take a copy of the daily disk home on a daily basis.

Notify all vendors when disaster strikes. Postpone deliveries and possibly make payment arrangements for bills. As an extra note, have an engraved sign in the window or on the bottom of the door, stating "In case of an emergency, please notify . . ." That will ensure that someone from the office is notified immediately. You should have certain emergency telephone numbers at home and in your car. Having these numbers readily available will be of tremendous help when disaster strikes. The following is a list of people whose emergency telephone numbers you should have:

- Insurance agent
- Landlord
- Neighbors
- Emergency boarding-up service

- Staff at home
- Vendors, companies, and utilities
- Rental companies for furniture, equipment, and office space
- Public insurance adjusters

The physician pays top dollar to get excellent malpractice coverage, so don't skimp on this insurance; it is just as important!!

The Facility

OFFICE LEASES

Most private physicians are found to be leasing office space, as opposed to buying. Ownership ties up capital and severely limits options regarding the future. There are real estate brokers who work solely with health care professionals. These brokers specialize in commercial and professional space.

> **MANAGER'S ALERT**
>
> Never sign a lease without first having the attorney review it.

Leases for medical offices come with their own set of problems. Some brokers want signatures on leases that allow no sublet and assignment rights and provide no disability escape clause! Don't lease on impulse! Just because the office is in a pretty building doesn't mean it is the office for you. Evaluate the needs of the practice, the layout, and location you desire, and the price you can pay. Then have the broker meet and discuss these considerations. She or he will be able to find a space that fits your needs. Don't forget to inquire as to the stability of the owner of the building. The appropriate time frame for a relocation is about 1 year. Remember the discussion in Chapter 7 on the ramifications of the Americans with American Disabilities Act for an office. A "workletter," which allows for construction or reconstruction of the office space to meet the tenant's needs, is a necessary part of any lease. Costs of modifying the office vary, depending on the location of the office. Because skilled labor is involved in the modification of a medical office, the cost will be high no matter where the office is. Check with the landlord; many times, she or he will give a cash contribution or discount on monthly rent to help with the changes.

A "triple net lease" is a lease whereby the tenant pays her or his share of the building's utilities, maintenance expenses, and real estate taxes. This lease comes with strings attached, in that "maintenance expenses" can include repair or replacement of heating or air conditioning. Expensive!

Give the lease to the attorney for review before you sign it!

MOVING THE OFFICE

Everyone knows the hassles of moving. By using the concept of the moving team, your office can handle this project with ease. A staff member from each department is assigned the responsibility for her or his department and is a member of the team. The office manager keeps the employees advised at all times regarding changes in plans and their responsibilities. Each department representative plays a critical role in handling the issues that arise during this project.

- Management representative
  - Schedules meetings with members of the team, the office manager, and the architect.
  - Distributes memos to keep employees up to date regarding the move.
  - Asks employees for suggestions regarding the move and allows them to voice any concerns.
- Accounting/bookkeeping representative
  - Prepares budget for moving expense and new equipment purchases.
- Computer systems representative
  - Obtains lockable space from contractor for new equipment that is being delivered.
  - Arranges for computer vendor to move computer to new space and install it there.
- Facilities representative
  - Holds regular on-site meetings with the office manager, physician, and architect.
  - On the first day in the new place, posts lists for employees to write suggestions and problems.
- Administration representative
  - Leases laptop computer for easier note taking and documentation during the move.

BUILDING A NEW FACILITY

Growth and expansion are a way of life for a medical office. Practices grow, more physicians are hired, more office hours are needed, etc.

Pitfalls to Avoid

Even the most effective plan for building a new facility is likely to have some pitfalls. These pitfalls are generally

- Poor location
- Inadequate time to properly plan, design, and construct a building
- Lack of attention to future expansion
- Misunderstandings about costs

Location

One of the most difficult and frustrating issues is location. Land is expensive, growth is unpredictable, etc. Perception is a major problem when talking about sites of offices. Sizes of lots can be deceiving, and land may appear adequate when it is actually too small to allow growth. Parking is a main consideration when constructing a new office; each municipality has zoning regulations regarding parking. Some townships require a designated number of parking spaces per square foot of office space. A multistory building requires two stairwells and an elevator shaft, which eliminates much needed space. An elevator is also an extra added expense. Other site pitfalls include storm water runoff from the property, easements, height restrictions, and landscape requirements.

Time Allowance

Normally, no matter how much time is allotted for the building project, it will take longer. Planning and design can take as much time as the actual construction, if not more. Other time-consuming factors include:

- Searching for and actually purchasing the land
- Rezoning the land
- Obtaining approval from regulatory offices
- Allowing staff to review architectural drawings and cost estimates

Long-Term Perspective

Long-term needs are major considerations when building a new facility. Practice growth, additional services, an increase in physicians, expansion of surrounding areas, increased staffing, and space requirements need to be considered. When making these plans, it is best to project 5–10 years into the future.

Building Costs

Costs are always higher than expected. Inflation is almost never taken into consideration, and physicians tend to compare the costs of the new office to the costs of their homes. On a per-square-foot basis, the cost of a medical office is always more than that of any other building type. Costs are never clear-cut; it is always a guess as to what is included and what is excluded. The total project cost includes:

- Site work, such as excavation, paving, sidewalks, fencing, lighting, and curbing
- Fixtures, wall covering, and window treatments
- Architectural, engineering, and interior design fees
- Furniture and equipment

A design firm should be brought in to help the physician and the office manager with these decisions. Evaluate the firm's experience, references, reputation, and range of services before deciding to enlist its efforts. Make the firm aware of the office's budget so that planning takes it into consideration. A building design done quickly and with little thought will result in unnecessary costs, and inefficiencies. If the project is planned correctly and slowly, the medical office will probably be a more successful and productive office.

The Office Blueprint

The office manager's main objective when a new facility is being planned is to design an office that "works." This means that each area of the office allows the practice to run efficiently, increasing productivity and profits, while allowing the delivery of quality care.

Before sitting down with the architect, divide the office into sections, such as business, clinical, professional, and reception. Depending on the type of practice, there might be additional areas in the office, such as an anesthesia room. Once these areas have been identified, consult the employees of each area on the problems with the current design. Ask for ideas for how patient flow can be maintained and organization can be put into place. Make a list of everyone's ideas and then discuss each idea with the physician and the architect. Remember, the new office design should not repeat mistakes made in the current office. Do not be afraid to make major changes in the layout.

In addition, decide what present equipment will be kept and what will be purchased new. By using an office furniture template (Figure 11–5), you can draw the furniture in various ways to check on availability of space. Try not to waste space; if there seems to be dead space somewhere, use it as a closet or for some type of storage. An office can never have too much storage! There are also commercial design kits that can be purchased for this project. Remember to allow enough

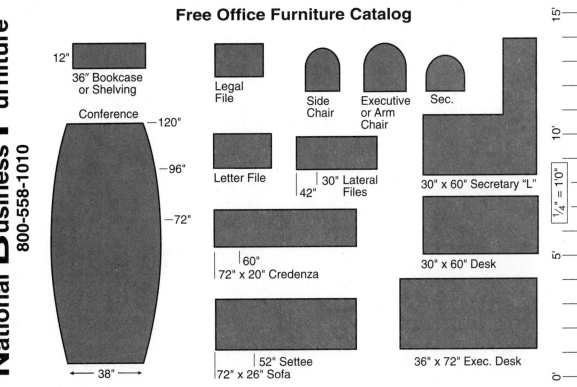

FIGURE 11–5. Template for arranging office furniture. (Courtesy of National Business Furniture.)

space for everyone to move around easily. The following are questions you might ask yourself at this time:

Do I want panel systems or individual desks in the business office?

Would I be better off with computer stations than with individual desks?

What type of filing requirements do I have in the business office?

What arrangements do I need to make for patient files? Do I want a record room?

Where will the employees eat?

What types of appliances will I need electrical outlets for in the kitchen/lounge area?

How many "dedicated" outlets will I need, if any?

Where will I put the copier? Will it be too noisy in certain areas?

Where will I put the computer? Will it be easily accessible to others? Will the printer be noisy?

How should the exam tables be placed? Is it easy for the physician to access the patient that way?

What is the best way to direct the flow of patient traffic?

Is the waiting room friendly?

Is there easy access to the receptionist's window?

Is the billing manager situated in a private area, so that patients can discuss financial matters?

Do we have enough storage areas for both clerical and clinical supplies?

Does the typist have an area free of background noise?

All of these questions and more come up when designing a new office. A good office manager addresses these questions before finishing the plans and moving in! Once the office is situated, it becomes much more difficult and costly to make changes. There are price wars going on all the time in the office furniture business. Don't hesitate to try to negotiate with office furniture sales people. Make sure everything is written down and both the supplier and the office have a copy. Don't rely on someone with a kind face saying, "Don't worry about that, I'll take care of it!" Many a nice relationship has soured over verbal deals such as these. Office furniture such as desks, chairs, computer stations, filing cabinets, bookcases, and credenzas can be found in catalogs at discounted prices. Check on shipping costs and the availability of the items before deciding to take this route.

DON'T MOVE . . . SPRUCE UP!

When the office size and location are suitable for the practice's needs, a coat of paint and some new furniture can change a rather dull office into a "showplace." Redecorating not only is less expensive than moving, but it has been proven to increase employee morale and therefore productivity.

The first thing to focus on when redecorating an office is the reception area. This is where the patients get their first impression of the practice and spend a lot of time. Soft wall colors, subdued wallpaper, tasteful pictures, healthy plants, and a quiet sound system with soothing music can do a world of good for a medical office. If the carpeting is poor, replace it. There are great new commercial carpets available that give that "warm and fuzzy" feeling to patients as they arrive at the office. Never buy couches. People generally do not like to sit next to others. They will always pick single chairs when choosing where to sit in the reception room. The best chairs are ones with arms that are approximately 18 inches deep and no deeper. Deep chairs are difficult for patients to get out of! Magazine racks are a better bet than magazines arranged on a table. Magazines on a table always look messy, no matter how hard the staff try to keep them neat. Televisions are always a good bet in a reception area. Patients can watch the news or other shows, and will forget about the time passing. Remember to keep the volume low so as not to disturb other patients. Studies have found that placing a television in a reception room decreases the number of complaints from patients in the reception room. The number of seats in the waiting room should be for three times the average number of patients seen in an hour. This will accommodate the drivers, family, and friends of patients, along with patients who have chosen to arrive an hour early for their scheduled appointment.

REVAMPING OF PRESENT SPACE

Limited remodeling and expansion can be done with a minimal amount of mess and can make employees and physicians happier. With just the smallest changes, patient flow and office efficiency can increase. By simply moving walls and decreasing space where it is not needed, you can open up additional rooms. For instance, by shaving off square footage on three exam rooms, a clinical room can be created for patients undergoing electrocardiograms and other special procedures that do not require much room. By creating this space, the exam room becomes free for the next patient. Revamping does not have to mean the moving of walls; it can be done

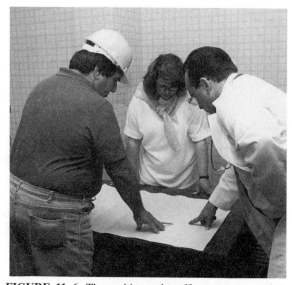

FIGURE 11–6. The architect, the office manager, and the physician should meet to establish the best design for the office.

simply by remodeling existing space and reorganizing. Getting the most from the office space is the most important issue. By using a space designer and/or an architect, major changes that will enhance practice productivity can be accomplished (Figure 11–6).

Be Humble . . . Apologize

When an office manager admits to a mistake, it becomes a positive experience for both the employee and the office manager. If you never admit to a mistake, you give the impression of inflexibility and snobbiness. This hard-core approach to mistakes is no longer considered the right way to manage. The office manager of the 1990s must soften up and admit mistakes. For instance, if you blame someone for taking a file and then find it in your attache case, you should simply say, "I'm sorry I blamed you. I found it."

> **MANAGER'S ALERT**
>
> Make sure all furniture to be delivered is delivered into the office itself. Make sure that this is stated clearly at the time of purchase. Some companies state they deliver only to the door. Delivery into the room will cost extra.

The staff will appreciate your honesty when you admit to a mistake, which in turn will build teamwork and cooperation in the office. No one is perfect; we all make mistakes. A good manager does not worry about saving face.

Professional Societies

MEDICAL GROUP MANAGEMENT ASSOCIATION

The Medical Group Management Association (MGMA) is a valuable source of information and services for medical office managers, administrators, and hospital management personnel. It supplies up-to-date statistics regarding the business side of medicine and advises individuals on national and global developments. The MGMA has developed a strong network that can aid an office manager in the areas of

- Library resources
- Management consulting services
- Group practice insurance plans
- Government relations resources
- Placement services
- Educational programs

You can contact the MGMA at the following address:
Medical Group Management Association
1355 South Colorado Boulevard, Suite 900
Denver, CO 80222-3331

PROFESSIONAL ASSOCIATION OF HEALTH CARE OFFICE MANAGERS

The Professional Association of Health Care Managers (PAHCOM) is an organized association that caters to small medical groups and solo practices. This organization supplies office managers with

- Salary surveys
- Educational topics
- Newsletters
- Changes in legislation

PAHCOM's published newsletter has valuable articles that will help you with the day-to-day operation of the medical office. For membership information, contact them at

Professional Association of Health Care Office Managers
Suite 102
2929 Langley Avenue
Pensacola, FL 32504-7355

References

Associated Regional Accounting Firms. *First, Stop the Bleeding.* Norcross, GA: Author, 1993.

Astrachan, A. "Spruce up the Office—and Boost Your Earnings?" *Medical Economics,* January 1987, pp. 177-188.

Bernstein, A., & Rozen, S. *Dinosaur Brains.* New York: Ballantine Books, 1989.

Brown, S., Nelson A., Bronkesh, S., & Wood, S. *Patient Satisfaction Pays.* Gaithersburg, MD: Aspen Publications, 1993.

Buss, D. "Ways To Curtail Employee Theft." *Nation's Business,* April 1993, pp. 36-38.

Calano, J., & Salzman, J. "The Careful Manager's Guide to Snap Decisions." *The Office,* May 1988, pp. 86-87.

Calero, L. "An Office Relocation Needs a Project Team." *The Office,* April 1992, pp. 52-53.

Demos, M.P. "What Every Physician Should Know About the National Practitioner Data Bank." *Archives of Internal Medicine,* September 1991, pp. 1708-1711.

Dolan, M. "Building New Facilities—What Planners Need To Know." *Group Practice Journal,* March/April 1993, pp. 40-42.

Dupree, M. Leadership as an Art. New York: Bantam Doubleday Dell, 1990.

Farber, L. *Encyclopedia of Practice and Financial Management.* Oradell, NJ: Medical Economics Company, 1988.

Green, W. "How To Run a Really Good Meeting." *US News & World Report,* October 12, 1987, pp. 80-82.

Heller, W. "How Safe Is Your Bank?" *Physician's Management,* February 1992, pp. 149-170.

Jamison, K. *The Nibble Theory.* New York: Paulist Press, 1984.

Kahaner, L. "Security Systems: How To Pick the Best for Your Home and Office." *Physician's Management,* March 1992, pp. 175-188.

Ketchum, S. "Overcoming the Four Toughest Management Challenges." *Clinical Laboratory Management Association,* August 1991, pp. 246-263.

Lankford, N. "Copier Trends." *The Office,* January 1993, p. 60.

Lopez, J. A. "The Boss from Hell." *Working Woman,* December 1991, pp. 69-71.

LeBoeuf, W. "Writing a CV That Brings Interviews." *Medical Economics,* May 1992, pp. 127-130.

Le Gallee, J. "Copier Control Systems Do More Than Curb Waste." *The Office,* March 1992, pp. 61-88.

Mackenzie, A. *The Time Trap.* New York: American Management Association.

Murray, D. "Coping with Tougher Times, Save Big on Equipment and Supplies." *Medical Economics,* September 1993, pp. 55-66.

Page, L. "Lost in the Translation." *American Medical News,* February 1993, pp. 31-32.

Peoples, D. A. *Presentation Plus.* New York: John Wiley & Sons, 1992.

Pepper, J. "Coping with Copiers." *Working Women,* April 1990, p. 54.

Slomski, A. "Making Sure Your Care Doesn't Get Lost In Translation." *Medical Economics,* May 1993, pp. 122-139.

Smith, P. *Taking Charge: Making the Right Choices.* Wayne, NJ: Avery, 1988.

Spero, K. "Ten Ways To Evaluate an Accountant." *Physician's Management,* August 1991, pp. 138-150.

Tinsley, R. "Plan Ahead Before Merging Medical Practices." *Group Practice Journal,* December 1993, pp. 28-32.

Tomasko, R. *Rethinking The Corporation.* New York: American Management Association, 1993.

Yerkes, L. "Making the Most of a Management Consultant." *Physician's Management,* July 1992, pp. 97-106.

12

Outpatient Services and Ambulatory Surgical Centers

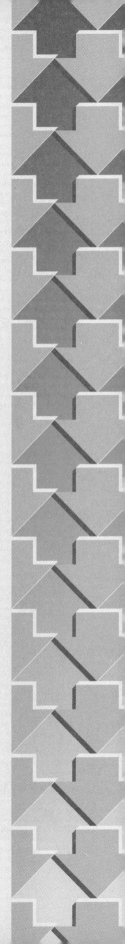

Outpatient Services

Physician Office Laboratories (POLs)
- *Types of Laboratory Tests Performed by POLs*
- *Tests Commonly Performed by POLs*

Ambulatory Care
- *What Ambulatory Care Is*
- *Hospitals, Ambulatory Surgery Centers, and Clinics*

- *Is Your Office Ready for Ambulatory Patient Groups?*
- *Cost Analysis of ASC Procedures*
- *Managing the ASC*
- *Facility Design and Development*
- *What Is a CON?*
- *Ambulatory Care Documentation and Form Structure*

Outpatient Services

Many forms of care are provided on an outpatient basis: x-ray exams, electrocardiograms, ultrasonography, CAT scans, laboratory services, physical therapy, and home care. The health care system today is undergoing massive "plastic surgery," shifting from hospital care to outpatient care and ambulatory services. This is creating an environment in which physician offices can thrive and offer a variety of services to patients. Office managers must be aware of the many services physicians can now provide patients, so that they can train their staff to be better able to assist the physician and the patient during medical care (Figure 12–1).

Outpatient testing has become increasingly popular in the 1990s. Americans thrive on medical testing as they strive to gain understanding of medicines, their own bodies, and wellness. People flock to health fairs, shopping centers, and drug stores in an effort to obtain free testing for various maladies. One survey found that in 1985, more than 20 million tests were performed at health fairs. This new type of patient, the "informed consumer," has created a demand for outpatient testing.

Hospitals are becoming involved with wellness promotion by holding wellness clinics in which preventive care is promoted. They offer senior citizens free blood pressure checks, low-cost eye exams, and free cholesterol checks. More sophisticated programs offer chest x-rays, mammograms, electrocardiograms (ECGs), and

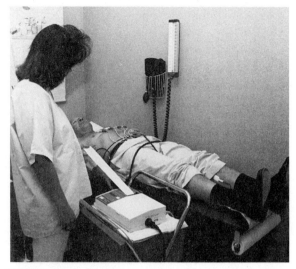

FIGURE 12–2. A patient presenting with chest pain is able to have an electrocardiogram in his physician's office.

Pap smears (Figure 12–2). The cost of having these more sophisticated tests done at a wellness clinic is minimal compared with what they would cost if a private physician ordered them. Most physicians do not see this as a threat to their patient load and invite these low-cost services for their patients. Reports of these tests can be sent to the family physician at the patient's request. Some hospital services are provided by hospital satellite facilities that offer a full range of primary care services for the patient. Clinics are being opened in deprived urban areas to assist in the medical care of patients. Physicians who do feel threatened by these clinics and satellites should reexamine their patient base to offer more services to offset this "competition." This can be done by adding an x-ray unit, a physician office laboratory, or physical therapy staff or by just being more available. Physician offices must remember that availability is one of the most important factors for patients when they are choosing a physician. Simply by extending weekday office hours or by adding Saturday hours, you can better accommodate your patients and make them more content with the office.

Defensive medicine is another reason for an increase in outpatient testing. Because of the medical–legal environment we have today, patients with simple cold symptoms will most probably find themselves receiving a battery of laboratory tests for that complaint. The most common reason for extensive medical testing is not to diagnose disease, but to protect the physician from the legal process of negligence.

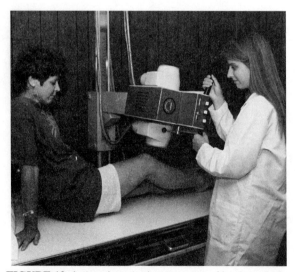

FIGURE 12–1. A patient receives an x-ray of her knee in the office of her orthopedic physician.

Physician Office Laboratories (POLs)

As a result of the government's plan for "Medicare prospective payment," many physician offices are setting up laboratories to perform preadmission testing in an effort to cut costs. The convenience to the patient and increased revenues that physician office laboratories (POLs) result in create a winning situation for everyone involved.

The Health Care Financing Administration reported that as of June 1993, there were 87,000 POLs in the United States (Figure 12–3). Most physician offices consider their testing equipment to be so user friendly and accurate that it can provide patient test results faster than the traditional hospital laboratories. This in turn facilitates better patient care, which is the main concern of physicians today. In addition, POLs have been found to perform less costly tests than those performed by most independent or hospital laboratories. When shopping for laboratory equipment, you should contact several vendors (Figure 12–4). Keep in mind that the main areas of concern are

- Ease of use
- Support
- Downtime
- Interaction capabilities
- Cost of equipment
- Cost of reagents/supplies
- Speed
- Maintenance costs

TYPES OF LABORATORY TESTS PERFORMED BY POLs

Five types of laboratory tests are performed by POLs:

- Screening tests
- Confirmatory tests
- Monitoring tests
- Stat tests
- Preadmission tests

A screening test is one that is performed for identification of a disease process. Screening tests are generally quick tests and are less expensive than most other laboratory testing. An example of a screening test is the "Mono-Spot" test for mononucleosis, which produces results within 5 minutes.

Positive screening tests are followed by confirmatory testing in order to diagnose the patient accurately. Confirmatory tests are more expensive and require more time for processing. They provide more specific information and are more complex in nature. An example of a confirmatory test is a test for hepatitis.

Monitoring tests are continuous in nature and follow the patient through the course of treatment. They differ from other tests in that they are always performed on patients for whom a diagnosis has already been made. An example of a monitoring test would be a complete blood count on a patient receiving chemotherapy drugs.

Stat testing is ordered on patients in emergency situations. They are most commonly used in the hospital setting. However, there are some instances in which stat tests are ordered in the physician's office. For example,

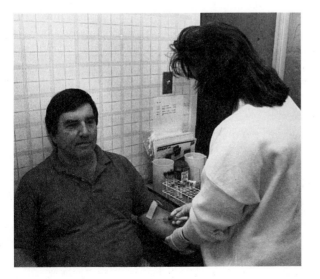

FIGURE 12–3. Patients can conveniently have their laboratory tests done in their physician's office when there is an in-office laboratory.

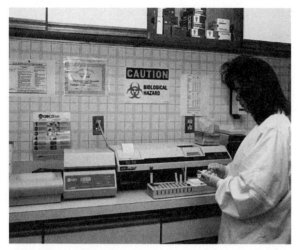

FIGURE 12–4. Physicians can obtain faster laboratory results for their patients when they have a laboratory in their office.

when a patient arrives at the office with severe diabetic symptoms, the physician needs a glucose stat.

A preadmission test is a nonurgent test that is required for the patient to be admitted to the hospital. Preadmission tests are also ordered for patients having outpatient surgery. These tests are screening tests designed to reveal any abnormality that could have an effect on the patient's hospitalization or procedure.

TESTS COMMONLY PERFORMED BY POLs

The tests most commonly performed by POLs are

- Multichannel tests and panels
- Routine urinalysis
- Complete blood counts (automated hemograms, red blood cells, white blood cells, hemoglobin, and hematocrit)
- Glucose
- Prothrombin time
- Partial thromboplastin time
- Sedimentation rate
- Pregnancy testing
- Rheumatoid arthritis
- Mono test
- Cholesterol

Ambulatory Care

WHAT AMBULATORY CARE IS

In the health care system as it currently exists, ambulatory care is exploding. This tremendous increase in ambulatory care is a response to the ever-changing needs of the modern population. Ambulatory care consists of the delivery of services without the inpatient factor—that is, the patient receives services from practitioners in a variety of settings without being admitted to a facility. That may sound scary and many would rather just call it "the walking patient." However, ambulatory care fits right into the mold of the managed care model, providing medical services in an ambulatory setting with less cost (Figure 12–5).

Ambulatory care can be preventive, primary, or secondary. Preventive care focuses on the wellness of individuals and their efforts to avoid disease. Primary care focuses on the daily, routine, basic care that individuals require from health care professionals. Secondary care is the care provided to ambulatory patients who require more specialized diagnosis and treatment.

HOSPITALS, AMBULATORY SURGERY CENTERS, AND CLINICS

Although most of the ambulatory care currently provided is provided in physician offices, an increasing number of services are being provided in hospitals,

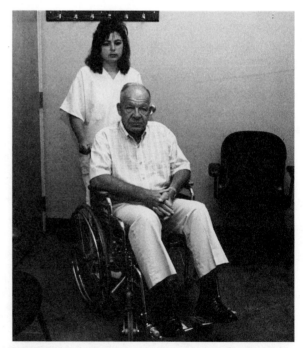

FIGURE 12–5. Having just completed a diagnostic procedure, a patient is wheeled out to his car to go home to rest for the balance of the day.

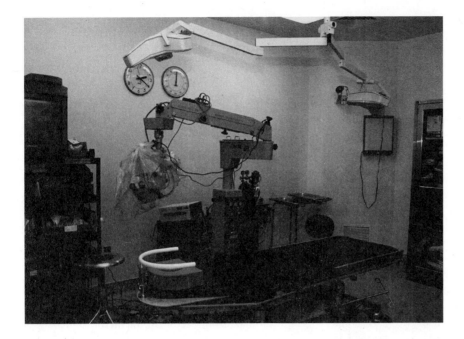

FIGURE 12–6. An operating suite in an ambulatory care center.

ambulatory surgery centers (ASCs), and clinics. Hospitals, through increased use of short procedure units (SPUs), are continually increasing the number of procedures they provide on a "same-day surgery" basis. Chemotherapy, blood transfusions, kidney dialysis, and many other services have joined the ranks of ambulatory care. Most hospitals have responded to the need for ambulatory services and have redesigned their facilities to further expedite the treatment of individuals with ambulatory care needs. By promoting ambulatory care, hospitals have positioned themselves in managed care to negotiate for both inpatient and outpatient services. This alone provides flexibility and opportunity for hospitals and managed care plans to effectively control costs.

The first ASC opened in Phoenix, Arizona. Its sole purpose was to provide "same-day" surgery care for patients who normally would be treated in hospital settings. It was completely independent of the hospital and provided a wide range of services (Figure 12–6). Colonoscopies, gastroscopies, bronchoscopies, thallium stress testing, cataract surgeries, laparoscopies, vasectomies, oral surgeries, arthroscopies, cartilige repairs, plastic surgeries, and many other services were provided (Figures 12–7 and 12–8). Some facilities are owned and operated solely by the physicians in a particular practice. Other centers have been opened by an affiliation of several groups of physicians (mostly different specialties), who have pooled their resources in an effort to provide quality care at less cost. These joint

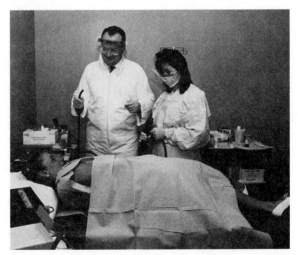

FIGURE 12–7. A patient prepares for a colonoscopy in the endoscopy suite of an ambulatory care facility.

ventures have combined their resources to design and construct facilities to meet the needs of the ever-growing community. Today, we even find hospitals that are involved in joint ventures with physicians to construct ASCs, in an effort to maintain their standing in the health care marketplace. Free-standing emergency centers have been popping up in every city to treat the emergency ailments that might arrive at their doorstep. These "Docs-in-a-Boxes" are relieving the

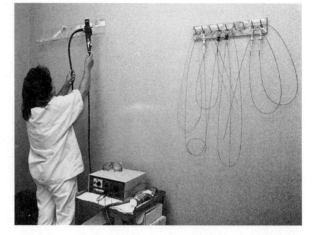

FIGURE 12–8. Staff taking care of equipment used in the endoscopy suite.

hospitals, emergency rooms of the nonemergency patients who normally would present there. They mainly provide primary care medicine and some additional emergency services. They are designed to handle the simple cuts, viral syndromes, and strains and sprains associated with daily community and family life. With society becoming more mobile and transitory, ASCs provide the type of patient care that is vitally needed.

The factors contributing to the rise of ASCs are increased revenues by way of facility fee reimbursement and the convenience to the physician and patient. More efficient appointment scheduling, the friendlier environment, and a desire for cost containment also factor into the equation. Physicians are constantly looking for ways to maximize their efficiency. Developing an ASCs can help them accomplished this while allowing them to continue to deliver quality care to patients. Quality assurance tends to be more thorough than in a hospital setting, and only patients whose health is generally good are scheduled for procedures in this facility (Figure 12–9). Any patient who might be considered at risk is scheduled to have her or his procedures performed in the hospital setting.

The result of this effort to make surgical procedures more user friendly has been to bring some patient groups knocking down the doors of ASCs. The success of this "mobile medical business" is based on many factors:

- The increased demand for outpatient surgeries by cost-conscious patients
- The increased desire of third-party payers to purchase services while remaining cost conscious
- Increased incentives from third-party payers for same-day surgeries
- More flexible physicians schedules, allowing for

increased productivity, which ultimately increases revenue
- Incentives from Medicare for the development of ASCs
- Easing of previously strict regulations for the establishment of ASCs

More than two million surgical procedures are performed in ASCs every year, and the number keeps rising (Figure 12–10). There are currently more than 1,700 ASCs in the United States today, providing surgical procedures that would cost 30% to 60% more if they were performed in the hospital operating room.

IS YOUR OFFICE READY FOR AMBULATORY PATIENT GROUPS?

Jumping Those Hurdles

Experience is always the best teacher. Because there have been many ASCs established throughout the country, it is best to learn from their experiences and try to avoid any unnecessary aggravations. There are a few basic steps that your office needs to take before jumping into the ASC arena:

- Determine the purpose of the facility.
- Discuss organizational issues and produce a business plan.
- Develop a team.
- Determine the location.
- Address construction issues.
- Consider costs.

Purpose of Facility

The first step is to identify the purpose of the development of the ASC. Is it being developed to increase the physicians' revenues, or is it being developed to provide the physicians with greater flexibility? Greater flexibility would allow physicians to become more productive, which would allow for additional patients to be seen. Greater flexibility would also give the physicians more leisure time. One of the most important and basic steps in this process is to identify the physicians' needs. After they have been established, you can begin assembling the building blocks necessary for this enormous undertaking.

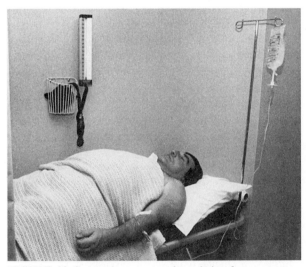

FIGURE 12–9. A patient naps as the sedation from a procedure wears off.

Organizational Issues

Having a qualified and informed individual to schedule all of the procedures performed at the ASC is imperative. This person is key to the success of the ASC. She or he should have working knowledge of the clinical side of the procedures being performed; knowledge of the physicians' preferences in sutures, equipment, anesthesia, etc; and awareness of the length of time necessary to perform each procedure (including cleaning and preparation of the room and the equipment). Having a highly competent person in this position should minimize turnaround time and thus maximize productivity.

A director can be appointed to oversee the operations of the facility, or this can be done by the office manager. In either case, the ASC should be constantly monitored for patient satisfaction, physician satisfaction, and cost containment. The director or office manager should be concerned with streamlining any task that hasn't already been simplified and should use automation whenever possible. Computers and efficient use of forms can eliminate the need to spend a lot of time on documentation.

Development of a Team

Teamwork is of utmost importance in the development of an ASC. Job descriptions must be precise, cross-training must take place, and staff's awareness of their roles in this process is imperative. Staffing should be analyzed with regard to the ASC schedule to ensure

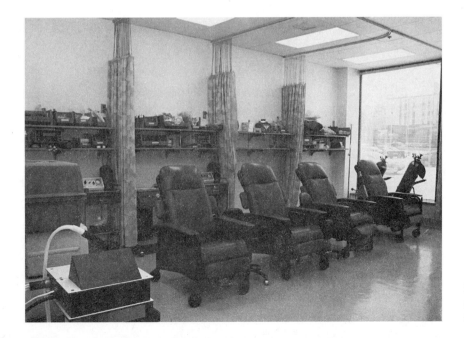

FIGURE 12–10. A recovery room in an ambulatory care center.

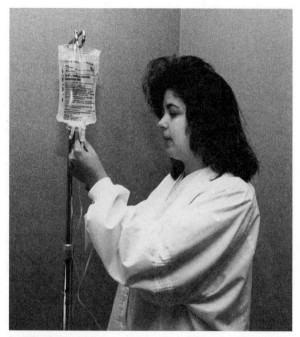

FIGURE 12–11. Preparation of an intravenous solution.

efficient patient flow coupled with quality care. Because supplies account for approximately 40% of the cost of operating an ASC, one team member should be designated as the supplies controller. This person would be responsible for

- Monitoring and maintaining the medical supply inventory.
- Standardizing equipment and supplies whenever possible.
- Monitoring supply charges to be sure they are captured.
- Negotiating price with various supply vendors.

Location

Where the ASC should be located depends heavily on whether the ASC will be used solely by the medical office developing it or will be opened for use by other physician groups. If others are involved, the site should be close to all participants and to the hospital. If the ASC is going to be used by only one physician group, choosing the location should not be a difficult task. It should be close to the office and the hospital. Other considerations should be parking, easy access, and traffic patterns.

Although one would think that patient demographics have a definite effect on this type of project, they really have little to no effect. Some will explain that the ages

of the patients in the practice, where they live, and their gender have an effect on the success of the ASC. However the commitment of the physicians to making the ASC successful is a more important consideration.

Construction

Before beginning the discussion of construction, it must be decided whether the facility will be applying for ASC certification. If certification is sought, there are extensive architectural regulations that must be followed. This, of course, increases construction costs; construction to meet the ASC requirements can go as high as $150,000 or more. It is best to use the expertise of a consultant to ensure that the proper steps are taken in complying with architectural regulations. Whether a new facility is being built or a previously owned facility is being renovated, it is important to comply with all of the architectural regulations if certification is sought.

Costs

The two largest variable costs that will be encountered in the operation of the ASC are personnel and medical supplies. (In Figure 12–11, a nurse prepares an intravenous solution for a procedure.) "Variable costs" mean just that—they are variable and therefore can be negotiated. The two largest fixed costs in the operation of the ASC will be rent (or mortgage) and equipment. Fixed costs are "set" costs, and no amount of negotiating will change them.

Sizing Up the Practice Before Taking the Leap

Before leaping into the world of the ASC, you need to consider what model the business will follow.

Model A

1 There are two to three physicians in the group.
2 A minimum of 100 procedures are generated each month.
3 The practice has a positive cash flow.
4 There are 1,500 to 2,000 square feet available for a procedure room.

Model B

1 There are three to five physicians in the group.
2 A minimum of 150 procedures are generated each month.
3 The practice has a positive cash flow.
4 There are 2,000 square feet per procedure room, and the facility has two rooms.

Model C

1 There are at least five physicians in the group.
2 A minimum of 200 procedures are generated each month.
3 The practice has a positive cash flow.
4 There are 3,000 square feet per procedure room, and the facility has three rooms.

The average cost of the setup of an ASC, including development, construction, and operation, ranges between $250,000 and $500,000 per procedure room. In most states, the project will take 12 months from start to finish. In a few states with more stringent regulations, the project could take as long as 24 months. If the conditions in Model A, B, or C cannot be met, it is not advisable to pursue the development of an ASC at this time.

Get a Consultant on the Job

It is a good idea to get help in the task of developing an ASC from professionals who have experience in this area. The business plan can be completed before the consultant is hired; this is not difficult to construct and will save the practice additional costs. During the development of the ASC, there are many factors that require excessive organizational skills and time management. The compliance with licensing offices is just the tip of the iceberg. The following are other areas where consultants can help in this major undertaking:

- The design
- Evaluation of equipment needed
- The obtaining of a contractor
- Negotiations of financial contracts
- Daily operations
- Negotiation of contracts with third-party payers
- Recruiting of professional personnel (physicians, certified registered nurse anesthetists, nurses, etc.)

Better consultants can help with all of the above and can coordinate the existing office personnel in daily, efficient operations once the project is completed. Some consultants provide ongoing facility management if needed. Consultants are available all over the country; contact the Federated Ambulatory Surgery Association, in Washington, DC, for list of competent consultants.

A consulting engagement that combines advice with a specific deliverable objective is referred to as "task orientation." In other words, an architect might be consulted regarding the feasibility of a specific location for an ASC. This same architect might be called on later to produce sketches and drawings of the proposed building. A broader consulting engagement, whereby the medical practice asks the consultant to address a variety of issues, is commonly referred to as a "comprehensive study." The goals of this study are not always related, and, in fact, most times they are not. Most comprehensive studies are multiissue studies.

COST ANALYSIS OF ASC PROCEDURES

One of the most challenging projects an office manager will ever face is the process of determining the cost of each case performed in the ASC. This analysis can be tedious, but its results are invaluable.

Start by making a list of all the items used for each procedure. Don't forget articles used for the administration of anesthesia (nasogastric tubes, IV fluids, etc.) if anesthesia is administered for the procedure. Now comes the "fun" part. Take this list and a big cup of coffee, and sit down to assign a cost to each item on the list. This is actually not a bad task, because it can be done simply by pulling the invoices for medical supplies. For instance, if you bought a bag of 25 nasal cannulas for oxygen, and the price per bag was $52.50, you know that the cost of each nasal cannula was $2.10. Do this with each item used in the procedure until a total item cost for the procedure is compiled.

Once you've tallied the total cost of the supplies used in the procedure, it is time to figure out the cost of the personnel involved in the procedure. This is an easy calculation. Take the monthly salary cost, including the cost of benefits, for all personnel, and divide this figure by the number of procedures done that month. For instance, if the monthly total personnel costs were $12,466 and there were 74 procedures performed that month, the personnel cost per procedure performed would be $168.46. To find out if this cost is "in line" with the personnel costs of other offices in the area, take the net revenue for the month and divide it into the monthly cost of the personnel; for example, $12,466/$38,982 = 32%. Personnel costs generally run between 15% and 25% of each dollar made. Thus in this illustration, personnel costs are running a little high.

You need to determine the total cost of supplies and personnel used for every procedure. By performing this calculation, you can assess the efficiency of the ASC and perhaps reevaluate what you're paying for supplies and your personnel needs.

MANAGING THE ASC

For the successful operation of the ASC, you must wear the hats of the following managerial positions:

- Organizer
- Financial manager
- Facilities manager
- Human resources manager
- Director of patient services
- Director of operations

As the organizer, you must develop a system of organization that ensures quality patient care, productive use of the physicians' time, efficient use of personnel, and reduced costs. You must continually review day-to-day operations for possible streamlining of procedures.

As the financial manager, you must be acutely aware of the financial operating systems of the facility. There must be in place a cash management policy; a system for collecting debt and managing accounts receivable; a continual audit of patient records to ensure accurate coding and billing; and, last but not least, a budget. This budget should provide the physician with such information as revenues and expenses, a cost analysis of services, and the projected costs of supplies and personnel. The financial needs of the facility are met with the following information:

- Income tax returns
- Information for income distribution
- Information for financial planning
- Information for decision making

This type of financial information is directly related to the control of the practice and is used for making practice growth decisions.

As the facilities manager, you are responsible for the physical operations of the facility, and this is an essential role. Consideration must be given on a regular basis to expansion, redesign, and renovation of the current facility. Such problems as parking, building access, and efficient patient flow require your attention. The need for replacement or additional equipment must also be assessed.

As the human resources manager, you must realize the importance of having highly trained and dedicated employees. On an ongoing basis, evaluate the number of employees to ascertain whether the facility needs additional personnel or whether revision of job descriptions can eliminate unnecessary personnel. "Rightsizing" the staff will create more efficient use of the facility. Share your management philosophies with your staff and make sure the "vision" of the facility envelopes employees in a positive environment. This role might also involve you in the procurement of physicians, nurse practitioners, physician assistants, and other skilled professionals. Physician recruitment can be aided by outside services that provide physicians on either a temporary or permanent basis.

As the director of patient services, you are ultimately responsible for any function that involves patient care. The umbrella of patient services covers

- Scheduling
- Patient referrals
- Support services such as laboratory tests, x-ray exams, ECGs, and physical therapy
- Patient education
- Medical records

Your role as director of operations involves you in the short- and long-term planning of the facility. You develop goals for the facility and make decisions regarding the facility in relationship to the needs of the community. In the health care environment, preparing for the future is an important responsibility.

FACILITY DESIGN AND DEVELOPMENT

Designing and developing an ambulatory care facility require much stamina and flexibility. You cannot appreciate the stress involved in such a project until you have been there. Before embarking on this project, find out your state's guidelines for the development of ASCs. Because health care regulations change so rapidly, it is imperative that you contact your state Department of Health for an up-to-date listing of design requirements.

WHAT IS A CON?

Many states require a certificate of need (CON) for Medicare certification of an ASC (Box 12–1). The CON is a leftover from the World War II days, when states imposed restrictions to minimize health care expenditures on facilities. In many states, these laws have not been updated. CONs are found today in 16 states, and some states, such as New York, strictly enforce these regulations.

To be eligible to bill for a facility fee to Medicare, the ASC must be Medicare certified. This certification hinges on fulfillment of the regulations of

- The state
- Medicare

- The state fire marshall
- The federal life safety regulations

Currently, there are approximately 29 states that allow Medicare certification (which means the facility can bill for a facility fee) without being licensed by the state. In such a case, the facility must be owned and used by the same physician group and can have no other owners or users. In the current climate of mergers and affiliations, it is advisable to obtain Medicare certification for the facility. Once the certification requirements are met, physicians can band together to share the use of the facility.

The state fire marshall and federal life safety regulations are strictly building related. These architectural guidelines must be met. Medicare will enforce these elements and will send surveyors to the site of the facility to interpret the guidelines and inspect the facility. This survey process is obtained by the federal government for the state Department of Health. In some states, where regulations are strict, these inspections often become impossible to pass.

Even in states that do not require a CON, it is generally in the best interests of the practice to apply for a state license. States that do not require specific need criteria put the burden on the practice to show a need for

an ASC. In reviewing Box 12–1, you will notice that Georgia is not listed anywhere. Georgia has complex rules and regulations regarding ASCs, and therefore its guidelines must be obtained even before the development process begins.

AMBULATORY CARE DOCUMENTATION AND FORM STRUCTURE

When developing an ASC, it is important to follow the documentation guidelines for each procedure performed. Generally, it is required that all medical records at an ASC contain the following forms:

- Consent for procedure
- History and physical form
- Anesthesia records:
  - Consent for anesthesia
  - Health history
  - Anesthesia record
  - Operative record
- Report of procedure
- Postprocedure instructions

These forms must be completely filled out, signed, and dated. Sample forms are provided in Box 12–2.

BOX 12–1. STATE BY STATE CERTIFICATE OF NEED (CON) REQUIREMENTS FOR AMBULATORY SURGERY CENTERS

States with No CON Requirements

Arizona	California	Colorado	Idaho
Indiana	Kansas	Louisiana	Minnesota
New Mexico	Texas	Utah	Wisconsin
Wyoming			

States with CON Programs That Do Not Cover Ambulatory Surgery

Arkansas	Florida	Nevada	New Hampshire
Oklahoma	Oregon	South Dakota	Tennessee

(Nevada does require a letter of intent in place of a CON)

States with No Specific Need Criteria

Alabama	Alaska	Connecticut	Hawaii
Iowa	Maine	Michigan	Montana
Nebraska	North Dakota	Pennsylvania	Rhode Island
South Carolina	Vermont	Washington, D.C.	

States That Do Not Require a CON (must be single specialty, physician owned)

Maryland	New Jersey	Ohio	Washington	West Virginia

BOX 12–2A. **PROCEDURE CONSENT FORM GASTROINTESTINAL SPECIALISTS, INC. CONSENT TO PROCEDURE**

NAME: _____

ADDRESS: _____

_____

1 I hereby authorize either _____ and such assistants as may be selected by him to perform a special diagnostic procedure in order to assist him in diagnosing my condition.

2 The procedure(s) necessary to treat/diagnose my condition (has, have) been explained to me by the physician and I understand it (them) to be:
Gastroscopy, Biopsy, or Heater Probe- passage of a flexible lighted instrument into the stomach, remove tissue/growth and cauterize blood vessels if needed.

3 It has been explained to me that during the course of the procedure, unforeseen conditions may be revealed that necessitate change or extension of the original procedure(s) or different procedure(s) than those already explained above. I therefore authorize and request that the above named physician, his assistants, or his designees perform such procedure(s) as are necessary and desirable in the exercise of his professional judgement. I understand that such conditions may cause a need for additional surgery, due to bleeding, perforation, or infection.

4 I have been made aware that there are risks and possible undesirable consequences associated with the treatment and diagnosis of my illness, including (but not limited to) severe blood loss, bowel perforation, infection, heart complications, blood clots, or death, that are attendant to the performance of any surgical procedure and I understand them. I am aware that the practice of medicine and surgery is not an exact science, and I acknowledge that no guarantees have been made to me concerning the results of the operation, procedure, or treatment.

5 The items listed above have been explained to me by Dr. _____ , and I understand and consent to them.

_____
(witness)

_____
(signature of patient/legal guardian)

(Courtesy of Gastrointestinal Specialists, Inc.)

BOX 12–2B. **HISTORY AND PHYSICAL FORM**

Gastrointestinal Specialists, Inc.
History & Physical Form

Age: _____ Sex: _____ Race: _____ S.M.W. _____

Allergies: _____

_____

_____

Purpose of Procedure: _____

_____

_____

_____

Chief Complaint: _____

_____

_____

_____

History of Present Illness: _____

_____

_____

_____

Past Medical History: _____

_____

_____

_____

Review of Symptoms: _____

_____

_____

_____

Family & Social History: _____

_____

_____

PHYSICAL EXAMINATION:

TPR: _____ BP: _____ Weight _____

_____

_____

_____

_____

_____

_____

_____

_____

_____

_____

_____

_____

_____

_____

_____

_____

_____

_____

_____

_____

_____

DIAGNOSIS: _____

_____

_____

Signature _____

(Courtesy of Gastrointestinal Specialists, Inc.)

BOX 12–2C. **ANESTHESIA CONSENT FORM**

R&P ANESTHESIA ASSOCIATES

B. Paul Stewart, CRNA, B.A.
Ronald Burkitt, CRNA

IMPORTANT INFORMATION—PLEASE READ

For your comfort and safety, your surgeon has requested a Certified Registered Nurse Anesthetist to be with you during your surgery to administer the necessary medications and monitor your vital signs. The anesthetist will meet with you the morning of surgery, review your history, and ask you questions about your medical health in order to select the appropriate anesthetic for you and the procedure you are about to undergo. He will also answer any questions you may have.

In the office operating suite there are generally two types of anesthesia which may be utilized. They are as follows:

1 Local anesthesia with IV sedation—This is the most common anesthesia in the office operating suite, and can be related to "twilight" sleep, where you are given a combination of medications which will make you very comfortable, and generally unaware of what is happening. For example, patients are usually able to respond if spoken to, but will be asleep during the procedure.
2 General anesthesia—In this instance, patients will be completely asleep, and in some cases where it is necessary to change the position of the patient, it will be necessary to place an endotracheal tube in the trachea (windpipe) to control the breathing.

In each case, the heart rate, blood pressure, electrocardiogram, arterial oxygen saturation, and respirations will be closely and continuously monitored by the anesthetist.

The anesthetist will remain with you throughout the procedure. After a suitable period of time, depending on the individual, you will be allowed to leave the facility in the company of a responsible adult. You will probably be sleepy and find that you will sleep for several hours after you return home. It is vitally important that you arrange to have someone with you for 24 hours after your surgery to help you to and from the bathroom, prepare liquids or soft foods for you to eat, assist with ice packs if ordered, and make sure you take your medications as they have been prescribed. You should not undertake any responsible activity, make any important decisions, or drive a car for a minimum of 24 hours after your surgery.

You may experience some mild nausea, sore throat, redness or bruising at the intravenous site, and a generalized feeling of being "washed out" for several days. Persistent or severe nausea and vomiting, bleeding, or severe swelling should be reported to the doctor immediately.

You should understand there is always a slight risk when you undergo surgery and anesthesia, and results cannot be guaranteed. If you have any further questions before the anesthetist meets with you, please do not hesitate to call Paul Stewart or Ron Burkitt. at the above telephone numbers.

AUTHORIZATION FOR ANESTHESIA

I hereby authorize and request R&P ANESTHESIA ASSOCIATES to administer the necessary anesthetics to _____ (Name) which, in their opinion, may be deemed appropriate for the surgical procedure to be performed by Dr. _____ (Physician's Name) on (Date) _____

I certify that the nature of the anesthetic procedures, including risks and possible complications, have been explained to me and that I understand the purpose of this authorization form.

DATE	SIGNATURE
DATE	WITNESS

(Courtesy of R&P Anesthesia Assoc.)

BOX 12–2D. **ANESTHESIA HEALTH HISTORY FORM**

R&P ANESTHESIA ASSOCIATES

HEALTH HISTORY

NAME OF PATIENT: _____

DATE OF BIRTH: _____ SEX: M F HEIGHT: _____ WEIGHT: _____

1 Are you allergic to any medication? Yes No. If yes, please list.

2 Are you taking any medications? Yes No. If yes, please list, and include over the counter preparations such as aspirin or antihistamines.

3 Do you smoke? Yes No. If yes, how many packs per day?

4 Do you drink alcohol? Yes No. If yes, how much?

5 Do you now, or have you ever used recreational drugs? Yes No. If Yes, when was the last time?
Such as: marijuana, cocaine

6 Do you have a history of any of the following?

Asthma	Yes	No	Hiatal Hernia	Yes	No
Bronchitis	Yes	No	Diabetes	Yes	No
High Blood Pressure	Yes	No	Seizures	Yes	No
Liver Problems (Hepatitis - Mono)	Yes	No	Cancer	Yes	No
Kidney Problems	Yes	No	Thyroid Problems	Yes	No
Rheumatic Fever	Yes	No	Arthritis	Yes	No
Bleeding Problems	Yes	No	Anemia	Yes	No
Ulcers	Yes	No	Fainting Spells	Yes	No
Heart Problems or murmurs	Yes	No	Glaucoma	Yes	No

7 Have you ever had any surgery? If so, please explain.

8 Have you or any member of your immediate family had any problems with anesthesia? If so, please explain.

9 Is there a chance you might be pregnant?

10 Are you under the care of a physician? If so, please list name and address:

11 How would you describe your present health? Excellent Good Fair.

12 Have you ever had a blood transfusion? Yes No.

13 Do you have any dentures, partial plates or capped teeth? Yes No.

14 Are you bothered by motion sickness? Yes No.

(Courtesy of R&P Anesthesia Assoc.)

BOX 12–2E. ANESTHESIA RECORD

ANESTHESIA   RECORD   PAGE

OPERATION _____

_____

DIAGNOSIS _____

ANESTHETIST _____

SURGEON _____

DATE _____ TIME X STARTED _____ TIME X FINISHED _ P.S. 1 2 3 4 5 E ALLERGIES _____

PRE-ANESTHETIC MED. & TIME _____
OR CONSENT: ☐ PATIENT IDENTIFIED ☐ PREMED. EFFECT
MEDICATIONS:

WEIGHT: PREPARATION
HEIGHT: I.V.
EST. BLD. VOL.   C.V.P.
                         Art.
Meal: L.P.
MONITOR: B.P. H.R. Resp. O_2
EEG.   TEMP.   EKG.

H/H 1

TIME														
O_2 L/min. (FIO_2)														
E.K.G.														
%SAO_2														
$ETCO_2$														

MAINTENANCE:

EQUIPMENT ☐

AIRWAY: NAT. O.P. N.P. MASK

INTUB: OT N.T. TRACH

TRAUMA:

SYMBOLS
: BP
• HR
RESPIRATION
○ SPONT
Ø ASSIST
⊕ CONTROL
◑ MECH
△ TEMP
x START ANES
• START SURG
⊗ END SURG
⊗ END ANES
◑ TO RR

VE

POSITION
INDEX

°C – 220
38 – 200
36 – 180
34 – 160
32 – 140
120
100
80
60
40
20
0

BOX 12–2E. **ANESTHESIA RECORD** *Continued*

URINE OUTPUT	ml	OTHER FLUIDS	
MEAS BLD LOSS			
E.S.T. BLD LOSS	ml	TOTAL BLOOD LOSS	
REPLACEMENT	ml		ml
	ml	TOTAL BLOOD REPL	
I.V. FLUIDS	ml		ml
	ml	**TOTAL FLUIDS**	
	ml		

AGENTS	TO R.R. ICU/PCU ROOM		
CONC/DOSE	CNS	AIRWAY	RESP
	AWAKE	NAT	SPONT
	SLEEPY	OP/NP	ASSIST
TECH/ROUTE	RESPON	INTUB	APNFIC
	UNCONSC	TRACH	
	BP	PULSE	

(Courtesy of R&P Anesthesia Assoc.)

BOX 12–2F. PROCEDURE FORM

PATIENT IDENTIFIED: _____

DIAGNOSIS: _____

SIGNIFICANT MEDICAL/SURGICAL HISTORY: _____

_____

ALLERGIES _____ GLAUCOMA _____ PACEMAKER _____

DIABETES _____ DENTURES _____ HEART DISEASE _____

CURRENT MEDICATIONS: _____

_____

SITE OF HEPLOCK OR IV STARTED: _____

PROCEDURE: _____ SITE OF CAUTERY RETURN PAD:_____

INSTRUMENT USED: _____ CONDITION OF RETURN PAD SITE:

	MEDICATION DOSAGE, ROUTE	TO BE GIVEN		SIGNATURE
		DATE	TIME	TITLE
START PROCEDURE: _____				
FINISH PROCEDURE: _____				
TIME OF DISCHARGE: _____				
ACCOMPANIED BY: _____				
MODE OF TRANSPORTATION: _____				

SPECIMENS: PATHOLOGY: _____

              CYTOLOGY: _____   MICROBIOLOGY: _____

BOX 12–2F. **PROCEDURE FORM** *Continued*

TIME	VITAL SIGNS	NURSES NOTES:

DATE: _____

SIGNATURE: _____
NURSE

_____

(Courtesy of Gastrointestinal Specialists, Inc.)

BOX 12–2G. **REPORT OF PROCEDURE**

Gastrointestinal Specialists, Inc.

Report of Procedure

PATIENT NUMBER: DATE:

SURGEON:

PREOPERATIVE DIAGNOSIS:

POSTOPERATIVE DIAGNOSIS:

OPERATION:

PROCEDURE:

(Courtesy of Gastrointestinal Specialists, Inc.)

BOX 12–2H. **POSTPROCEDURE INSTRUCTIONS**

POSTPROCEDURE INSTRUCTIONS FOR GASTROSCOPY

1 You may not eat for 20 minutes after the procedure.

2 You may not drive for 6 hours after the procedure.

3 You may be drowsy. Do not operate any dangerous machinery or lift any heavy machinery.

4 If you have a sore throat, you may use a throat lozenge or cough drop.

5 Report to us if you develop a fever, chest or abdominal pain, or black or bloody stools.

6 If you have any questions or problems, do not hesitate to call our office at 664-9700.

(Courtesy of Gastrointestinal Specialists, Inc.)

References

Erdman, Marshall and Associates. *Medical Office/Ambulatory Healthcare Facilities.* Madison, WI: Erdman, Marshall and Associates, 1993.

Erdman, Marshall and Associates. *Organizing, Designing and Building Medical Office/Ambulatory Healthcare Facilities.* Madison, WI: Erdman, Marshall and Associates, 1994.

Erdman, Marshall and Associates. *Planning, Designing and Constructing Group Practice Facilities.* Madison, WI: Erdman, Marshall and Associates, 1993.

Ross, A., Williams, S., & Schafer, E. *Ambulatory Care Management.* Albany, NY: Delmar Publishers, 1991.

Travers, E. *Managing the Physician's Office Laboratory.* New York: McGraw-Hill, 1994.

13

Business Systems and the Medical Office Manager's Financial Responsibilities

An Introduction to Accounting

Fra Luca Pacioli, a scholar, mathematician, and Franciscan monastery director who lived in the 15th century, is known as the "father of accounting." He was the first one given credit for using the double-entry bookkeeping method, which had already been in use among Italian merchants for two centuries. This double-entry model became the standard for accounting in the Western world.

To put it simply, accounting is the art of interpreting, measuring, and describing economic activity. It is called the "language of business." We live in a time of accountability, a time of multinational corporations, banks, buyouts, and the growing realization that health care is a business (just like anything else). The purpose of accounting is to provide financial information about an economic entity, such as a medical office.

An accounting system must be developed and implemented in order to communicate financial information. An accounting system consists of methods, procedures, and devices a business uses to keep track of its financial activities and to summarize them in an effort to make decisions. Three basic steps must be included in any accounting system: recording, classifying, and summarizing. *Recording* the daily office activities in terms of money is the first step. Any transactions that can be expressed in monetary terms must be entered into the accounting record. *Classifying* data into related groups or categories of transactions should be the second step. *Summarizing* the data in these categories is the third step in the process.

Cost accounting is determining what it costs the medical office to perform a particular service. For example, the office manager should know what it costs the office to do an x-ray exam. Cost accounting is valuable for understanding the cost of each procedure and the total cost to the office of a patient's visit to the office or the hospital. It is used to evaluate whether or not to participate in insurance plans. An insurance company's fee schedules can be compared with the costs of seeing the patient. The office can then decide whether to participate in the insurance plan.

Two Major Financial Statements: The Balance Sheet and Income/Expense Statement

The two financial statements most commonly used in the medical practice are the balance sheet and the income/expense statement.

THE BALANCE SHEET

The *balance sheet* is a financial statement showing the assets, liabilities, and owner's equity of the medical practice. Assets are the economic resources owned by the practice, liabilities are the debts or financial obligations of the practice, and owner's equity is the owner's residual interest in the practice. A *ledger account* is a device for recording the increases or decreases in one financial statement item, such as a particular asset, a type of liability, or owner's equity. A *ledger* is an accounting record that includes the ledger accounts, for all items included in the practice's financial statements.

It is important to understand the differences between debits and credits. *Increases in assets* are recorded by *debits,* and *decreases in assets* are recorded by *credits. Increases in liabilities and owner's equity* are recorded by *credits,* and *decreases in liabilities and owner's equity* are recorded by *debits*. The debit and credit rules are related to an account's location in the balance sheet. If the account appears on the lefthand side of the balance sheet (assets), increases in the account balance are recorded by left-side entries (debits). If the account appears on the righthand side of the balance sheet (liabilities and owner's equity), increases are recorded by right-side entries. Every transaction is recorded by two sets of entries; hence the system is called the double-entry system of accounting. Debit entries to one or more accounts and credit entries to one or more accounts make up this system. In the recording of any transaction, the total dollar amount of the debit entries must equal the total dollar amount of the credit entries. Journal entries must be made to record common business transactions. Each journal entry should include

1 The date of the transaction
2 The names of the ledger accounts affected
3 The dollar amounts of the changes in these accounts
4 A brief explanation of the transaction

THE INCOME/EXPENSE STATEMENT

The *income/expense statement* shows the cumulative profit and total expenses for the month. It also provides such information as employees' withholding and pension plan contributions. A sample statement should be itemized to include the following operating expenses:

Automobile
Collections
Contributions
Medical supplies
Office supplies

Professional dues and subscriptions
Education
Travel and entertainment
Insurance
Interest
Licenses and taxes
Telephone
Utilities
Rent/mortgage
Salaries
Payroll taxes
Accounting/legal services
Maintenance
Refunds to patients
Refunds to managed care
Miscellaneous

By using this format, the office can keep track of expenditures and will notice a trend in increases or decreases easily. Other expenditures that might be added to this statement are

Equipment and improvements
Employee taxes paid
Employee taxes held
Employee contributions withheld
Employee contributions paid
Personal draw on account

This conclusion of this statement specifies the

Total charges
Starting balance
Total deposits
Total expenditures
Ending balance

How to Read a Statement of Retained Earnings

If the income/expense statement reveals the office's performance during a period, and the balance sheet shows a picture of the office at the end of that period, shouldn't that picture reflect that performance? It does. The net income for the period is added to the equity account called *retained earnings* to show that profits are reinvested into the company. Any profits paid to the physician owners as dividends reduce retained earnings. Although this account reflects reinvested earnings, it does not represent cash. It is possible for an office with a growing clientele to experience financial problems. This is one reason why the office manager should have an understanding of the mechanics of cash flow.

Cash Flow Statements

The cash flow statement reveals not only the increase or decrease in the collected cash for that period, but the accounts, by category, that caused that change. To read and understand a cash flow statement, you must start at the bottom of the statement, where the increase or decrease in cash and the beginning and ending balances are revealed. It is important to understand the office's cash balance and how it changed during the periods that are being reviewed. Next, look at the total change in cash caused by the three major activities presented on this statement: operating, investing, and financing. To understand the medical office's daily cash flow fully, you need to analyze the increases and decreases in cash caused by changes in the working capital accounts and the revenue and expense accounts. Cash flows from operating activities can be presented using either the direct method or the indirect method. In the direct method, cash inflows and outflows are summarized for major categories, including the following:

- Cash received from customers
- Cash paid to employees and suppliers
- Cash paid for interest
- Cash paid for taxes

Although the direct method is a more intuitive approach to understanding cash flows from operating activities, it is the indirect method that is seen in most annual reports. The indirect method lists net income followed by a series of adjustments to remove the effects of accrual accounting. The first adjustment is to add back depreciation expense, because it is a noncash expense that was subtracted when determining net income. This subtotal is then added or subtracted to the cash that was created or consumed by the working capital accounts. It is in these accounts that cash seems to appear and disappear mysteriously. The resulting cash flow from operating activities is one of the most important indicators of the company's performance. From this brief review of the statement of cash flows, you should have a general sense of

- The amount of cash created or consumed by daily operations, including the cash effect from changes in working capital accounts
- The amount of cash invested in fixed or other assets
- The proceeds from the sale of stock or payments for dividends
- The increase or decrease in cash for the period

Because each of the financial statements presents a different focus on the practice's financial health—financial position versus operating performance versus cash flow—you must review them all to get a complete comprehensive picture.

Financial Ratios Tell the Story

Financial ratios provide statistics and information that allow you to evaluate how well the medical practice is doing and compare it with other practices in the same specialty or the same geographical area. You can also tell how well individual physicians are doing. You convert raw numbers from the current year's and prior years' financial statements into different ratios that highlight different financial characteristics, such as profitability and liquidity. However, before you rely completely on specific ratios, remember these words of advice: Avoid drawing a strong conclusion from any one ratio and refer back to the specific accounts involved in the statements to see if the numbers confirm what the ratios suggest.

ACCOUNTS RECEIVABLE RATIO

The *accounts receivable ratio* is a formula for measuring how fast outstanding accounts are being paid. This analysis gives you useful pictures of the status of collections and of probable losses. The longer past due an account receivable becomes, the greater the likelihood that it will not be collected in full. The accounts receivable distribution is one of the most important thermometers of the health of the practice. A practice that has good billing and insurance habits will show an accounts receivable distribution that looks like this:

Current	31–60 days	61–90 days	91–120 days	Over 120
75%	10–12%	6–7%	4–5%	5%

These figures are percentages of the total balance, and they will vary depending on the type of practice and on the payer mix the practice has. You can use the accounts receivable ratio in office meetings to show either the inefficiency or efficiency of the billing department.

$$\frac{\text{Total accounts receivable}}{\text{Monthly receipts}} = \text{Dollar turn around}$$

For example, if your office had a total accounts receivable of $130,000, with a monthly receipt of $63,000, the accounts receivable ratio would look like this:

$$\frac{\$130,000}{\$63,000} = 2.06\%$$

$$2.06\% \ (\% \text{ of month}) \times 30 = 61.8 \text{ days}$$
is the turnaround time for payment of an account.

COLLECTION RATIO

The *collection ratio* is a financial calculation that shows the percentage of outstanding debt collected. This is a good tool for instructing and motivating the collection department. This ratio is as follows:

$$\frac{\text{Total receipts}}{\text{Total charges}} = \text{Collection ratio (unadjusted)}$$

For example, if the total receipts were $30,000 and the total charges were $40,000, the unadjusted collection ratio would be as follows:

$$\frac{\$30,000}{\$40,000} = 75\% \text{ Collection ratio (unadjusted)}$$

The *adjusted collection ratio* takes into consideration the adjustments of

- Medicare
- Medicaid
- Workers' Compensation
- Managed care
- Other adjustments

The adjusted collection ratio for the preceding example would be as follows:

Total receipts = $30,000
Add:
Medicare Adj $2,000
Managed Care Adj $3,000
Medicaid Adj $1,000
                            $6,000 + $30,000 = $36,000

$$\frac{\$36,000}{\$40,000} = 90\% \text{ Collection ratio (adjusted)}$$

BILLING RATE

The *billing rate* is an indicator of the average billing per patient. This is calculated by dividing the total billing per month by the total number of patients per month.

$$\frac{\text{Total billing}}{\text{No. of patients}} = \text{Average billing per patient}$$

For example, if the total billing for that month was

$318,000 and the total number of patients for that month was 3,700, the ratio would look like this:

$$\frac{\$318,000}{3,700} = \$85.94 \text{ average billing per patient}$$

SALARY RATE

The *salary rate* is an indicator of the average amount of money a physician makes on a patient.

$$\frac{\text{Total salary}}{\text{Total patients}} = \$ \text{ per patient}$$

For example, if Dr. Smith earned $40,000 in one month for seeing 525 patients, the salary rate for Dr. Smith would be as follows:

$$\frac{\$40,000}{525 \text{ patients}} = \$76.19 \text{ per patient}$$

OVERHEAD RATIO

The *overhead ratio* shows the cost of the office overhead on a monthly basis. By taking the total expenses, subtracting the physician benefits, and then dividing by the adjusted receipts, you can calculate the overhead. It is very important to monitor this figure not only monthly, but also on a year-to-date basis. This makes it easier to see a trend in overhead increases.

$$\frac{\text{Total expenses} - \text{Physician benefits}}{\text{Adjusted receipts}} = \text{Overhead \%}$$

Physician benefits consist of

- Medical insurance
- Auto expense
- Meals and entertainment
- Salary expense
- Travel and lodging

For instance, a sample overhead ratio would look like this:

Physician benefits:		
Medical insurance	$	500
Auto expense	$	500
Meals and entertainment	$	250
Salary expense	$	8750
Travel and lodging	$	0
		$10,000

$$\frac{\$45,500 - \$10,000}{\$40,000} = 88.7\% \text{ overhead expense}$$

COST RATIO *Profit*

To calculate the cost of performing a procedure or service in the office, divide the total expenses for 1 month by the number of procedures performed that month. The ratio is as follows:

$$\frac{\text{Total expenses}}{\text{Total no. of procedures}} = \text{Cost per procedure}$$

For example, if the total expenses were $4,800 for 1 month and the total number of procedures for that month was 24, the ratio would look like this:

$$\frac{\$4,800}{24} = \$200 \text{ cost per procedure}$$

REVENUE RATIO

To calculate the *revenue ratio*, divide the total revenue by the number of procedures performed in any given period. The ratio is as follows:

$$\frac{\text{Total revenue}}{\text{Total no. of procedures}} = \text{Revenue per procedure}$$

For example, if the total revenue was $7,200 and the total number of procedures was 24, the ratio would look like this:

$$\frac{\$7,200}{24} = \$300 \text{ revenue per procedure}$$

PROFIT RATIO

The *profit ratio* is the amount of profit after total overhead and expenses are met. The ratio is as follows:

Total revenue − Total costs = Profit
$300 − $200 = $100 profit on each procedure/service

Cost Analysis

The cost, revenue, and profit ratios are used in many medical offices to evaluate the financial profitability of providing certain services in the office. For instance, an ophthalmologist might want to perform cataract surgery in her or his office. After arriving at the total revenues from providing this service in the office and subtracting the total costs of providing this service in the office, the ophthalmologist can determine whether the margin is enough to make it profitable. Some offices use the cost, revenue, and profit ratios to determine whether simple laboratory studies or x-ray exams should be done in their offices. By using these three ratios, the office is performing what is called a *cost analysis* in business.

Cost analysis is a very important aspect of the practice. It involves research and tedious amounts of work to determine exactly how much it costs the practice to provide a service. This same analysis is used by companies when they are deciding on the price to charge for a product they have produced and marketed. Two cost factors are involved in cost analysis: fixed costs and variable costs. *Fixed costs* are costs that do not change during a short period of time. Examples of fixed costs are mortgage payments, equipment lease payments, rent, depreciation of equipment, and insurance payments. *Variable costs* are costs that change regularly. Examples of variable costs are medical supplies, office supplies, electricity bills, billing services, and laboratory and x-ray services.

The cost factor of each patient begins when she or he enters the office. There are administrative costs associated with the cost of maintaining the patient's records and sending bills to the patient. There are support personnel costs that arise from the care that the nurse or technician provides the patient. There is the cost of the capital equipment—supplies such as laboratory machines, gauze dressings, and alcohol pads—used on the patient. Let's not forget the cost of the physician. The physician cost is made up of the cost of malpractice insurance, the cost of interpreting tests, the cost of diagnosing the condition, and the cost of implementing treatment. Many office managers—and physicians, for that matter—do not completely understand how much it costs the physician to see a patient in the office. By calculating and reviewing cost analyses, the office obtains information necessary to set fees and to market its services. Cost analyses help determine profit and monitor the practice's performance.

General practitioners and family practice physicians typically spend more on overhead than do such specialists as anesthesiologists and radiologists. Box 13–1 lists the overhead expenses of some specialists.

It can cost the office many dollars if you wait until the end of the year to check on practice trends. A practical and easy way to control the office's finances is to estimate the expenses and income for the next year. This can be done annually, quarterly, or even monthly. The expense categories listed in Box 13–1 can be used as a guide.

Flash Reports

A *Flash Report* is a series of calculations that can aid you and the physician in the financial management of the practice. This report should be distributed on a monthly basis to all physicians in the practice and should be discussed at monthly meetings. It can be used as a tool in taking the pulse of the practice. It shows trends in practice growth, expenses, and revenues. A sample Flash Report is shown in Box 13–2.

Steps in an Accounting System

1 Record transactions in a cash journal.
2 Post information into ledger accounts.

BOX 13–1. **MEAN OVERHEAD EXPENSES BY SPECIALTY**

Specialty	Payroll	Auto	Rent	Malpractice	Medical Education	Supply
Family practice	18.9%	1.9%	6.0%	2.6%	1.0%	4.1%
OB/GYN	13.6%	1.7%	6.1%	8.1%	1.1%	2.5%
Psychiatry	6.7%	2.4%	5.4%	1.6%	1.4%	1.6%
Anesthesia	5.7%	2.1%	2.0%	8.7%	1.4%	0.8%
Pediatrics	18.0%	2.1%	6.8%	2.5%	0.8%	4.8%
Internal medicine	14.4%	1.9%	6.1%	2.4%	0.9%	2.1%
General surgery	11.3%	1.9%	4.9%	7.0%	1.1%	1.5%

BOX 13–2. **SAMPLE FLASH REPORT**

Flash Report for _____ (month) _____

Total number of patients   _____

Total number of new patients   _____

Total charges   _____

Total deposits   _____

Billing rate   _____

Collection rate (unadjusted)   _____

Collection rate (adjusted)   _____

Salary rate   _____

Accounts receivable ratio   _____

Overhead ratio   _____

3 Prepare a trial balance.
4 Prepare financial statements.

In most computerized medical offices, Steps 2 through 4 are done automatically by the computer.

Profits are the bottom line for every office and what every physician wants to know. Economists define *profits* as the point at which the business is better off during a specified period of time. Accountants like to call profits "net incomes" and define them as the excess of the price of services rendered over the cost of rendering those services during a specific period of time. The dictionary defines *profit* as a "valuable return." However you define it, it is the most important segment of the business side of the practice!!

Types of Medical Accounting Systems

Various types of accounting systems exist, so it is important for you to recognize the needs of the office and how they may be met by the use of different systems. The three most common systems are

1 Pegboard systems
2 Single-entry systems
3 Double-entry systems

Not all medical offices have the same needs, and even

though these three systems are based on the same principles, they differ somewhat in application.

PEGBOARD SYSTEM

The pegboard system not only is easy to operate, but makes the possibility of employee dishonesty less likely. It provides control over collections, payments, and charges. It provides a "running balance" on patient accounts and is easily used by office personnel. The initial cost of using this system might be higher than the initial cost of using other systems, but the ease of use and the control that it provides speak for themselves. To use this system, a pegboard and specially printed forms must be purchased. This pegboard is generally made of metal or plastic and contains a series of pegs down its left side for holding the forms in place. This system is a "one write" system. That is, by placing the forms in the correct manner on the board, the user writes an entry on the daily sheet, an entry on the patient ledger card, and a "walk away" statement for the patient (showing the amount paid and the amount outstanding) all at the same time. The use of this system also eliminates errors that result from the need to make repetitive entries (Figure 13–1).

SINGLE-ENTRY SYSTEM

The single-entry system is one of the oldest methods of accounting used in the medical office. It is more cumbersome than the pegboard system, because it involves the use of three accounting records. These

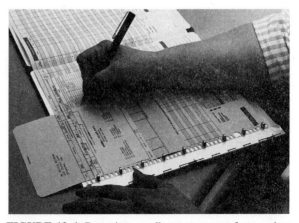

FIGURE 13–1. Preparing a walk-out statement for a patient using a pegboard system.

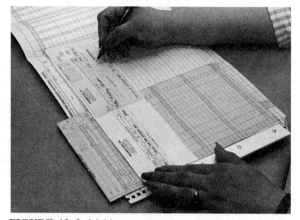

FIGURE 13–2. Making an entry into the accounts payable book using the pegboard system of bookkeeping.

records are a cash journal, a day sheet, and an accounts receivable ledger.

Columnar paper can be useful when the office chooses this system. Columnar paper allows you to record charges, receipts, and payments made to the physician for her or his services. A ledger card is kept for each patient or her or his family for the recording of accounts receivable transactions. In the single-entry system, each entry is written separately, which becomes not only tedious, but time-consuming. Moreover, there are no built-in controls in this system, which opens many avenues for employee dishonesty (Figure 13–2).

DOUBLE-ENTRY SYSTEM

The double-entry system is not as popular as the pegboard and single-entry systems. To use this system correctly, personnel must be trained in simple accounting and bookkeeping procedures. This system is based on the accounting principle that assets equal liabilities and capital. Each and every time a transaction is entered, it must be entered on both sides of the equation, and all transactions must remain in balance at all times. Control is built in with this system; however, its complicated procedures make it less likely to be used in a medical office.

How to Choose an Accountant

Whom to hire as an accountant is one of the most crucial decisions the medical office manager makes. Be aware of the needs of the office and of all candidates available before deciding on an accountant for the office. It was once thought to be beneath a physician to consider her or his practice a business, and physicians perceived the business aspect of medicine as a hindrance. Few still think so today. However, perhaps as a carryover from the old days, many physicians view accountants simply as number crunchers and do not use their talents to the fullest. You can open the physician's eyes, if necessary, and help her or him choose an accountant who will strive for the maximum return on all the hard work the physician, you, and the staff do. *Never* just hire a friend, neighbor, or former classmate of the physician—or a friend of anyone's, for that matter. An accountant is nothing less than a business investment. Choose the best!

Before beginning the search for an accountant, you need to determine the goals of the practice. Does the physician anticipate growth? Look to retire? Simply wish to skate by for the coming years? The physician who is looking for practice growth requires an accountant with expertise in business development and marketing. The physician who is facing retirement requires less financial planning (because most of this should already be done) and needs fewer accounting services. Discuss in detail with the physician her or his priorities and goals for the practice to help in evaluating an accountant.

QUALITIES OF A GOOD ACCOUNTANT

A good accountant *is well versed in basic accounting knowledge.* She or he is able to answer such simple questions as "Should we lease or purchase a photocopy machine?"; "Should we incorporate?"; and "What is the best method for obtaining financing?" It is good to know in advance the range of advice the accountant will be able to provide the office.

A good accountant *interviews you as you are interviewing her or him.* That is, the accountant wants to know and understand how your office works. The good accountant wants a list of the office's priorities so that it is easier to focus on relevant issues. An accountant who is really on the ball wants to know the source of the office referrals. It is important to position the office so that it generates business in the manner in which the physician wants it to. Is the patient base referred by other doctors or the result of high visibility in the community?

A good accountant also *wants to know the physician's future plans on a personal level.* Does the physician plan to run for political office in the future? Is the physician's main goal in life to be an old-time "horse and buggy"-type doctor? Some physicians want to broaden their careers by devoting time to lecturing, networking, and serving on various boards, both professional and community based.

A good accountant *has expertise in the intricacies of the medical profession.* Check candidates' references to see if they have other clients in the health care profession. Ask candidates whether they are familiar with the problems associated with medical billing. Do they have an understanding of third-party billing? Do they understand coding and how it affects reimbursement?

A good accountant *not only prepares monthly statements, but sits and explains these statements to you and the physician in a language you can understand.* These reports become a valuable tool in troubleshooting. An easy way to understand accounting procedures is to think of a balance sheet as a snapshot of the financial condition of the practice on a particular day. A balance sheet is a financial statement that indicates what assets the business owns and how those assets are financed in the form of liabilities or ownership interest. An income statement can be considered a video of the practice's financial condition over a particular time period. An income statement is a financial statement that measures the profitability of the business over a period of time. All expenses are subtracted from services to arrive at a net income. There are a variety of reports for example, an aged trial balance and an income statement analysis, that should be run monthly. The good accountant explains what the various reports tell you about the practice. This accountant wants to see a financial statement so that she or he can analyze the whole picture, not just its parts.

A good accountant *is knowledgeable about salaries, hiring and firing issues, health insurance plans, Workers' Compensation, and disability.* You should be able to look to the accountant for advice when you are shopping around for health insurance for the employees. The accountant is not expected to know everything there is to know about each subject; however, she or he should know the basics and know where to go to get help if needed in these areas.

The good accountant *can be consulted every time there is new equipment to be bought.* By way of a cost–benefit analysis, the accountant will tell you whether the ultimate benefit of the purchase will justify the cost.

The good accountant *is well versed in retirement plans.* The physician will want a feasibility study done,

with plans to install and carry out the necessary steps for retirement. If the accountant does not have expertise in financial planning, she or he should be able to recommend someone who does. Information regarding profit sharing and pension plans is highly important to most medical offices. The accountant should recommend the appropriate plan for an office of your size, number of employees, and cash flow.

A good accountant *is aware of how all new tax laws affect the medical office and thinks over the office's tax situation and offers recommendations in a proactive way.* Tax laws are too complex for there to be a black-and-white answer to every question. They are subject to the interpretations of business owners and the IRS. The physician and the accountant should have similar philosophies regarding the interpretation of tax laws. Conservative or aggressive, the accountant should be in tune with the physician's general philosophy about taxes and understand how much creativity the physician wants her or him to use. As an example, whereas the uncreative accountant sees the physician's family members as dependency exemptions, the creative accountant sees them as avenues for income splitting to reduce taxes. It's not good to be *too* conservative. Ask candidates how many of their clients have been audited by the IRS. If the answer is none or very few, the candidate may be too conservative. In addition, be wary of any accountant who seems more intimidated by the IRS than the office is. There is a difference between a conservative accountant and an accountant who is afraid to have her or his work examined.

There are three ways to handle a tax situation, and two of them are the wrong ways! The first is to lower your taxes and improve your cash flow. The second way is to overpay your taxes. The third way is to be challenged by the IRS and lose. The second and third ways should not even be considered! Meetings with the accountant should take place not only at tax time, but on a regular basis throughout the year. You and the physician should be continually informed of financial, business, and tax strategies. Monthly financial statements should show a clear picture of the practice as well as serve as a springboard for ideas on how to improve the bottom line of the practice, such as by lowering your taxes.

ACCOUNTANTS' FEES

The more contact the office has with the accountant, the higher the bills will be. When the bills reflect the quality of work done, the physician should authorize payment of these services. In general, an accounting firm will bill for services on an hourly rate commensurate with the level of the professional who performed the work. These fees can range from $65.00 to $250.00 an hour, depending on the complexity of the work done and the status of the accountant within the firm. A senior partner will come with a higher price tag than a new associate (Figure 13–3).

How to Choose a Financial Advisor

It is never an easy task to decide whom to trust with the profits. Financial advisors come in various shapes and sizes; however, there are a few questions to ask that should help the selection process.

"Tell me about your firm. How long have you been in business?"
"What is your professional background?"
"What qualifies you to advise me on these subjects?"
"Describe your typical client."
"What is your investment philosophy? Is it conservative or aggressive?"
"Who handles the money in your household?"
"Do your clients rely solely on you for advice?"
"Do your clients do a lot of their own homework?"
"How often do you speak with your clients?"
"How do you interact with your clients' other professional advisors?"
"What sets you apart from others in your field?"

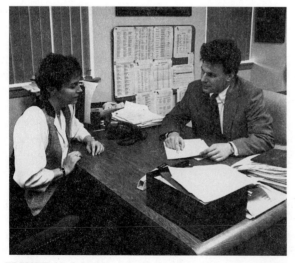

FIGURE 13–3. Having a good working relationship with the accountant is important.

"Why do you want to do business with me?"
A financial advisor should want to understand the needs of the practice and meet them. She or he should always be there to guide the office in decision making and answer all questions that are raised. The most important concern is that the financial advisor have the same philosophy as the office.

Banking on the Right Bank

The first bank in the United States opened in 1791 in Philadelphia. At one time, there was no doubt that a bank was a stable institution; however, since 1986, the stability of all banking institutions has varied. Considering that since 1986, 1,000 banks in the United States have failed, you should evaluate all possible banks before choosing the bank for the practice. To protect the office from losses by choosing an unstable bank, you can now call VERIBANC at 1-800-442-2657 to receive a report on the financial stability of each bank you are considering. VERIBANC is a bank rating and analysis firm in Massachusetts that reports any adverse financial conditions that might be found in a banking institution.

In 1992, there were 10,673 banks in the United States. Of them, 25 were insolvent, 199 were nearly insolvent, and 224 were "troubled." A bank that is insolvent is one whose liabilities are greater than the reasonable market value of its assets. With the cost-containment measures being imposed on the health care profession today, the last thing the medical office wants to deal with is a troubled bank. The five most stable states for banking are Iowa, Pennsylvania, Michigan, Alabama, and Illinois. The five worst states for banking stability are New Hampshire, Connecticut, Rhode Island, Massachusetts, and Washington, D.C. You can also find out about problems with banks simply by reading articles in local newspapers regarding poor financial performance, management shake-ups, or regulatory examinations.

Choosing the Correct Bank Account

Banks offer a variety of services that can be used by the medical office (Figure 13–4). They offer four basic types of accounts: checking accounts, savings accounts, money market accounts, and CDs. Although most banks offer the same types of accounts, be sure to read the fine print when choosing the account for the office. To open

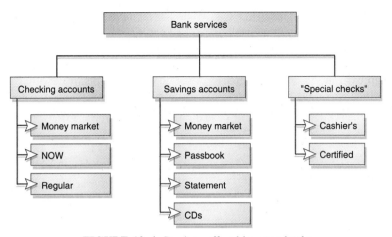

FIGURE 13–4. Services offered by most banks.

the office account, the physician should appear at the bank branch that has been selected with the following items: money to deposit into the account, personal identification, a business license (some banks also ask to see a medical license), and her or his social security number or tax ID number.

Checking Accounts

Checking accounts are the backbone of the banking system today. Most people now use checks to pay their bills. In fact, an average family writes approximately 20 checks in a month. When a staff member deposits a check into the office account, it is sent to the bank of the patient who wrote the check. The bank then takes money out of the patient's account and transfers it to the office account. How soon the office account will be credited depends on where the patient's bank, or the insurance company's bank, is located. To be safe, always allow 2 to 5 days for the amount deposited to become available. Figure 13–5 shows the path of a check once it is issued to the physician's office.

If a staff member writes a check in error and the office wishes to stop payment on it, the bank will issue a "stop payment order" on the check for a fee. Most banks will ask that the office manager, or appropriate person, sign the appropriate form in person. Some banks will allow individuals to arrange a stop payment order over the telephone. (Having a good working relationship with

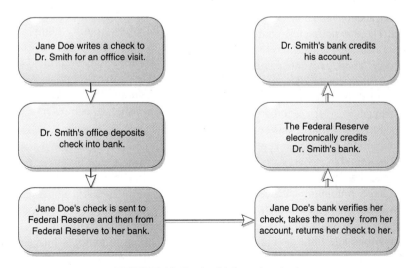

FIGURE 13–5. The lifeline of a check.

personnel at the bank comes in handy at times like this. Make sure that you become well known in the bank in which the office does its business.) The stop payment order is good for 6 months in most banks.

If there is not enough cash in the office account to cover a check that the office wrote, the bank can refuse to pay on it. The office would be charged a fee (between $12.00 and $35.00) for checks returned, and the individual to whom the check was issued will also be charged a fee.

The best way to avoid overdrafts on office checks is to apply for overdraft protection. This will prevent embarrassing situations with vendors and others if your bookkeeper should happen to make a mistake. The bank would automatically transfer the necessary funds to cover the check. Overdraft protection saves the office money, embarrassment, and aggravation. Keep in mind that chronic bouncing of checks can affect the office's credit rating.

If a patient issues the office a bad check, the same fees apply. Some banks will not charge the practice's account if a patient's check is returned to her or him for non-sufficient funds.

TYPES OF CHECKING ACCOUNTS

The three most common types of checking accounts are

1 Regular checking accounts
2 NOW accounts
3 Money market accounts

Regular checking accounts allow the office to write as many checks as necessary. The bank charges a fee for each check written on the account and a fee for monthly service on the account. There is no interest paid on the account. *NOW accounts* also allow the office to write as many checks as necessary. These accounts pay a small interest on the balance in the account. These accounts generally come with added incentives, such as free traveler's checks, no annual fees for credit cards, and sometimes discounts on loans. These accounts generally require that a certain minimum balance be kept in the account at all times. *Money market accounts* provide the office with an interest rate that changes on the basis of market conditions. A large minimum balance is required, and the fees for going below this balance can be severe. Some money market accounts limit the number of checks that may be written and limit the number of transfers per month.

The *minimum balance* is the smallest amount that can be kept in an account to qualify the account for certain benefits, such as reduced fees or free checking. Some banks define the minimum as the combined amount in all of your accounts. If the office can take advantage of minimum balance options, it will save money. Ask your local bank what its requirements are.

THE ANATOMY OF A CHECK

Checks are an everyday part of any type of business, including the medical office. More than 90% of the payments received in the medical office are checks. No one ever attends a course on "How To Write a Check" or "The Components of a Check." There are three different kinds of information found on the front of a check. Some information is preprinted on the check, some is handwritten on the check, and some is printed on the check during processing at the bank. Figure 13–6 shows a drawing of a check. The following is a list of the parts of the check.

1 The name and address of the owner of the check
2 The date the check was written
3 The check number
4 The bank ID number
5 The name of the person to whom the check was written
6 The amount that the check was written for
7 The name of the bank on which the check was drawn
8 A memo area where the reason for the check can be noted
9 The signature that authorized the transaction (it must correspond to the bank card that was signed)
10 The check routing number (identifies the bank and the Federal Reserve in the area)
11 The check number, printed again when the check was processed
12 The amount of the transaction is printed at time of processing, so computers can scan it for accuracy

Staff should be trained to make sure that a check is filled out completely by the patient before they accept it. Always make sure the patient has signed the check. There are times that patients are so distracted that they forget to sign the check. Some patients will even write out the check, sign it, and then close their checkbook and leave the office with the check in their checkbook. It is important to treat the financial part of the visit as carefully as the clinical part.

CHECK ENDORSEMENT

The endorsement of the check is an important step when accepting a check from a patient. The purpose of the endorsement is to transfer the rights in the check to another individual. The first step employees should take when accepting a check from a patient is to stamp the back of the check with a stamp reading "For Deposit Only" and possibly the account number of the office checking account.

Patients may present the office with a check from a third-party payer that they would like to sign over to the office. This can be done, but certain steps must be followed for proper endorsement of this check. The patient, or guarantor, first signs the back of the check in ink. Then, under her or his signature, the patient writes "Pay to the order of" and the physician's name. The check may then be accepted by the office.

> **MANAGER'S ALERT**
>
> NEVER accept a postdated check from a patient. If this situation arises, have the patient date the check with the date of the visit, place the check in an envelope on which is written the date the check can be deposited, and place the envelope in a locked drawer until the date on the envelope.

CHECK NO-NO'S

- Do not accept checks with corrections on them. Ask patients to issue another check if they made an error when writing the first one.
- Do not accept a check marked "Payment in Full" if the check does not pay the account in full. Legally, you would not be able to collect the remaining balance.
- Accept checks only for the exact amount owed for the services rendered.
- Do not cash a check for a patient.
- Do not accept an out-of-town check unless it is from a family member of one of your patients.

BAD CHECKS

Some checks that are issued to a physician's office do not clear the bank for one reason or another—a mixup in bookkeeping on the patient's part, information missing from the check, or a stop payment order. In any case, the bottom line is that the office does not receive payment for that service. Banks will hold a check for 3 to 5 days before clearing it for deposit into the account. If you should call the bank to inquire about the balance of the office's account, the bank will generally offer two amounts: the balance and the currently available balance. The balance is the amount that has been deposited by the office. This should match the deposit slips. The currently available balance is the amount of the checks that have already cleared and whose funds are now available. The difference between these two figures is

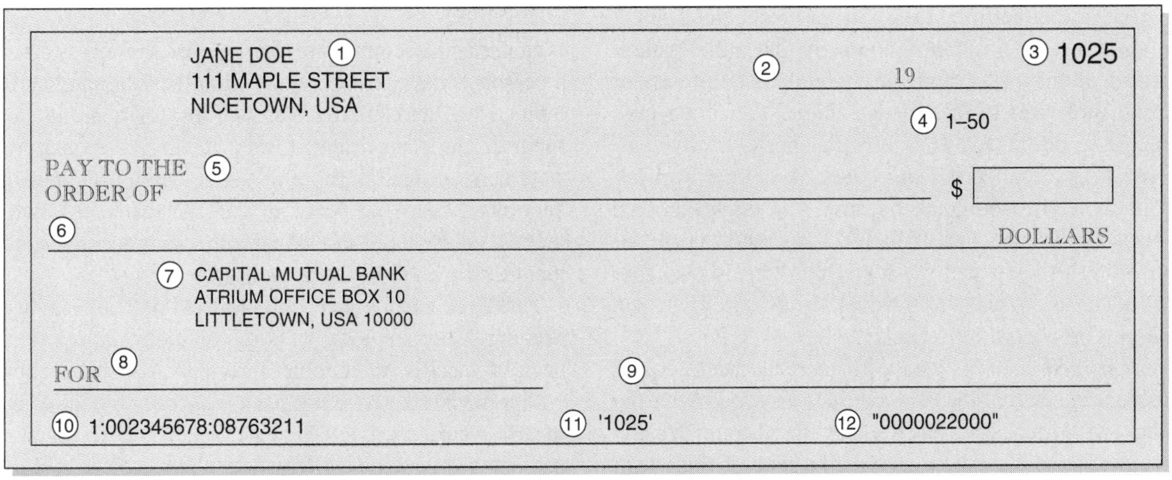

FIGURE 13–6. The parts of a check (see text for explanation of numbers).

the amount of the checks that have not yet cleared the bank, making the funds unavailable until they clear.

How long it takes a check to clear the bank depends on whether

1 The check is drawn on the same bank that the office uses.
2 The check is drawn on a local bank.
3 The check is drawn on an out-of-town bank.
4 The check is drawn on an out-of-state bank.

If the check is drawn on the same bank that the office uses, the check amount will become available immediately. If the check is drawn on a different bank in town, the funds should be available no later than 2 days from the date of deposit. If the check is drawn on an out-of-town bank, it is usually cleared in no later than 3 days. If the check is drawn on a bank in a different state, it is generally cleared within 5 days. Legislation in 1987 reduced the amount of time that a bank can hold a check to a maximum of 7 days from the date of deposit, but most banks clear a check within 5 days.

FROM THE AUTHOR'S NOTEBOOK

When a patient issues a bad check, it is always a good idea to note that event either in the financial section of the patient's chart or in the computer.

SPECIAL CHECKS

There are times when a business check is not enough, and a certified check or cashier's check must be used; if the insurance company pays the patient instead of the office and the amount that the patient has to turn over to the office is large, the office may request to be paid with a certified check. A *cashier's check* is also called a *bank check*. A cashier's check is guaranteed to be good, because it is drawn against a bank's own account. It includes a carbon copy for the office to keep with its records. There is a charge for a cashier's check; however, it is less than the charge for a certified check.

A *certified check* is also a guaranteed check. It is a business check that the bank certifies as good. After the check is written, the bank freezes the account for the amount of the check and stamps the face of the check with the word "certified." There is a fee associated with the purchasing of a certified check.

MANAGER'S ALERT

Once a cashier's check or certified check reaches its destination, you cannot put a stop payment order on it.

Traveler's checks and money orders also fall into the category of special checks. The office would not have any reason to purchase these checks; however, many patients use a traveler's check or money order to pay for services in the office. Provide the front-desk staff with information about these checks, so that when they appear, the staff understand them.

Traveler's checks are used by individuals who are traveling. They are issued by auto clubs, banks, and credit cards and come in various denominations. The purchaser must sign each check at the time of purchase and then again in front of the person to whom the purchaser is giving it for payment. Some patients pay their bills at the office with money orders. These are generally patients who do not have checking accounts. Money orders are to be accepted as cash. There is no risk involved in accepting money orders, and they should be included on the deposit slip as cash.

Types of Savings Accounts

There are three types of savings accounts:

1 Statement accounts
2 Passbook accounts
3 Money market accounts

Statement accounts are the type of savings account a person makes deposits on, withdraws from and earns interest on, and all the transactions for a month are reported on a statement. (Some banks issue quarterly statements instead of monthly statements.) If the person also has a checking account with that bank, the statement savings would show on the checking account statement that is received each month.

Passbook accounts are the old tried-and-true savings account. They are not very common today, most having been replaced with statement savings accounts. People with a passbook account have a passbook that they take to the bank each time they conduct a transaction involving the account. When they leave the bank, the transaction, be it a deposit or withdrawal, has been recorded in the passbook. The frequency with which interest is added to the account depends on the number of transactions conducted.

Money market accounts are savings accounts with checking incorporated into them. There is a limit on the number of checks that can be written each month. Money market accounts pay the most interest as long as a certain minimum balance is maintained.

Many savings accounts can be tied into checking accounts to provide overdraft protection. Savings accounts do not pay as much interest as CDs or money market funds, but the money is more "liquid," in other words, easy to retrieve if needed on short notice.

Do You Know Where Your Petty Cash Is?

Petty cash is a problem in many offices. Money is kept in a petty cash box, and no one is accountable for it. The size of an office's petty cash fund is determined by several factors: the size of the office, the types of purchases made, and the frequency with which it's replenished.

The secret to successful petty cash funds is to appoint one staff member to be accountable for all transactions. This person can be you or one of the other staff members. A voucher system should be used for all transactions. In other words, a balance should first be established. Generally, if large purchases are not made with petty cash, a balance of $75.00 to $100 is more than adequate. When a staff member finds it necessary to make a purchase from petty cash, she or he must present a slip for the amount spent. This slip should specify the date and the item purchased. If it does not, the petty cash attendant must write this information on it. At the end of the month, the slips are totaled and presented to the bookkeeper or physician, who in turn writes a check to petty cash to replace the amount spent. An example is as follows:

Total starting amount	$75.00
Purchases: Coffee, cream, sugar	$10.61
Extension cord	$ 2.79
Lightbulbs	$11.34
	$24.74

Slips totaling $24.74 are presented to the bookkeeper. The bookkeeper writes a check for $24.74 to petty cash, the check is cashed, and the money is placed in the petty cash fund.

Some offices use petty cash to purchase stamps. This is not a good idea, because it causes too much activity in the petty cash fund. Stamps should be bought with a separate check. This creates a paper trail and makes tracking easier.

Interest Calculations

Interest is calculated in one of three ways:

1 Day of deposit to day of withdrawal
2 Average daily balance
3 Lowest balance

In the day-of-deposit-to-day-of-withdrawal system, interest is earned every day the money is in the account. In the average-daily-balance system, interest is paid only on the average balance for the period of time the money is in the account. In the lowest-balance system, interest is paid only on the smallest balance during the period of time the money is in the account. For instance, if your bank was paying 6% interest using the day-of-deposit method and you made a deposit of $2,000 and a withdrawal of $1,000, your ending balance would be $1,000 + $12.00 in interest. If your bank paid 6% interest and used the average-daily-balance method and you deposited $2,000 and withdrew $1,000, your balance would again be $1,000 + $12.00 in interest. However, with the lowest-balance method, at 6% interest, your $2,000 deposit and $1,000 withdrawal would leave a balance of $1,000 + $6.00 in interest.

> ### MANAGER'S ALERT
>
> Be sure to check with the bank to see when it pays interest. Some accounts are credited on a quarterly basis, and if you withdraw before the quarter ends, you lose all the interest for that period.

Electronic Banking

The innovative banking methods available today allow the medical office to do its banking with the ease of a phone call. With electronic banking, the office can have its loan payments, mortgage or lease payments, insurance payments, and payments of utility and vendor bills automatically deducted from its checking account. When a bill arrives at the office, the bookkeeper simply calls the bank to authorize the payment of the bill directly from the office's checking account. Large

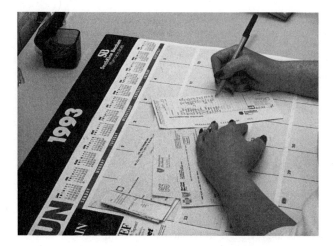

FIGURE 13–7. Preparing the daily deposit slip.

offices find this especially helpful. You must sign a consent form to authorize the automatic payment of these bills.

> ### MANAGER'S ALERT
>
> With electronic banking, it is often difficult to keep track of when bills are being paid and, therefore, difficult to maintain the appropriate balance in the account at the appropriate time. Always weigh the benefits against the risks before authorizing an electronic banking system.

Direct Deposits

The office might want to consider direct deposit for its employees. Direct deposit can be used for payroll, pensions, and Social Security payments. The amount is automatically deposited into the appropriate account on the designated day. The office simply files an application with the government or pension broker to arrange for electronic credit. The bank will do the rest. The employees may want the ease of direct deposits for their paychecks.

Night Depository

To maximize the office's cash flow, you should make sure that bank deposits are made on a daily basis. You can do this by using the night depository or going to the bank on a daily basis. Most medical offices use a night

DATE _____ 19 ____		
	DOLLARS	CENTS
CURRENCY		
COIN		
CHECKS		
1		
2		
3		
4		
5		
6		
7		
8		
9		
10		
11		
12		
13		
14		
15		
16		
17		
18		
19		
20		
21		
22		
23		
24		
25		
26		
PLEASE ENTER TOTAL		

TOTAL ITEMS

3–1
310

Checks and other items are received for deposit subject to the provisions of the Uniform Commercial Code or any applicable collection agreement.

DEPOSITS MAY NOT BE AVAILABLE FOR IMMEDIATE WITHDRAWAL

FIGURE 13–8. Sample deposit slip.

depository. To make night deposits, you need to buy a night deposit bag from the bank. The charge is about $25.00 and provides you with a reusable bag, a key to lock the bag, and a key to open the night depository at the bank. Some banks are now offering only disposable bags for nightly deposits, which can be costly. Try to avoid a bank with this type of system. These charges can run as much as $10.00 a week!

Preparing the Deposit Slip

The bank will appreciate it if the office knows the proper way to prepare the deposit slip (Figure 13–7). First, the cash should be counted and double-checked. The amount is then written on the deposit slip under "cash." Next, the checks should all be listed by inserting the bank number on the deposit slip in the block preceding the area where the amount of the check is written. Then the check amount is filled into the next block. An example of a deposit slip is shown in Figure 13–8.

References

Benson, R. *Professional Practice Builders.* Novato, CA: McVey Associates, 1993.

Berger, E. "Ten Questions To Help You Choose a Financial Advisor." *Executive Female,* May/June 1993, p. 58.

Bobryk, J. "Make Your CPA Accountable." *Physician's Management,* June 1992, pp. 109-127.

Cleverley, W. *Essentials of Health Care Finance.* Gaithersburg, MD: Aspen, 1993.

Farber, L. *Encyclopedia of Practice and Financial Management.* Oradell, NJ: Medical Economics, 1988.

Meigs, W. & Meigs, R. *Accounting: The Basis for Business Decisions.* New York: McGraw-Hill, 1987.

14

The Hospital

What is a Hospital?

The oldest hospital in the United States, Pennsylvania Hospital, was founded in Philadelphia in 1756. The definition of *hospital* is "a charitable institution for the needy, aged, infirm, or young where the sick or injured are given medical care."

Today's Physician–Hospital Relationship

As everyone is aware, the practice of medicine has changed a lot in the last two decades. A climate of curtailed inpatient admissions and reimbursements is driving individual physician practices into extinction and making it imperative for group medical practices and hospitals to rely on each other if they wish to thrive. Managed care policies are forcing the formation of key alliances between hospitals and clinics, between group medical practices and ambulatory surgical centers, and between health maintenance organizations (HMOs) and clinics. Hospitals and physicians are forming groups to negotiate better contracts with managed care companies. Hospitals are involving their medical staff in strategic decision making and are finding ways to accommodate the practical needs of physicians, including providing support for outpatient facilities.

The rise of managed care has made patient satisfaction the shared goal of hospitals and medical practices. Both hospitals and medical offices are striving to deliver quality care to each patient, to increase patient safety and comfort, and to improve the accuracy of diagnosis and treatment.

Attributes by Which Hospitals Are Classified

Hospitals can be distinguished by a number of different attributes:

- By the type of ownership they have (private or government)
- By the type of problems they treat (for example, tuberculosis or hypertension)
- By whether they play a role in physician education (teaching hospitals)
- By the average length of patients (short term or long term)
- By the type of medicine provided (medical or osteopathic)
- By the size of the institution (number of beds)

Hospital Ownership

There are three types of hospital ownership: government or public, voluntary, and proprietary.

GOVERNMENT OWNERSHIP

Government ownership refers to federal, state, or local government ownership of a hospital. Examples of federally owned hospitals are

- Veterans Administration hospitals
- Hospitals owned by the Department of Defense (for example, Bethesda Naval Hospital in Bethesda, Maryland, and Walter Reed Army Hospital in Washington, DC)
- Federal prison hospitals, owned by the Department of Justice
- Hospitals owned by the Department of Health and Human Services (Gallup Indian Medical Center in Gallup, New Mexico, and St. Elizabeths Hospital in Washington, DC)

The federal government operates military hospitals for the sole purpose of treating military personnel and their families.

Every state operates a hospital system designed specifically to treat the mentally ill or mentally retarded. These hospitals are used by state residents who cannot afford the care at another hospital. Some states also operate hospitals for the treatment of specific chronic illnesses, such as tuberculosis. Other state-owned hospitals are state university medical school hospitals and state prison hospitals.

VOLUNTARY OWNERSHIP

Voluntary ownership refers to private, nonprofit ownership of a hospital. Examples of voluntary hospitals are

- Hospitals owned by churches (for example, the Sisters of Mercy hospitals owned by the Roman Catholic Church)
- Shriners hospitals
- HMO hospitals (for example, the Kaiser-Permanente Hospital)

PROPRIETARY OWNERSHIP

Proprietary ownership refers to private, for-profit ownership of a hospital. Proprietary owners of hospitals range from corporations to individuals.

Types of Hospitals

TEACHING HOSPITALS

A teaching hospital is a hospital that has a physician residency training program. It has an agreement with a medical school to provide student physicians the clinical experience necessary for completion of their degree. Teaching hospitals also provide clinical experience for nurses and allied health personnel.

COMMUNITY HOSPITALS

A community hospital has a very broad definition. A community hospital is a hospital that serves a particular locality and/or is open to anyone, as opposed to being open only to particular patient groups. Community hospitals are generally nonteaching hospitals. A community hospital takes the name of the town or locale in which it is located. Some examples of community hospitals are Monroe County General Hospital, Doylestown Hospital, and Suburban General Hospital (Figure 14–1).

OSTEOPATHIC HOSPITALS

Osteopathic hospitals were started for the sole purpose of allowing osteopathic physicians to treat and hospitalize patients. Now osteopathic hospitals are found to have a mixed staff, that is, both medical physicians and osteopathic physicians. An osteopathic physician is one who is trained in osteopathy, a medical discipline founded by Andrew Taylor Still that is based on the theory that the body is capable of making its own remedies when its structure is normal. Practitioners of this discipline use the same medicinal, physical, and surgical methods of diagnosis and treatment that medical physicians use, while maintaining the importance of normal body mechanics and manipulation. As seen in Figure 14–1, Suburban General Hospital is not only a community hospital, but an osteopathic hospital as well.

MEDICAL HOSPITALS

Medical hospitals are not found much today. These hospitals allow only medical physicians to practice

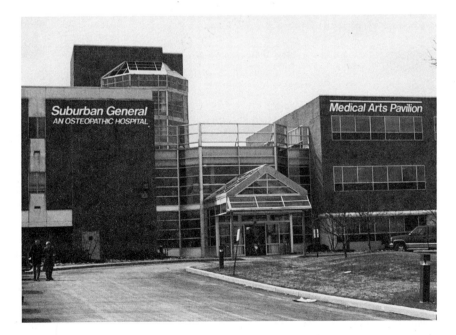

FIGURE 14–1. Suburban General Hospital is a local community hospital in the suburbs of Philadelphia, Pennsylvania.

within them. In other words, they are closed to osteopathic physicians. Medical doctors are trained in the diagnosis and treatment of disease and treat with medicine, therapies, and surgeries.

SPECIALTY HOSPITALS

Specialty hospitals provide care only for patients with a particular type of disease, for example, tuberculosis, orthopedic disease, or ophthalmologic disease. An example of a specialty hospital is the National Hospital for Orthopedics and Rehabilitation, located in Arlington, Virginia.

MEDICAL CENTERS

Medical centers consist of either one hospital or several hospitals that have come together as a complex in a geographical area. Medical centers are often associated with a medical school or university. They are generally known for their expertise in certain types of medical care, such as pediatric care or urgent care.

TERTIARY CARE HOSPITALS

Tertiary care hospitals are mainly university hospitals and work with the most complex of patients. Many of their patients are referred by other hospitals for special care.

PRIVATE HOSPITALS

A private hospital is one that is owned by an individual, a group of individuals, or a corporation. Examples of private hospitals are

- Kaiser Foundation Hospital
- Shriners Hospital for Crippled Children
- Sisters of Mercy Health Corporation
- American Medical International

Private hospitals are becoming increasingly popular as various HMOs and religious groups get involved in health care. Some private hospitals are owned by corporations for the care of their employees. A private hospital may have for-profit or nonprofit ownership. A nonprofit, or voluntary, hospital is one that is formed for the purpose of providing hospital care to the members of a group or community. A for-profit hospital is one that is owned by a physician, group of physicians, or corporation for the care of their patients.

GENERAL HOSPITALS

The general hospital is the most common type of hospital and accounts for the most admissions. A general hospital is run by a Board of Governors, which generally has 5 to 15 members. This Board is divided into subgroups, such as the Executive Committee, the Finance Committee, and the Fundraising Committee. One of the functions of the Executive Committee is to approve physician appointments to the staff. The hospital administrator is appointed by the Executive Committee and is responsible for the appointing of department heads. The components of the hospital are

Medical staff
Nursing services
Medical departments
Support services
Administrative services

The Internal Structure of the Hospital

The hospital's governing body is the Board of Trustees, which is made up of approximately 20 members. They meet once a month, abide by their own bylaws, and elect their own officers. The Board is divided into various committees, one of which is the Executive Committee. The Executive Committee is responsible for appointing the hospital administrator, the physicians, and other health care professionals to the medical staff.

THE MEDICAL STAFF

The medical staff consists of physicians, dentists, podiatrists, and psychologists. A medical staff can be open or closed. When it is open, any physician can apply and, after approval, be admitted to the staff. When it is closed, the hospital is not allowing new physicians on the staff at that time.

There are several types of hospital staff membership open to physicians. When you are recredentialing the physician, it is important to know in what capacity she or he wants to be on the staff. The categories available to the physicians are

Active staff—regular membership
Associate staff—physicians who are new on the staff or who do not want admitting privileges

Consulting staff—physicians who are allowed to consult but cannot admit

Courtesy staff—physicians who are allowed to use the hospital only on occasion

Emeritus—physicians who are retired from the active staff

House staff—residents

Honorary staff—physicians of notoriety who are not heavily involved in the hospital

Each category carries with it regulations according to the bylaws of the hospital. It is important for you to be aware of the rules and regulations associated with each type of staff membership so that the physician complies with them. Failure to comply can mean termination from the staff.

The medical staff has an elected president, vice president, secretary, and treasurer. It is also composed of the following committees:

Executive Committee

Joint Conference Committee

Utilization Review Committee

Credentials Committee

Tissue Committee

Medical Records Committee

Pharmacy Committee

Infection Committee

The Executive Committee is made up of the various chiefs of service: medicine, surgery, anesthesia, etc. It is responsible for making decisions regarding the medical staff and hospital. The Joint Conference Committee is a combination of members of the governing board and the officers of the medical staff. The Utilization Review Committee is responsible for reviewing all charts to establish validity for admission to the hospital. The Credentials Committee consists of appointed physicians from the staff to review the applications of all current and new physicians for membership to the staff. The Tissue Committee is responsible for reviewing surgeons' performance by checking specimens submitted. The Medical Records Committee is responsible for making sure proper documentation is on all the charts and that the appropriate signatures are obtained. The Pharmacy Committee reviews on a regular basis the drug formulary that is set up at the hospital. Changes are made at various times to update the types of pharmaceuticals carried in the hospital pharmacy. The Infection Committee reviews all diagnoses of contagious diseases among the patients and monitors the hospital's infection control procedures.

DEPARTMENTS WITH WHICH THE MEDICAL OFFICE INTERACTS CLOSELY

The hospital is organized into different departments that function together to provide the highest quality of care for patients. These departments are as follows:

Department of Nursing

Department of Medicine

Department of Surgery

Department of Pathology

Department of Radiology

Department of Physical Therapy

Department of Anesthesiology

Dietary Department

Department of Medical Records

Department of Human Resources

Department of Social Services

Department of Central Supply

Department of Housekeeping

Department of Physical Plant Operations

Department of Security

Department of Emergency Medicine

Department of Nursing

The Department of Nursing is the largest department in the hospital. The medical office deals directly with floor nurses when the physician has patients in the hospital. Nurses can be found not only on the floors, or units, of the hospital, but also in operating room suites, recovery rooms, nurseries, delivery rooms, cardiac rehabilitation areas, and wellness units. The chain of command in the Department of Nursing is as follows:

Director of nursing

Nursing supervisor

Head nurse/department head

Registered nurse

Licensed practical nurse

Nurse's aid

Ward clerk

The medical office will most likely have relationships with the registered nurses, licensed practical nurses, and ward clerks. If the office or physician has an unresolved problem with any of the nursing staff, it is appropriate for you or the physician to contact the nursing supervisor or director of nursing. Problems will be quickly resolved at that point.

Department of Pathology

Another department important to the medical office is the Department of Pathology. This is the department that performs tests on patients' blood, urine, and various other parts of the body. The Department of Pathology is generally divided into further departments. The medical office commonly interacts with the following departments:

Chemistry Department
Hematology Department
Bacteriology/Microbiology Department
Cytology/Histology Department
Blood Bank
Immunology Department

The Chemistry Department analyzes the blood for abnormalities involving the liver, pancreas, heart, kidney, thyroid, muscle, gallbladder, etc. A chemistry analyzer performs all these tests on one small sample of blood or serum. The Hematology Department analyzes the blood for abnormalities and anemias. The Bacteriology/Microbiology Department analyzes bacteria and their growth. The Cytology/Histology Department prepares tissues removed during surgery for analysis and prepares bodily fluids for detection of cell changes. The Blood Bank maintains blood and blood products for patients who need transfusions. The Immunology Department studies the function and structure of the immune system.

FROM THE AUTHOR'S NOTEBOOK

Always have a professional contact in the laboratory and radiology departments. This contact may come in handy when you need to schedule a patient for a test on a day on which there is no opening. It is easier to ask favors if you have already cultivated a relationship with someone in that department. It is nice to treat your contacts to lunch once in a while to show that you appreciate their help.

Department of Radiology

The Department of Radiology is another department in the hospital that interacts closely with the medical office. This department performs x-ray studies of various parts of the human body. It reports such abnormalities as fractures, dislocations, masses, organ enlargements, ulcers, and any other abnormality seen on x-ray film.

Department of Physical Therapy

The Department of Physical Therapy helps patients' rehabilitation from both injury and illness. These very gifted people patiently help disabled patients learn to walk and talk again and relearn various other motor skills that are necessary.

Patients who have suffered a stroke or been in an automobile accident are referred to this department. Even patients with chronic back pain can benefit from their services of hot packs, cold packs, and massage.

Department of Anesthesiology

The Department of Anesthesiology maintains patients under anesthesia during minor and major operations. They also administer certain pain-relieving treatments for patients who require pain relief from nerve blocks, etc.

Personal Patient Services

A variety of personal services are available to patients in today's hospitals. The hospital has become as service oriented as a hotel! It understands that if it does not provide these services, patients will schedule their testing and hospitalizations at other facilities that do provide them. Some personal services provided in the hospital today are

- Pastoral care
- Communication services
- Hair care services
- Automatic teller machines
- Gift shops
- Newspapers and book carts
- Televisions
- Notary public services
- Meals for visitors
- Valet parking
- Coffee and donuts in outpatient waiting areas
- Transportation services
- Voice-to-voice communication system for patients living alone
- Pet therapy
- Community health education services
- Sibling visiting

Hospital Accreditation

Every hospital must meet certain standards set forth by a professional association. The major accrediting body is the Joint Commission on Accreditation of Health Care Organizations (JCAHO). In 1917, the Third Clinical Congress of Surgeons of North America decided that a system of standardization of hospital equipment and wards was needed. The JCAHO was formed in 1951 by the American College of Surgeons, American College of Physicians, American Hospital Association, American Medical Association, and Canadian Medical Association. The Canadians withdrew in 1959 and formed their own association.

The JCAHO develops standards and provides advice to hospitals about meeting them. It also accredits long-term nursing care facilities, psychiatric facilities, and ambulatory care facilities. Accreditation by the JCAHO is required if the facility wishes to be reimbursed for services. Many insurance plans will not provide reimbursement to facilities that do not have accreditation through JCAHO. Educational grants and federal funding also hinge on this accreditation. Because of this agency, your office might occasionally receive panicky phone calls from a person in the hospital's medical records department stating that the physician finish hospital charts, because they are being inspected the following day. This inspection is critical to the operations of the hospital.

Diagnosis-Related Groups

In 1980, a system of prospective reimbursement for hospital services that was based on diagnosis-related groups (DRGs) began to be used by the state of New Jersey. This system was used by all payers—Medicare, Medicaid, Blue Cross, and all other insurance plans. In 1983, this system was phased in nationwide under the Social Security Amendments of 1983. In this system, payment for care is fixed at a certain amount, regardless of whether the actual costs of the care are over or below that amount. Each DRG is given a relative cost weight by which the dollar amount to be paid is determined, based on national cost averages. In other words, if Mrs. Smith was in the hospital for 5 days with pneumococcal pneumonia and Mr. Comer was in the hospital for 7 days with pneumococcal pneumonia, both bills would be paid at the same rate, regardless of the number days hospitalized.

Professional Standards Review Organizations

Hospital Professional Standards Review Organizations (PSROs) were mandated in 1972 by the Social Security Amendment of 1972. The PSRO was to be an association of physicians who reviewed professional and institutional services covered by the Medicare and Medicaid programs. It was intended to monitor both the cost and quality of care. Hospitals delegated their PSRO review functions to their utilization review committees. Because their effectiveness was not clear, PSROs were replaced in 1982 by Peer Review Organizations (PROs).

Peer Review Organizations

The Tax Equity and Fiscal Responsibility Act of 1982 led to the creation of PROs to review the cost and quality of Medicare services on a regular basis. There were 54 PRO regions designated, one for each state; the District of Columbia; and Puerto Rico, the Virgin Islands, and the Pacific Territories. The major differences between the PSROs and PROs are that the PROs are statewide and their activities are carried out under performance-based contracts with the U.S. Department of Health and Human Services.

References

Pozgar, G. *Legal Aspects of Health Care Administration.* Rockville, MD: Aspen Publications, 1990.

Wilson, F., Neuhauser, D. *Health Services in the United States.* Cambridge, MA: Ballinger, 1985.

15

Medical Marketing and The Community

Marketing—It's Everywhere

Marketing is found everywhere in our economy and affects everyone. Marketing is more than just a business activity; it is something that almost everyone participates in, whether in the role of marketer or customer. Marketing can be defined as the process of developing and selling ideas, goods, and services that satisfy customers, using the principles of pricing, promotion, and distribution. Service marketing falls into the category of marketing of intangible products that offer financial, legal, medical, recreational, or any other benefits to the consumer. Throughout this chapter you will often see the words "patient satisfaction" and "consumers." The concept that patients are consumers who must be satisfied is the core concept of marketing in the healthcare field.

Service Marketing

Service marketing has four unique characteristics:

Intangibility—The consumer cannot evaluate what is being marketed with sensory means such as sight, hearing, touch, or taste.

Inseparability—Performance of the service cannot be separated from consumption, which means that the consumer must be present at the time the service is performed.

Perishability—Services cannot be stored.

Heterogeneity—Performance of the service can vary.

There are five major classifications of services:

Profit—Nonprofit or profit

Customer type—Consumer or organization

Labor and equipment needs—Labor based or equipment based

Customer contact—A high or low degree

Provider skill level—Professional or nonprofessional

Obviously, health care falls into the last category, provider skill level, which presents a couple of marketing challenges. First, services that are based on a high level of skill are hard to prove, even after the service is performed. This requires that consumer education be an integral part of the marketing scheme, because the benefits of some skilled services may be unclear to health care consumers. Second, services involving higher skill levels usually encounter more regulation from professional organizations. For example, health care professionals' services are regulated by the government and influenced by such groups as the American Medical Association.

Advertising Isn't the Same Thing as Marketing

One important factor for the office manager to realize is that advertising and marketing are not the same thing. Marketing involves analyzing both the practice and its potential market. Only after this analysis is completed is an advertising campaign started. Physician offices that go straight into advertising before doing marketing are wasting money and not being effective.

There are two types of marketing: external and internal. External marketing is the type that we see, the advertising of, for example, Dr. Jones's Chiropractic Clinic. Even more important than external marketing is internal marketing, that is, what the office is doing to promote itself.

Internal Marketing

Internal marketing consists of

1 Patient satisfaction
2 Patient satisfaction surveys
3 Referring physician surveys
4 Patient education programs
5 Patient information handbooks

It is crucial to understand what can be done from inside the medical practice to make the practice grow. Internal marketing is the most important marketing that can be done in a medical office.

PATIENT SATISFACTION

It is a well-known fact that patients are the foundation of all medical practices. They are the base that health care professionals build on. What is this buzzword "patient satisfaction"? How is it defined? There are a variety of books and articles on the subject, and each defines it differently. Patients themselves define it differently, because each person's needs are different. No generic statement can be made about patient satisfaction; patients must be satisfied one by one.

Patient satisfaction is made up of quality medical care and quality service:

Quality Medical Care + Quality
Service = Patient Satisfaction

All physicians are sure they are providing their patients with the best possible medical care; however, are they providing top-notch service?

Patient satisfaction rewards the practice with

- Increased productivity
- Increased profitability
- Increased patient referrals
- Increased employee morale
- Increased collection rate
- Decreased employee turnover
- Decreased risk of malpractice

Patient dissatisfaction results in losses for the practice. Leonard Abramson, president of US Healthcare, a large managed care company, once said, "Dissatisfied patients have feet—they'll walk away!" Statistics have shown that the revenues lost through the loss of one patient are $238,000 over the life of a practice. Patients who fail to keep appointments (many times as a result of dissatisfaction) range from 19% to 52%, which of course, directly affects the practice revenues. Not only is that patient lost, but any referrals that the patient might have made in the future are also lost. It is a good practice to send patients a thank-you note when they refer patients to the office. A note like the one shown in Box 15–1 can be used.

The need to provide good service is not news to American businesses, which have long recognized the importance of service. Companies like Federal Express, the Ritz-Carlton, Wal-Mart, and Disney have prided themselves on providing excellent customer service in a very competitive society. Health care facilities are now realizing that they, too, are businesses. Many health care institutions, such as Prudential, US Healthcare, Cleveland Clinic, and Hospital Corporation of America, have begun to recognize the importance of the "customer satisfaction" credo and are now in the process of establishing patient satisfaction programs. Some insurance companies are now rating the physicians who participate in their plans. Members are sent patient satisfaction forms and asked to complete them fully. Statistics are compiled from these forms, and "report cards" on the physicians are sent to members. On these report cards, physicians are graded on appropriateness of care; cost of care; outcomes of care; and, of course, patient satisfaction. Today's patients are more educated and quality oriented than were the patients of the past. They want service and quality care for their dollar!

There are several areas in which a patient can become dissatisfied with a medical office:

- Telephone communication
- Appointment scheduling
- Environment
- Comfort
- Convenience
- Interaction
- Service orientation
- Dignity
- Parking

BOX 15–1. REFERRAL THANK-YOU LETTER

Dear

   Today it gave me great pleasure to serve someone you referred to our office. I know how important it is for the friends and family members of our patients to get encouragement to come to us for their health care needs. When someone is looking for a doctor, that person wants to know that the doctor and staff are competent and that he or she will receive personalized attention.

   Thank you for your trust in me and our office staff to meet these types of needs when you recommend others to our office. It means a lot to me personally.

   If you have any health questions or concerns, please feel free to call our office at any time. Also, if there is anything we need to know to improve our ability to serve you, I hope you will be direct in telling me your suggestions. I value your perspective on my work and know that there may be others you will send for diagnosis and treatment.

   Thank you again for recommending my office. I value your participation in our practice.

Wishing you the best of health,

- Quality
- Follow-up
- Referral physicians
- Patient perception

There is an exercise you can do with the employees at a staff meeting that will increase their awareness of the various things that can go wrong for a patient during an office visit. Have the staff call out the steps a patient takes when she or he arrives at the office door, and have a staff member serving as the secretary write each step down on a piece of paper with a sticky edge. For instance,

1 The patient enters the office,
2 The patient registers with the receptionist,
3 The patient sits in waiting room,

and so on.

Line the pieces of paper across the wall of the office. Then have the staff talk about what could go wrong at each step of the way. Write each possibility on a piece

of sticky paper, and place everyone's suggestions directly under each step. You might end up with many pieces of paper. Remind employees that the purpose of this exercise is not to poke fun at the office, but to point out what incidents would turn the patient away from any office. When some office managers have tried this exercise with their staff, some staff have taken offense, thinking co-workers are talking about them. See Figure 15–1 for an example of how to set up this exercise. Figure 15–2 shows some of the things that can go wrong at various stages in the office visit, creating a dissatisfied patient.

To bring about patient satisfaction, physicians and staff must be willing to change their attitudes toward health care. It is important that you understand the value of improving practice processes and interactions with patients. Some office managers have always recognized that efficiency and consistent service create patient satisfaction and, thereby, practice success. Other office managers have always been more businesslike and have viewed good service as simply a business principle. Change is part of life, professional life no less than personal. Today, people have choices in many areas of their lives, including their health care. Patients, as well as insurance companies, are making choices every day that will affect the future of health care. The successful office accepts change, putting patients and their needs first and constantly striving for patient satisfaction.

THE PATIENT SATISFACTION FORM

The smart office manager obtains feedback from patients to make sure that the office is doing a good job. A Patient Satisfaction Form can be designed and distributed to patients to complete. The form can be distributed in various ways:

- The form can be handed to patients on a clipboard in the waiting room.
- Patients can be handed the form as they exit and asked to mail it back to the office.
- Patients can be asked to complete the form while they are in the waiting room and place it in a box there.
- Have the form printed on a post card with a flap so that it can be taken home by patients and easily mailed back with privacy maintained.

A sample Patient Satisfaction Form is shown in Box 15–2. It can be copied and used as is or changed to better meet the needs of your practice.

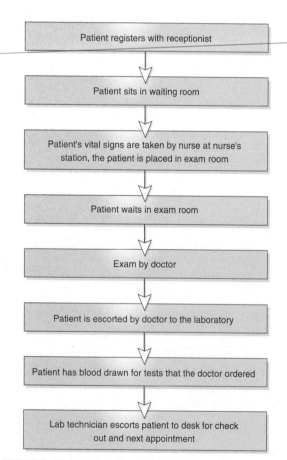

FIGURE 15–1. Patient flow chart for the medical office.

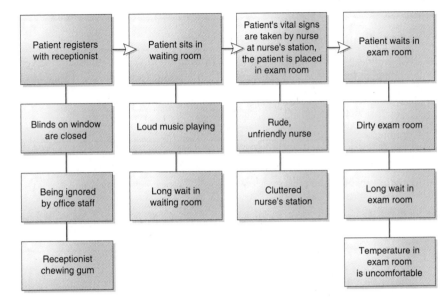

FIGURE 15–2. Things that should not occur during patient flow.

THE REFERRING PHYSICIAN SURVEY

Referring physicians are an important factor for the practice. If the practice for which you work is a specialty practice, referring physicians may be its lifeblood. One of the most important responsibilities of the medical office manager is to be aware of any problems that might occur between your office and the referring physician's office. A solid working relationship should be in place at all times. The referring practice's happiness (satisfaction) is a critical issue for the specialist practice. Some offices send surveys to their referring physicians to find out how they can better serve their needs. A more productive approach is for you to visit each referring physician's office, speak with the office manager to establish a common ground, and inquire about any problems that might be occurring between offices. This information can be extremely helpful for both practices. You can then take a *minute* (doctors are always busy and will appreciate your recognition of this fact) of the referring physician's time to introduce yourself and ask how your office can better accommodate her or his needs. A Referring Physicians Satisfaction Sheet is shown in Box 15–3 for copying or customizing.

PATIENT EDUCATION PROGRAMS

Patients love to read about illnesses! Whether it is their own or someone else's, they are often intrigued by various different illnesses. Patient education is an important part of patient satisfaction and is also monitored by the insurance companies. They want their patients to be well informed and find that patients are more at ease when procedures and illnesses are explained thoroughly. Brochures and pamphlets can be purchased through a variety of vendors, but you might want to compose educational materials relating specifically to your office. For instance, an orthopedist might offer a pamphlet entitled "Saving Your Back . . . How To Lift Properly." A pediatrician's office might offer a pamphlet entitled "How to Choose a Qualified Day Care." Patient education materials from a gastroenterology office are presented in Boxes 15–4 and 15–5.

THE *PATIENT INFORMATION HANDBOOK*

A *Patient Information Handbook* can be fun to design and can be a valuable tool when used correctly. This handbook contains a wealth of information regarding the practice: its hours, how appointments are scheduled, where its offices are located, etc. The staff can hold regular meetings to develop this manual. Everyone's input is important! Distributing the *Patient Information Handbook* to patients can eliminate many phone calls from patients. Many misunderstandings can be eliminated because patients have their handbook to refer to regarding office policies and procedures. These handbooks can either be mailed to new patients before they arrive at the office or handed to them on their first visit to the office (see Appendix for one office's *Patient Information Handbook*).

BOX 15–2. SAMPLE PATIENT SATISFACTION FORM

tell us about ourselves . . .

Please rate our office by using the following grading system. Circle 4 for very satisfied, 3 for satisfied, 2 for adequate, 1 for inadequate. You are very important to us; please help us to help you!

Were we able to give you an appointment in a timely manner?

    4 3 2 1

Comments: _____

_____

Once in our office, were you seen in a satisfactory period of time?

    4 3 2 1

Comments: _____

_____

Was our staff pleasant and eager to help you?

    4 3 2 1

Comments: _____

_____

Did you have any problems with our billing department?

    4 3 2 1

Comments: _____

_____

Did your family doctor receive a report from us?

    4 3 2 1

Comments: _____

_____

Were you satisfied with your total experience in our office?

    4 3 2 1

Comments: _____

_____

Did you have trouble finding our office?

    4 3 2 1

Comments: _____

_____

Would you recommend this office to others?

    4 3 2 1

Comments: _____

_____

Suggestions: _____

_____

BOX 15-3. **REFERRING PHYSICIAN SATISFACTION SHEET**

Date: _____

Name of Referring Physician: _____

Name of Office Manager: _____

Appointment Scheduling: _____
_____
_____

Patient Comments: _____
_____
_____

Referring Physician Staff Comments: _____
_____
_____

Did you receive a patient report in a timely manner? _____
_____
_____

Referring Physician Comments: _____
_____
_____

How can we improve our service to you? _____
_____
_____
_____
_____

General Comments: _____
_____
_____
_____
_____
_____
_____
_____
_____

BOX 15–4. PATIENT EDUCATION MATERIAL ON COLONOSCOPY

What is a Colonoscopy?

You will be asked to lie on the exam table and turn on your left side. The doctor will examine your rectum with a gloved finger and then insert the flexible colonoscope tube gently into your rectum. He will advance the tube slowly through your colon, examining the lining thoroughly. You may feel some abdominal cramping from the air that the doctor injects into your colon. You may also be asked to change position slightly to help the passage of the scope.

Biopsies (tiny bits of tissue) may be taken for microscopic examination, but these should not cause you any pain or discomfort.

The colonoscopic examination takes about 20 minutes to 1 hour. After the procedure, you will be moved to a quiet room to rest until the effect of any medication wears off. You may feel some bloating from the air that remains in the colon. You may be more comfortable if you expel this air, but it is not advisable to force this.

It is very important that you be escorted home after the examination and that you remain home resting until the next day.

BOX 15-5. PATIENT INSTRUCTIONS FOR COLONOSCOPY PREPARATION

You are scheduled for a colonoscopy on:

_____

Do not take any food or liquid by mouth after midnight the night before the procedure.

You may take your medications with a sip of water the morning of the procedure.

The day before the procedure, you should maintain a clear liquid diet. This can include jello, tea, clear broths, or apple juice.

On _____, start to take *Golytely*. This is one gallon of fluid. Drink one glass (8 oz) every 10 to 15 minutes until the entire contents have been consumed.

Report to the office at Community General Hospital, Suite 20, on:

_____ at _____.

Because you will probably receive an anesthetic, it is important to bring someone with you to drive you home.

If you have any questions, please call the office at (115) 222-3500.

NO-COST AND LOW-COST MARKETING TOOLS

Use the patient billing statement to your advantage! At the bottom of each statement, print a message that will bring you patients. For example, at the bottom of the July statement, print the message "Don't forget about your children's back-to-school physicals!" This can be a standard message for a family practice or pediatrician's office for its July billing. An August statement from an internist's office can read, "Flu season is approaching, call for your flu shot today!" An ophthalmologist billing statement for any month could read, "Glaucoma is a silent stealer of eyesight—have your eyes checked!" Another internist's office could print the message "Hypertension is the silent killer. When did you have your blood pressure checked last?" You can develop a set of messages that can automatically be input by other staff members on each month's bill. This is a great way to get patients into the office and thereby increase revenues. It takes only a few minutes to implement this system, and it doesn't cost any more in postage or stationery, yet it can be very productive. If you are like almost every office today, you have a computer system—so why not use it?

You might want to suggest to the physician that she or he hold monthly lunches for the practice's referring physicians. This is a good way for the physician to develop rapport with referring physicians whom she or he doesn't see often. The lunch can be a simple buffet at a restaurant near the hospital. Monthly lunches with referring practices can be held on a staff level also. It never hurts to build good working relationships with your referring practices. These staff luncheons can be held in the office and can be either catered or potluck. Give the other office's staff members a tour of the facility, and perhaps point out any new equipment that was just purchased for special procedures. The staff will undoubtedly pass this information on to their physician when they return from lunch!

The diploma is a marketing tool in its own quiet way. One office covered a complete wall with the physician's diplomas. The massive "wall hanging" of diplomas and certificates looked very impressive. Patients commented on how smart the physician must be. Other offices choose to scatter the physician's diplomas and certificates around the exam rooms for patients to look at while waiting for the physician. Evaluate your office and decide which arrangement will work best. Whichever way you decide to do it, make sure that the physician's diplomas are in a highly visible place in the office.

Cooperative Marketing . . . A Concept for the 1990s and Beyond

The health care field is currently in a phase of incredible change: hospital mergers, declining reimbursement, hospital closings, medical practice mergers, layoffs, and hiring freezes. It is very difficult to compete in today's society as a single medical office. A first-class marketing and advertising campaign is needed. There's one problem with a first-class marketing and ad campaign, however. It costs a fortune! As a result, some practices are looking into the concept of "cooperative marketing." This concept can be an important tool for solo practitioners and group practices alike. It allows physicians to engage in marketing activities with other physicians and institutions, while keeping their practices independent. Participating in community health fairs, forming joint ventures, and opening a free-standing ambulatory care center are just some of the activities that can be shared. The power that group marketing provides allows the delivery of quality care in cost-effective ways. Independent offices who join in cooperative marketing keep a strong presence and thrive with little to no sacrifice. By participating in cooperative marketing, the office can tap into a wider range of resources and can successfully compete with large offices and practices that have resulted from mergers.

An obstacle to cooperative marketing is the fear of collaboration that many physicians feel. This fear is the result of the tough competition for grades and facilities they experienced all through medical school.

There are some very important questions that you must ask to determine whether cooperative marketing is right for your office.

Are the physician's services different from those of other physicians in the same type of practice?
Does your office do any special procedures that are not provided by other offices?
How do most of your new patients hear about the practice? Are they being referred? If so, by whom?
Do the majority of your patients come from a certain zip code?
Can your office afford to become involved in a marketing plan?
What new services can your office add that might benefit new patients?
How much time can your office give to a marketing plan?
What type of return are you looking for?
What services, if any, might your patients need in the future that your office can provide?

Cooperative marketing plans work best when they are accompanied by a long-range plan. The physician should be asked what type of long-range plans she or he has for the office. These plans and the physician's personal agenda can have a decisive influence on how aggressive the marketing plan should be. Call other office managers who work closely with your office to ask whether they have a marketing plan. It is crucial for you to be aware of what the competition is doing and to determine whether these efforts might be something that your office should be undertaking.

One way in which the office can use the cooperative marketing plan is to join in a cross-referral venture with other offices. This is a much more complex system than the referral programs that are now in place. The physicians in a cross-referral system should clearly define one another's duties and obligations while maintaining an open and honest relationship with one another. All offices involved should train their staff to make them aware of the specific referral procedures that must be followed. An example of a joint marketing venture would be the mailing of brochures to prospective and existing patients to describe any special services that the office might provide.

As an example of cooperative marketing, several physician offices may join together to create a community newsletter and share the cost of producing it. A family practice might contribute an article on ear infections and the upcoming swimming season, an OB/GYN practice might submit an article advising women on breast cancer and the importance of mammography, an allergist's practice might submit an article on the approaching allergy season, and an orthopedist's practice might contribute a piece on the many injuries being treated because of "in-line" skates. Other issues that are community oriented are cataracts, glaucoma, colon cancer, and vasectomies. It is important that each cooperative marketing plan be designed to serve the specific needs of the community the offices want to target. Organizing and implementing such a program can be a big job for the office manager. Local hospitals, community organizations, and the Chamber of Commerce can be called on for guidance and humanpower. Don't hesitate to call them!

Sharing is a unique concept in a medical office and will probably bring the physician right to her or his feet when you start to discuss it. It actually is a very clever way to increase services at no extra cost for the patients. All patients love the concept of one-stop shopping! They are happy to have an appointment and their laboratory work done in one office and then walk next door for an x-ray exam. Sharing is the concept of sharing special services and technologies between offices. Billing services, legal services, and a variety of other services can be shared. By sharing their technologies,

offices can obtain state-of-the-art equipment and share the expense. Cooperative marketing is the only way some physicians can become involved in a highly professional, yet affordable marketing plan. In today's competitive health care field, cooperative marketing can mean the difference between an office that is just treading water and an office that is swimming briskly upstream.

How to Market Your New Physician

Successful marketing of the new physician is a major impetus to the growth of the practice. It is important to keep in mind the cost of marketing this new physician ... don't spend more than the office can really afford. Weigh the benefits of several marketing plans before choosing one to use. Marketing of the new physician does not have to consist of big-ticket items such as a professionally designed and written announcement. There is a certain amount of printing fees that the office will have to absorb; however, the peripherals can be cut to an acceptable level. The following are a few ways that you can introduce a new physician to the community.

- To properly introduce the new associate, send out an announcement that you either designed on the computer or bought as a standard item through a catalogue. Be sure to mention any special skills or education the physician might have. Send the announcement to physician members of the hospital staff, departments in the hospital, and some community members. Other professionals to mail the announcement to are pharmacists, optometrists, opticians, dentists, psychologists, and solo physical therapists. It might also be beneficial to mail the announcement to any local community organization and the Chamber of Commerce. It is a relatively inexpensive way to introduce the new physician and at the same time advertise the practice.
- Have a copy of the announcement printed in the local newspaper for about 2 weeks. Perhaps the newspaper could do a human interest piece on this new addition to the practice. Some offices purchase local radio advertising to introduce their new associates. Television spots are unnecessary and expensive.
- Arrange for the new physician to meet area social and community organizations. Advise the new

physician that it would be prudent for her or him to join the local medical society and any other community group, such as the American Cancer Society, the American Red Cross, the Diabetes Support Group, etc. Have the new physician visit pharmacies and dentists in the area to introduce her- or himself.

- You might want to enlist the expertise of a public relations firm to help you promote the new physician. The firm can provide you with tips on how to market the physician successfully, and the cost is not outrageous. It might be a nice way to try out this firm for future use in marketing the practice.

Geoecometric Marketing

If nothing else, the term itself is impressive! Just as patients today are shopping around for physicians, physicians should be selecting the best candidates for their services. With geoecometric marketing, physicians can reach their ideal patients, using whatever selection process they choose. This type of marketing was developed by Sansum Medical Clinic in Santa Barbara, California. When the ideal patients for a specific practice are targeted, good outcomes and patient satisfaction are a sure bet. This marketing style has proven to bring in patients who require more sophisticated diagnosis and treatment, and therefore increased practice revenues.

It is no secret that there are more than 500,000 private physicians in the United States and that the reimbursement provided by insurance companies is shrinking. This is what is called "pressure." The basis on which geoecometric marketing is founded is that certain characteristics identify the most desirable prospective patients. These characteristics encompass patient demographics such as age, sex, income, and education. In addition, there are certain motivational factors that cause people to do what they do. Those who are predisposed to take advantage of personalized service and can afford to do so are widely dispersed throughout the population. These patients can be found, however, by accessing a wide range of databases. It is imperative to analyze data concerning major disease categories within prescribed groups. Often, this research will identify for the office a new service niche that it can fill.

As an example, one office purchased a mailing list from a magazine on fine dining and sent mailings regarding nutrition and diet and the services that the office provided along those lines. The goal of this office was to introduce itself to this targeted group of individuals. A mailing of 250,000 marketing pieces was done each quarter. The information in the marketing piece was designed to trigger responses. That is, an offer was made for interested individuals to be placed on a regular mailing list to receive the office's newsletter. This office received between 4% and 24% returns on their mailings; the average on normal mailings is 1%. This marketing strategy has demonstrated that professional-services marketing can be cost-effective and can lead to an increase in revenues. The key to the success of this marketing is establishing positive, long-term relationships and maintaining the correct patient mix.

Advertising

Gone are the days when a physician didn't dare advertise, for fear of being thought unprofessional and unethical. Although there is still a slight stigma to medical advertising, most physicians now advertise. This doesn't mean that every medical practice has to advertise, however. Depending on the type of practice, advertising can be a great help or a waste of money. If the practice is a specialty practice such as cardiology or urology, the majority of the patients seen are referred by other physicians. However, if the practice is a family medicine, internal medicine, or plastic surgery practice, many patients will seek out the practice. They do this by getting recommendations from family, friends, and co-workers; by looking in the Yellow Pages or the local newspaper; by asking a physician referral service, or by jotting down the name of a practice advertised on the radio. Physicians who use elaborate advertising techniques generally do not recover the costs of such advertising. The physicians who are most involved with advertising are those who want to promote special services or products. For example, a physician with expertise in sports medicine may do extensive advertising to gain public awareness.

COMMUNITY INVOLVEMENT

One of the best ways to advertise the practice is to get the physician involved in the community. If the physician joins any social or civic organization, she or he will become known. As an example, one family practice physician agreed to become the physician for the school football team. It was not long before many players were coming to the office for non-football-related ailments and bringing their families with them. Have the physician volunteer at Little League games or join an adult softball team in the community. The physician might also want to organize a local chapter of a health organization in her or his specialty, such as the American Liver Foundation, the Diabetes Association, the American Cancer Society, the American Lung Association, or the Ileitus and Colitis Foundation. If the physician is interested in the arts, she or he might find involvement in a local theater group or museum more than just creatively rewarding. By volunteering to speak to local community groups, such as the community garden club, the local nurses association, or the Moose or Elks club, or providing a free lecture once a month at the local hospital on topics associated with her or his specialty, the physician will also benefit the practice.

The local newspaper might want to do a feature story on the new physician in town, especially if it is a small town. Maybe the physician has an interesting side to her or his personal life that can be mentioned, such as teaching blind persons how to ski or repairing old violins. This makes great reading and human interest material. The new physician should visit the pharmacies in town and introduce her- or himself. Building rapport with pharmacists is a good idea. They refer many customers to physicians—why not your practice? A good office manager is constantly making time in the physician's schedule for promotional aspects of the practice. Schedule Tuesday's appointments to end a little early so that the physician can go to the pharmacy to introduce her- or himself. Making the physician aware of the importance of this type of marketing might be a challenge; however, it can be one of the most important aspects of your job as medical office manager!

AN ADVERTISING PLAN

An advertising plan for the practice should be made and maintained. This plan should have specific objectives, based on the physician's goals for the practice. What exactly does the physician want to accomplish with this campaign? There are many different reasons for advertising:

- An OB/GYN physician wants to discontinue the OB part of the practice.
- A physician who will be retiring soon wants to maintain a steady flow of patients without much growth.
- A young family practice physician wants to build her or his practice and is looking for the possibility of growth within the practice.

THE MEDIUM

After the objectives of the advertising are clear, it is necessary to decide the medium in which to advertise:

- Local newspaper
- City magazine
- Radio
- Direct mail
- Television
- Telephone book

Newspapers and Magazines. Most physicians will choose to advertise in the local newspaper and/or city magazine. Newspapers get the best coverage, whereas city magazines might cater to the well-to-do.

Radio. Radio advertising is a bit more costly and narrows down the audience somewhat. An all-news station would be the best bet for the money, because this type of station gets the most listeners. The office would have to decide when and how many times the advertisement should be aired. Should it be aired during the morning rush-hour, when people are anxiously listening for traffic reports? Should it be aired in the evening, when people are home cooking dinner? These questions are best answered by the radio station. Ask for statistics regarding advertising and the targeting of certain individuals.

Direct Mail. Direct mail allows the office to target a certain type of people or certain zip codes. This can be done inexpensively or expensively, depending on how direct mailings are targeted and the quality of the paper and printing used.

Television. Television is very expensive, doesn't target many people well, and is out of the financial reach of most medical offices. The addition of air time, ad agencies, and preparation of material can be costly.

The Yellow Pages. The Yellow Pages of the local telephone book offer a variety of options to physicians' offices today. Studies have found that the public views the Yellow Pages as the most appropriate advertising medium for health care professionals, with the highest praise going to physicians who provide a lot of information in their listing. It has been found that 84% of people who "let there fingers do the walking" through the Yellow Pages follow up their research with action. Few physicians today can afford not to have an overt presence in the Yellow Pages directory.

A listing in the Yellow Pages can be simple or elaborate, depending on the philosophy and needs of the practice. The following are a few possible types of Yellow Pages Listings:

- A listing of the physician's name, address, telephone number, and specialty in the alphabetical listings

- A listing of the physician's name, address, telephone number, and specialty, with the physician's name and specialty in bold print, in the alphabetical listings
- A listing of the physician's name, address, telephone number, and specialty in the alphabetical listings, coupled with the same listing in a specialty section of the Yellow Pages
- An in-column ad of one-eighth, one-fourth, or one half of a page, with additional information such as hours, special procedures, etc.
- A display ad ranging from one column to a whole page
- An in-column ad with two-color printing

The in-column ad is a relatively modest way of providing information about the practice. It has the advantage of relatively low cost while setting the practice apart from other listings in the section. This type of listing can be made distinctive through the use of a practice logo. The display ad has become the norm for many large group practices in metropolitan areas of the country. This ad can be extremely helpful to potential clients, telling them such things as what medical problems the practice specializes in and services it offers, what payment options are available, and whether the practice takes Medicare assignment or will file insurance. It can also explain the appointment policy along with the hours of the physician(s). A small map can even be included in the ad to aid patients in their search for the office.

THE AD AGENCY

Ad agencies are another possibility for the medical office to consider. If your office decides to use an agency, make sure that it has experience with health care advertising. Check the fees carefully before hiring the agency, because there can be hidden costs, such as paying the person who writes the copy, the person who places the ads, the person who sits and works with the printer, etc. Find out from the agency just how the fee structure is set and make sure everything is written down in the contract.

Selling the Practice's Services

The first step in selling a practice is marketing. This includes advertising, newsletters, seminars, direct mail, and mall and health fairs. Some practices even go as far as key chains and refrigerator magnets. As a medical office manager, you need to sell the practice's services just as a salesperson sells cars. Know your product! That is what they teach you in sales school. The same goes for a medical practice. You should have the knowledge to be able to discuss in detail everything about the practice and sell it.

The areas where the practice should be marketed are

- Insurance companies
- Local companies in the area
- Churches
- The community

Companies today are looking to cut insurance costs and provide wellness care to their employees. This is an area where the physician's office can do marketing easily and effectively. Make appointments with the benefits managers at local companies to propose that the office provide wellness and social programs for their employees. This is a great practice booster. Some programs that you might want to suggest are

- Stress management
- Nutrition and diet
- Weight reduction
- Alcohol awareness
- Drug awareness
- Women's health issues
- Smoking cessation programs
- AIDS awareness
- CPR
- Fitness and exercise
- Wellness (high blood pressure, high cholesterol, etc.)

This is a benefit not only to the physician, but to the company, because employees' morale is raised when the company institutes programs for their general well-being. This can be done at low cost through the company with a high yield in employee satisfaction.

The Practice Newsletter

The practice newsletter can be either a goldmine or a ton of useless rock! A well-done practice newsletter generates income by attracting new patients and providing the proper amount of media exposure. With today's focus on patient satisfaction and education, the newsletter can be a handy means of providing professional information to patients in a friendly way. It can contain valuable information regarding the practice and its policies, which can save time for the office staff. The down side is that, depending on the demographics of the practice, some newsletters go unread.

PERSONALIZING THE NEWSLETTER

You need to decide on the type of information that will be included in the newsletter and on the format of the newsletter. The newsletter should look as though it is unique to the practice. It should convey the feeling that it was developed strictly for the education of the patients in your office. This will give a sense of personalization, which is a very big issue these days. The following are some tips on how to keep the newsletter on a personal level:

- Write the newsletter exclusively for your practice, not to appeal to a wide range of practices.
- You, as the office manager, should control the content.
- Write stories that reflect your physician's or office's personal philosophy.

You and your staff can easily put together a one-page newsletter on the computer or word-processing unit. This entails simply typing the copy and formatting it on the computer. You can then print it out onto colored paper. Fold the paper in thirds, staple it at the top, stamp it, and apply an address label generated by the computer. There is no need for costly printing, typesetting, and designing services.

To make sure the newsletter looks professional, use a good desktop publishing program (such as Word-Perfect) and a good printer (not a dot matrix printer). Make sure to pick a vibrant-colored paper to catch the reader's eye. Look at magazines and newspapers for ideas on format and content. If the newsletter cannot be produced in the office without looking shoddy, have it done professionally.

You also need to commit to producing the newsletter on a regular basis. Decide whether it should be released on a monthly, bimonthly, or quarterly basis and set up a year's schedule of production dates based on that. If it cannot be done on at least a quarterly basis, it should not be done. Don't be afraid to repeat certain important information—repetition pays.

The following are some tips for producing a newsletter for your practice:

1 Keep it dignified, professional, and honest.
2 Stimulate inquiries by discussions in the newsletter regarding certain symptoms of illnesses.
3 Define the goals of the newsletter.
4 Be sure to reflect the practice—let the newsletter mirror your perception of the practice.
5 If you or your staff are unable to write engaging articles, seek professional writing help.
6 Make the message subtle—give important facts about the practice along with health information.
7 Have the physician give her or his thoughts on certain medicines and treatments.
8 Be committed to the newsletter. Send it on a regular basis and keep in mind that it isn't advertising; it's marketing!
9 Mail the newsletter first-class, to keep it apart from junk mail. Be sure to put the return address on the top left corner.
10 Consider mailing the newsletter to others besides the patients—for example, to pharmaceutical reps, the media, hospital departments, community organizations, etc.
11 Leave copies of the newsletter in the waiting room for new patients to pick up.
12 Ask patients what they are interested in so that it is easier to pick topics for discussion.

GETTING THE MARKETING EDGE WITH THE NEWSLETTER

You may want to get involved with another office for the purpose of sharing the expense of the newsletter. It is also an opportunity to get greater exposure and can be a practice builder. By splitting the costs of the newsletter, each office gets more pages and more information for less. For instance, the joining of an OB/GYN practice with an expectant-mothers group could be a perfect match. Even such specialists as a cardiologist and an ophthalmologist can create a newsletter that works for everyone.

If you're working for a small, struggling practice, you might check with the local newspaper to see if it is interested in running your newsletter as a community awareness article.

Most American companies today are concerned with the wellness and education of their employees. They might be interested in helping to finance your newsletter as a service to their employees. They may agree to help finance the newsletter if their employees receive copies of it when it is distributed. This can act as a growth tool, because some employees may wish to come to see the physician who wrote that great article in last month's newsletter!

There are various ways to use the newsletter to benefit both the community and the practice. Every community has bulletin boards. Mount copies of the newsletter on the bulletin board with staples or tacks so that individuals can easily take one. The newsletter can also be exhibited at health fairs and screenings in pharmacies, stores, and shopping malls. Place copies of the newsletter in adult day care centers, senior centers, and any other community buildings. Ask local nursing homes if you can place some of your newsletters in their waiting areas. Make copies available to schools, libraries, and medical supply stores. Offer copies of the newsletter to referring physicians for their waiting rooms and offer to place their newsletters in yours. This becomes a win–win situation for both offices.

The Managed Care Factor

"We must plan for the future, because people who stay in the present will remain in the past."
—Abraham Lincoln

Today, medicine is moving in the direction of managed care. This is having an enormous effect on the medical office and the practice of medicine. Many offices where patients have been treated for years are now finding that many employers' decision to change insurance companies has snatched these patients from the practice and placed them under the care of a physician who is participating in the particular plan the employer joined. This is a traumatic situation not only for the patient, but also for the office. Two issues have resulted from the continued growth of managed care:

1 The need for physicians participating in managed care plans to understand that patient satisfaction is critical to the success of the medical practice
2 The need for the physician and staff to understand the importance of a healthy relationship between the patient and the physician

Confidence, trust, honesty, protection, and *care* are words for the physician's office of the 1990s to live by. The combination of these qualities with quality clinical care is what leads to success in today's practice. To establish whether your office is ready for managed care, there are a few questions you and the physician need to ask yourselves:

Are you willing to accept capitation?
Do you understand its cost structure?
Are you willing to accept the outcomes of managed care?
Do you measure your utilization rates?

Is patient education a strong component of your practice?
Are efforts to ensure patient satisfaction an integral part of your practice?
Do you have quality management procedures in place?
Do you have the capability to assess potential networks?
Do you have a practice strategy in place?

If you answered yes to all of these questions, your office will be better prepared to face managed care.

Quality Service

FACTORS THAT INFLUENCE PATIENTS' ACTIONS

Creating rapport with patients is easily done once they reach the office, but what about the external factors that can influence patients' actions before they reach the office? These factors are

- Word-of-mouth information from other patients
- Newspapers or TV ads
- Word-of-mouth information from co-workers
- Comments by other physicians

In a medical office, there are three concepts to deal with:

1 Patient expectation
2 Patient experience
3 Patient perception

Patient expectation refers to patients' expectations regarding what will take place during an office visit. *Patient experience* is the circle of events that actually took place during the office visit. *Patient perception* is how the patient rates the office visit. Remember, the staff's perception of how the office visit went can be very different from the patient's perception of how the office visit went. Touch is very important in the outcome of an office visit. Patient's must feel they are cared for.

Experience + Needs + Communication = Expectations
Perception → Expectations = Satisfaction
Expectation ← Perception = Dissatisfaction

ELEMENTS OF QUALITY SERVICE

The word *quality* means "a degree of excellence." Your office's main goal should be to ensure that each patient feels that she or he received high-quality service.

There are four key elements to the delivery of quality service:

1 The customer—Without the customer, or patient, there is no need to strive for quality service. There is also no need for the staff to come to work!
2 Staff commitment—Without the commitment of the office manager, the physician, and the staff, quality service will fall by the wayside.
3 Patient expectations—If the office does not attempt to fulfill the patients' expectations, it stands no chance of satisfying patients.
4 Continuity of service—Quality service requires consistency.

These four elements result in patient satisfaction, staff motivation, professional fulfillment, and the success of the practice.

The Consumer

It has always been difficult for medical practices to see patients as consumers. The reality is, that patients are indeed consumers, consumers who are shopping for a service. They must be thought of in that respect. Everyone who works in a medical office knows that some patients are demanding, annoying, pushy, and loud; others are understanding, pleasant, easygoing, and intelligent; and others are timid, softspoken, naive, and lacking in knowledge. Too many offices think of and talk about patients as diseases, saying, for instance, "The peptic ulcer in Room 1 needs lab work." This type of chatter in an office shows that there is no personalization present, that the patient has been pigeon-holed into a disease category. That "peptic ulcer" in Room 1 has a name; it is Mrs. Bancock, an intelligent older lady with a grandson in medical school.

Staff Commitment

Commitment to quality service must start at the top. The physician must make the first commitment to the patient before the staff can make any type of commitment. A commitment is a pledge to provide a certain course of action. It carries with it a certain depth and sincerity. This commitment must be total; in other words, everyone on the staff must be 100% commited to providing quality service to the patient. As the office manager, you are considered the physician's surrogate when it comes to management issues, and this must be conveyed to all employees.

The Basics of an Office Manager's Commitment

There are a few fundamental practices you should follow closely to facilitate commitment to quality service. You should

- Have a solid vision.
- Have conviction in what the office is doing.
- Be visible.
- Learn and grow every day.
- Reward staff for a job well done.
- Develop a plan and review the progress of the office once a year.

A Commitment Exercise

You may want to do the following commitment exercise at one of the regularly scheduled staff meetings. Hand a legal pad to each employee and ask her or him to respond to the following questions:

- What business are we in?
- Why are we in this business?
- Who are our patients?
- Who should our patients be?
- What are the expectations of our patients?
- How can we meet the expectations of our patients?
- What type of image do we want to portray?

Remind the employees that there may be more than one answer to the questions. They should feel free to write down all possible answers. The questions should be answered honestly, and this exercise can be done confidentially if staff members wish. You might want to ask the physician to answer these questions also and then compare answers. The results may be interesting.

This exercise can also be done with a flipchart or blackboard. It can be a brainstorming session, in which employees call out answers to the questions, and all answers are written down to be discussed at the end of the session. Brainstorming is a method of encouraging free thinking and creative ideas within a group. During brainstorming sessions, make sure all employees are given time to think about the issue or question. Remind them that no ideas are stupid! There can be no criticism and ideas should focus on processes, not people. Ideas should be spontaneous, and shy employees should be encouraged to participate.

Patient Expectations

It is important that the communication between the physician, the staff, and the patient is clear. After all, if staff are unaware of what the patient wants and needs, it is impossible for them to provide satisfaction. Many employees know the patients well and are aware of their needs and expectations. Employees who are not in tune with patients must try harder to understand patients' needs and make an effort to satisfy them. These expectations must be evaluated and immediately acted on. Complaints commonly lodged by dissatisfied patients are

"I had to wait 2 hours before I was seen!"

"I had to put on that paper gown and sit in a cold exam room for 25 minutes, waiting for the doctor to come in!"

"The doctor kept getting interrupted by the telephone!"

"The doctor ordered all these tests and never told me what was wrong!"

"The doctor wasn't listening to me! He acted like he didn't care about what I was saying!"

"All that office was worried about was the money!"

"The doctor never returned my telephone calls!"

"The nurse was talking to another nurse about her date last night, instead of concentrating on giving me my shot!"

Expectations differ from patient to patient. Various factors affect what a patient expects of an office visit: the patient's age, the patient's sex, the patient's mood that day, the patient's problem, the patient's personal life, the time of day, the day of the week, etc. In other words,

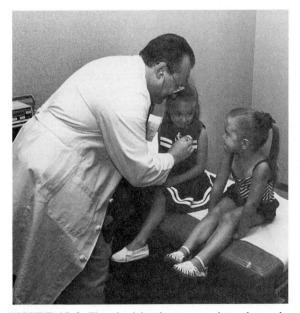

FIGURE 15–3. The physician keeps two sisters happy by allowing them to be together for their visit.

there is no standard for patient expectations. You can, however, get to know patients, in order to have a better idea of what their needs may be. Understand patients' needs, be flexible, and gently manage unrealistic expectations through patient education. In Figure 15–3, a physician is obliging sisters who wish to be seen by the physician together.

Continuity of Service

Continuity means "persistence without essential change." By instituting a continuity system, you ensure that quality service is given continuous, consistent attention. Someone once said that continuity is service that gets better day after day. Continuity does not mean that no change can take place. It requires flexibility and continuous watching. Continuity of service means continuing to do the very best that can be done for the patient, while constantly looking for ways to improve. You cannot institute this system of continuity alone; it requires the commitment of the physicians and staff to succeed!

OBSTACLES TO QUALITY SERVICE

The office as a whole must believe in quality service, not just as a currently fashionable topic of discussion, but as an attitude change. The office's commitment to this philosophy will be the driving force that makes it work. Deep commitment to quality service is a sure route to a successful practice! Some of the roadblocks to the delivery of quality service are

- Lack of commitment
- Doing too much too soon
- Misplaced priorities

MAKING TEAMWORK WORK

A team is a set of interpersonal relationships serving to achieve established goals. They function as individual members of the team interact. The essential elements of effective teams are

- Positive interdependence
- Individual accountability
- Face-to-face interaction
- Collaborative skills
- Group processing

Positive interdependence is the perception that one member of the team is linked with others in such a way that she or he cannot succeed unless the others do and vice versa. One person's work benefits the others', and the others' work benefits that person. It is the belief that everyone sinks or swims together.

Individual accountability is present when the performance of each team member is assessed to inform the group and increase the others' perceptions.

Face-to-face interaction is the perception that a team member's efforts and participation are needed, and this perception increases as the size of the team decreases.

Collaborative skills must be taught just as technical skills must be taught. Team members must be taught the precise social skills for high-quality collaboration and must be motivated to use them.

Group processing is the group's ability to make decisions and describe what member actions were helpful.

Six Processes Necessary for Teamwork

There are six processes that must take place for teamwork to be effective:

1 The team is given the opportunity to create and identify the issues. It must have the collective knowledge to envision the office's needs.
2 The team members gather information regarding the issue.
3 The team analyzes the information and prioritizes it.
4 The team plans a course of action.
5 The team leader implements the plan.
6 The process is evaluated to ensure that goals have been met.

Teamwork ensures the delivery of quality service, efficiency of operations, decreased stress, and confidence. Don't forget to include the physician in the practice team. She or he is the team's owner, and you are its coach. It is important to stress to the employees that all members of the team must work together, from clinical personnel to billing personnel to front-desk personnel. They must form a cohesive bond whereby everyone strives to work together as efficiently as possible.

Benefits of Teamwork

Teamwork yields high gains in both productivity and social areas. It is one of the most important factors in creating a friendly office. It has been proven that patients are happier in an office where all staff work together toward a common goal. Employees working together accomplish so much more than employees

working independently of one another. Some of the benefits of teamwork are

- Increased office morale
- Satisfied patients
- Increased quality of work
- Increased productivity
- Open communication
- Better organization and scheduling
- Easier cross-training
- Decreased staff turnover
- Happier physicians
- Positive working environment
- Increased revenues

Dealing with the Employee Who Is Not a Team Player

If you find that an employee refuses to be a team player, give serious consideration to replacing that employee with one who will be a team player. The last thing an office needs is a negative attitude among employees . . . replace that person quickly! There is something about negativism; it seems to spread quickly throughout an office, turning a hard-working, happy office into a waking nightmare.

Rallying and Rewarding Team Members

Make your employees feel needed and reward them for a job well done. Everyone—the patients, the physicians, and the employees—likes to feel important. If the employees and physician feel important, it will trickle down to the patients, providing them with satisfaction. Show the employees that you care about them. Recognize their individual accomplishments and their contributions to the team. Listen to them, support their ideas, and value what they contribute to the general working of the office. Don't make them feel that they are working in a threatened environment. Don't use threats to get jobs done . . . you won't like the results. Remember, it's nice to be nice. A good office manager manages without resorting to threats. She or he rallies employees to work together; motivates them; encourages them; and, most of all, believes in them. A good manager stresses the common thread among them: the desire to achieve. The last thing a manager should hear is "That's not my job" or "Well, we've always done it this way." These are the phrases that send office managers through the roof. Help employees build confidence in themselves and each other. Show them that a little effort to adapt to change will lead to big rewards. Give them clear expectations, guidance, and the resources to be able to affect change. Be a cheerleader, cheering your team on to success!

STAFF SATISFACTION

Staff have certain basic needs: good benefits, pleasant work environment, and competitive salaries. They also have another agenda of needs: recognition, appreciation, and participation.

A Happy Staff = A Happy Office = Happy Patients

Everyone wins in this situation. Every type of motivation works on someone at some time. It sometimes take the proper mix of ingredients to provide staff satisfaction:

- Appreciation of their work
- Job security
- Good working conditions
- Loyalty from the management
- Competitive salaries
- An understanding office manager
- Participation in office decisions

Management expert Frederick Herzberg, has stated that there are six factors that influence job satisfaction:

1 Achievement
2 Recognition
3 The work itself
4 Responsibility
5 Advancement
6 Growth

There are also some extrinsic factors that affect job satisfaction:

1 Company policy
2 Supervision
3 Work conditions
4 Salary
5 Relationship with peers and subordinates
6 Status
7 Personal life
8 Security

Employees should have positions that are meaningful and enriching. According to Herzberg, the best form of motivation is the kind that gets people involved with what they do, making them feel that their efforts result in worthwhile contributions to the organization. Encour-

age your employees to provide ideas on change that would benefit the office. When an employee offers a valuable suggestion or changes, reward her or him. There are various ways to reward employees for achievement:

- An instant reward, such as a plant, flowers, or a gift certificate
- An incentive reward, such as immediate verbal recognition, a letter of thanks, or business cards for staff members
- Success celebrations, such as a half day off with pay or a gift certificate for two at a local restaurant
- Team incentives, such as buying lunch for the office or having a casual-dress day once a week
- Financial rewards, such as salary increases, bonuses, increase in benefits, and a reduced work-week

Staff who feel appreciated are more productive, create an environment of calm, and do the very best they can for the office. It has been proven that others are inspired by people who show passion for and conviction in their work. People respond to enthusiasm and to positive feedback. This type of atmosphere spills over onto the patients, and the office becomes a warm, friendly, and caring place to be.

A WORD ABOUT COMPETENCE

Unlike the patients of the past, today's patients shop around for their doctors. They use stiff criteria when shopping for their doctors, and their main concern is the skills and competence of both the physician and the staff. Be aware that patients today judge not only the physician, but also the staff. Every patient contact that the staff has is very critical. *Courtesy* is the key word. Many patients' unhappiness with a practice has its roots in dissatisfaction with the office staff. If patients feel neglected or become annoyed by the office staff, they will not bother with meeting the doctor.

THE IMPORTANCE OF A MISSION STATEMENT

What should be mentioned in a mission statement? Each practice has its own ideas about what it should address in its mission statement: quality care; quality service; coordinated care; responsiveness to needs; enhanced quality of life for the patient; recognition of the roles of patients, insurance companies, hospitals, staff members, and physicians in care; the need for a competent and trained staff; and the importance of wellness care. A mission statement should be developed on the basis of the practice's answers to the following questions:

1 What is our purpose?
2 Who are our principal users?
3 What is distinctive about our practice?
4 What are our principal market segments?
5 What are our principal services, present and future?
6 What philosophical issues are important to our future?
7 What has changed about our practice in the last 3 years? In the last 5 years?
8 What is likely to be different about our practice in the next 3 and 5 years?
9 What are our principal economic concerns, and how are they measured?

You should display your office's mission statement, or vision, and make it available for patients to read. Some offices have their mission statement professionally printed and framed and hang it in each exam room. Some offices hang it in the waiting room. Others have it printed on the back of their appointment cards. All offices should make their mission statement a part of their patient handbook. This is a great internal marketing tool and should be used anywhere possible. This statement serves as the foundation for the practice to grow on. It shows commitment to the patients, commitment to the practice, and commitment to community service. This statement says who you are, what you are, and where you intend to go. A sample mission statement can be seen in Box 15–6.

BOX 15–6. A SAMPLE MISSION STATEMENT

Quality patient care and patient satisfaction are the main goals of our practice. We believe the enthusiasm and efficiency of our staff are key segments in the obtaining of these goals. Because of our commitment to quality patient care, we hire staff that share in our commitment by exhibiting motivation, cooperation, productivity, and care. The physicians and staff at Central City Cardiology share in that commitment, which reflects the philosophy and direction of our practice.

References

Adler, W. *"A No Cost Marketing Campaign Saved My Practice."* Medical Economics, February 22, 1993, pp 60-65.

Bovee, T. *Marketing.* New York: McGraw-Hill, 1992.

Brown, N., & Bronkesh, W. *Patient Satisfaction Pays.* Gaithersburg, MD: Aspen Publications, 1993.

Johnson, J. *Joining Together.* Englewood Cliffs, NJ: Prentice Hall, 1987.

Kahaner, L. *"Ten Tips for Creating a Successful Patient Newsletter."* Physician's Management, July 1992, pp 123-127.

Kaye, E. *"Practice Newsletters."* Group Practice Journal, May/June 1992, pp 108-109.

Trigg, D. *"Reaching Ideal Patients Through Geoecometric Marketing."* Group Practice Journal, April/May 1992, pp 60-61.

Wood, S. *"The Promotional Cornerstone."* Group Practice Journal, September/October 1988, pp 43-52.

Appendices

APPENDIX A

Sample Employee
Pension Plan Booklet

ARTICLE I
PARTICIPATION IN YOUR
PLAN

Before you become a participant in the plan, there are certain eligibility and participation requirements that you must meet. These requirements are explained in this section.

ELIGIBLE EMPLOYEES:

All of your employer's employees are considered eligible employees and may participate in the plan, once they meet the eligibility and participation requirements. This is with the exception of members of a collective bargaining unit and nonresident aliens.

ELIGIBILITY REQUIREMENTS:

You will be eligible to participate in the plan on the first entry date after you have attained age 20.5, completed 6 months of service, and been credited with 1,000 hours of service during the eligibility computation period.

The eligibility computation period is the 12-month period that begins with the date you were hired. If you don't meet the service requirements during the first year following your date of hire, the eligibility computation period becomes the plan year. You may then meet the requirements during any plan year.

ENTRY DATES:

Participation in the plan can begin only on an entry date. Your first entry date will be the first day of the next plan year, January 1, after you meet the eligibility requirements.

REHIRED EMPLOYEES:

If you satisfied the eligibility requirements before you terminated employment, you will become a participant immediately on the date you are rehired, if your rehire date is on or after your first entry date, as defined above. Otherwise, you will be eligible to participate on the next entry date.

If you had not yet satisfied the eligibility requirements at the time you terminated employment, you must meet the eligibility requirements as if you were a new employee.

ARTICLE II
CONTRIBUTIONS

EMPLOYER CONTRIBUTION:

Each year, your employer will make a contribution to the plan on the behalf of the eligible plan participants. In order to receive the employer's contribution, you must have worked 1,000 hours during the plan year and be employed on the last day of the plan year. If you do not meet the hours requirement or are not employed on the last day of the plan year because you have become disabled or died, you will still receive a contribution.

The amount of the employer's contribution is 10% of your total compensation plus 5.7% of your compensation in excess of a fixed level amount. The fixed compensation level is defined as the Social Security wage base in effect on the first day of the plan year.

For example, you might receive 2% of your total pay plus another 2% of pay in excess of the fixed level. If your pay was $20,000 and the level amount was $10,000, your share would be:

$$\$20,000 \times .02 \text{ plus } (\$20,000 - \$10,000) \times .02 = \$600$$

If the level amount was $10,000 and your compensation was $9,000, your share would be:

$$\$9,000 \times .02 = \$180$$

OTHER REQUIRED CONTRIBUTIONS:

In certain situations, your employer may be required to change the amount of the contributions to the plan. If the plan is top-heavy (see Article IX), your employer may have to take corrective action. This action could result in either a reduction in the contributions for the highly compensated participants or an additional employer contribution.

ARTICLE III
VESTING

The term "vesting" refers to the percentage of your employer contribution account that you are entitled to receive in the event of your termination of employment.

If you terminate employment before you meet the requirements for retirement **(see Article VII),** the distribution from the employer account will be limited to the vested portion. Your vesting percentage grows with your years of service. **Article VI** explains how years of service are credited.

VESTING SCHEDULE:

Years of Service	Percent Vested
Less than 1	0
1 but less than 2	0
2 but less than 3	20
3 but less than 4	40
4 but less than 5	60
5 but less than 6	80
6 or more	100

You will also become 100% vested at normal retirement, if you become disabled or if you die. See **Article VII** for information on retirement, disability, or death.

ARTICLE IV
SERVICE RULES

YEAR OF SERVICE:

You will earn a year of service for vesting if you are credited with 1,000 hours of service during a plan year. However, if you are credited with 1,000 hours during your first year of employment, you'll earn a year of service for vesting. You cannot earn more than one year of service credit during any plan year, though. Years of employment prior to age 18 will not be considered in determining your years of service.

If you terminate employment and are later rehired by the employer, your years of service after reemployment may be added to the years of service you had accumulated when you left. In order for the two periods of service to be added together, you must return to work within 5 years of your termination date.

HOURS OF SERVICE:

You will be credited with the actual number of hours you work for service and vesting purposes.

BREAK-IN-SERVICE RULES:

For vesting, a break in service occurs whenever you fail to complete at least 501 hours during the plan year. Thus, in any year in which you work less than 501 hours (approximately 3 months), you will incur a break in service.

However, in certain circumstances, your plan is required to credit you with 501 hours, even though you didn't actually work 501 hours. This is primarily if you take time off to have, adopt, or care for a child for a period immediately following birth or adoption. You will receive this credit only for the purpose of determining whether you have incurred a break in service and not for receiving additional credit for a contribution or for vesting.

ARTICLE V
COMPENSATION

Throughout this summary plan description, the words "compensation" and "pay" are used to define contribution amounts. "Pay" or "compensation" means the total wages paid to you by your employer for the plan year.

In no event shall compensation in excess of $200,000 (as adjusted for changes in the Consumer Price Index: $209,200 for 1990) be taken into account for any participant in this plan.

Your compensation for the first plan year in which you participate shall be your compensation from the employer from the time you became a participant through the end of the plan year.

ARTICLE VI
PARTICIPANTS' ACCOUNTS

Under the money purchase pension plan, your employer contributions are placed into investment accounts, which are credited with gains and losses at each valuation date. The valuation date for your pension plan occurs on the anniversary date.

FORFEITURES:

In addition to contributions, the employer contribution account is credited with forfeitures if they occur. "Forfeitures" are amounts that could not be paid to terminated participants because they were not 100% vested when they separated from service with the employer.

ROLLOVER AND VOLUNTARY ACCOUNTS:

Your plan may allow employees who had retirement accounts with a previous employer to transfer the previous account balance to your plan. This is a segregated "rollover" account, and it is always 100% vested. In order to avoid taxes on your "rollover" money, you must transfer the money from your old plan to this plan within 60 days after receiving the money.

Also, your prior plan (if any) may have allowed you to make voluntary after-tax contributions to your plan. (You can no longer do this under this plan.) If you elected to make voluntary contributions under the prior plan, you also have a "voluntary" account.

INVESTMENTS:

All of the money deposited into the plan by your employer will be invested by the trustees.

The trustees are fiduciaries of the plan, which means that they have a responsibility to you to invest the plan assets prudently.

CREDITING YOUR ACCOUNTS WITH GAIN OR LOSS:

Each investment account is credited with investment gain or loss as of each valuation date. Earnings or losses are allocated on the basis of the ratio your account balance bears to the total account balances of all participants in the same investment. You are then credited with that percentage of earnings or losses.

ARTICLE VII
BENEFITS UNDER YOUR PLAN

NORMAL RETIREMENT BENEFITS:

The normal retirement age for the plan is the later of age 65 or your age on the 5th anniversary of your participation in the plan.

Your normal retirement date is the first day of the month coincident with or next following the date you reach normal retirement age.

At your normal retirement date, you will be entitled to 100% of your account balance. Payment of your benefits will begin as soon as practicable after you've retired **(see Article VIII).**

LATE RETIREMENT BENEFITS:

If you decide to work past your normal retirement date, you can defer payment of your benefits until your retirement date. Payment of your retirement benefits will commence as soon as practicable following your late retirement date.

DEATH BENEFITS:

Should you die before retirement, your spouse or beneficiary will be entitled to 100% of your account balance.

If you are married at the time of your death, your spouse will be the beneficiary of your death benefits, unless you otherwise elect in writing on a form to be furnished to you by the plan administrator. IF YOU WISH TO DESIGNATE A BENEFICIARY OTHER THAN YOUR SPOUSE AS YOUR BENEFICIARY, YOUR SPOUSE MUST CONSENT TO WAIVE HIS/HER RIGHT TO RECEIVE DEATH BENEFITS UNDER THE PLAN. YOUR SPOUSE'S CONSENT MUST BE IN WRITING AND WITNESSED BY A NOTARY OR A PLAN REPRESENTATIVE.

If you are married and die before retiring, your spouse's benefits will usually be paid in the form of a "preretirement survivor annuity," a life annuity for your spouse. The amount of the annuity will depend on your account balance at the time of your death. Also, your spouse may be able to select another form of payment, depending on the options available at the time of your death.

If you want to designate someone other than your spouse as your beneficiary, you have the option of waiving the preretirement survivor annuity, with your spouse's consent. This waiver can be made at any time after the beginning of the plan year in which you reach age 35. The administrator will provide you with a detailed explanation of the preretirement survivor annuity before you reach age 35. This explanation will be given to you at some point during the 3-year period beginning on the first day of the plan year in which you reach age 32, or during your first 3 years of participation if you enter the plan after age 32. In order to receive this information in a timely manner, you should inform the plan administrator when you reach age 32.

If your spouse has consented to a valid waiver of any rights to the death benefit, or your spouse cannot be located, or you are single at the time of your death, then your death benefit will be paid to any beneficiary you may chose. The plan administrator will supply you with a beneficiary designation form.

Since your spouse has certain rights under your plan, you should immediately inform the plan administrator of any changes in your marital status.

DISABILITY BENEFITS:

Should you become permanently disabled while a participant under this plan, you will receive 100% of your account balance. "Disability" means a medically determinable physical or mental impairment that may be expected to result in death or to last at least a year and that renders you incapable of performing your duties with your employer. A determination of disability will be made by the plan administrator in a uniform, nondiscriminatory manner on the basis of medical evidence.

If it is determined that you are disabled, your payments will begin on or before the anniversary date following the date you were determined to be disabled.

BENEFITS UPON TERMINATION:

If your employment is terminated for any reason other than those set out above, you will be entitled only to that portion of your employer accounts in which you are vested. (You are always entitled to 100% of the account balance of any voluntary contribution money you contributed to your plan.)

"Vesting" refers to the percentage of your account balance you are entitled to at any point in time. For each year you remain a participant in the plan, you become vested with a higher percentage of your employer account balance (see Article III).

If your benefit is over $3,500, you may at your option, and with your spouse's consent, request the plan administrator to distribute your benefit to you before your retirement date. However, you must incur a break in service before you can receive a distribution.

If your benefit is $3,500 or less, the plan administrator may distribute your benefit early. No spousal consent is needed for distributions of $3,500 or less.

DISTRIBUTIONS DUE TO A DOMESTIC RELATIONS ORDER:

In general, contributions made by you or your employer for your retirement are not subject to alienation. This means they cannot be sold, used as collateral for a loan, given away or otherwise transferred. They are not subject to the claims of your creditors. However, they may be subject to claims under a qualified domestic relations order (QDRO).

The administrator may be required by law to recognize obligations you incur as a result of court-ordered child support or alimony payments. The administrator must honor a QDRO which is defined as a decree or order issued by a court that obligates you to pay child support or alimony, or otherwise allocates a portion of your assets in the plan to your spouse, child, or other dependent. If a QDRO is received by the administrator, all or portions of your benefits may be used to satisfy the obligation. It is the plan administrator's responsibility to determine the validity of a QDRO.

TAXATION OF DISTRIBUTIONS:

The benefits you receive from the plan will be subject to ordinary income tax in the year in which you receive the payment, unless you defer taxation by a rollover of your distribution into another qualified plan or an IRA. Also, in certain circumstances, your tax may be reduced by special tax treatment such as "5-year forward averaging."

In addition to ordinary income tax, you may be subject to a 10% tax penalty if you receive a "premature" distribution. If you receive a distribution upon terminating employment before age 55 and you don't receive the payment as a life annuity, you will be subject to the 10% penalty, unless you rollover your payment. There is no penalty for payments due to your death or disability.

The rules concerning rollovers and the taxation of benefits are complex; please consult your tax advisor before making a withdrawal or requesting a distribution from the plan. The plan administrator will provide you with a brief explanation of the rules concerning rollovers, if you request a distribution that is eligible for a rollover.

ARTICLE VIII
BENEFIT PAYMENT OPTIONS

There are several different payment options available under your plan. The method of payment you will receive depends on your marital status at the time you receive payment, as well as the elections you and your spouse make. All payments under your plan are "equivalent." This means that, after making adjustments for longer or shorter periods, or for payments continuing to a beneficiary or spouse after your death, all payments are actuarially equal to one another.

If you have been married for at least one year at the time of your retirement, the normal payment option under your plan is 50% joint and survivor annuity. That means if you die before your spouse, your spouse will receive, after your death, 50% of the benefit you were receiving at the time of your death. You may elect another joint and survivor annuity, or you may elect another form of payment, with your spouse's consent. However electing another option will affect the payments made to you and your spouse. You should consult your tax adviser before making any election.

If you are not married (or have not been married for at least one year) at the time of retirement, or if you and your spouse reject the joint and survivor annuity, you may choose to receive payment in the form of a lump-sum distribution of your total account balances, a life annuity, or any other form of payment that may be permitted under your plan, at the time of your distribution. Consult your plan administrator for other options of payment.

When you are near retirement, the plan administrator will furnish you with explanations of the joint and survivor and life annuities. You will be given the option of waiving the joint and survivor annuity during the 90-day period before the annuity payment is to begin. If you are married and decide to waive the joint and survivor annuity, your spouse must consent to the waiver. Your spouse's consent must be signed before a notary public or a plan representative. Any waiver you make can be revoked later. However, your spouse cannot revoke his/her consent to the waiver without your permission. The plan administrator will provide you with the necessary forms to waive the joint and survivor annuity.

The plan administrator may delay payment to you for a reasonable time for administrative convenience. However, unless you choose to defer receipt of your distribution, the plan must begin your payments within 60 days after the close of the plan year following the latest of:

1 the date on which you reached your normal retirement age,

2 the 10th anniversary of the year in which you became a participant in the plan, or

3 the date you terminated employment with the employer.

In any event, the law requires that your distributions begin no later than April 1 of the year following the date you reach age $70\frac{1}{2}$ (the date 6 months after your 70th birthday).

ARTICLE IX
TOP-HEAVY RULES

A plan becomes top-heavy when the total of the key employees' account balances make up 60% or more of the total of all account balances in the plan. Key employees are certain highly compensated officers or owners/shareholders.

If your plan is top-heavy, plan participants who are not "key" must receive a minimum contribution. This minimum contribution is the smaller of the percentage of pay contributed by the employer to key employees, or 3% of your compensation. If the employer contribution allocated to your account for the top-heavy year is equal to or more than this minimum contribution, no additional employer contribution would be needed to meet the top-heavy rules.

ARTICLE X
MISCELLANEOUS

PROTECTION OF BENEFITS:

Your plan benefits are not subject to claims, indebtedness, execution, garnishment, or other similar legal or equitable process. Also, you cannot voluntarily (or involuntarily) assign your benefits under this plan.

LOANS:

Loans under this plan are not permitted.

AMENDMENT AND TERMINATION:

The employer has reserved the right to amend or terminate your plan. However, no amendment can take away any benefits you have already earned. If your plan is terminated, you will be entitled to the full amount in your account as of the date of termination, regardless of the percent you are vested at the time of termination.

PENSION BENEFIT GUARANTY CORPORATION:

The Pension Benefit Guaranty Corporation (PBGC) provides plan termination insurance for defined benefit pension plans. In your money purchase pension plan (a defined contribution plan), all of the contributions and investment earnings are allocated to participants' accounts. PBGC insurance is not needed and does not apply.

CLAIMS:

When you request a distribution of all or any part of your account, you will contact the plan administrator, who will provide you with the proper forms to make your claim for benefits.

Your claim for benefits will be given a full and fair review. However, if your claim is denied, in whole or in part, the plan administrator will notify you of the denial within 90 days of the date your claim for benefits was received, unless special circumstances delay the notification. If a delay occurs, you will be given a written notice of the reason for the delay and a date by which a final decision will be given (not more than 180 days after the receipt of your claim.)

Notification of a denial of claims will include

1 the specific reason(s) for the denial;
2 reference(s) to the plan provision(s) on which the denial is based;
3 a description of any additional material necessary to correct your claim and an explanation of why the material is necessary; and
4 an explanation of the steps to follow to appeal the denial, including notification that you (or your beneficiary) must file your appeal within 60 days of the date you receive the denial notice.

If you or your beneficiary do not file an appeal within the 60-day period, the denial will stand. If you do file an appeal within the 60 days, your employer will review the facts and hold hearings, if necessary, in order to reach a final decision. Your employer's decision will be made within 60 days of receipt of the notice of your appeal, unless an extension is needed due to special circumstances. In any event, your employer will make a decision within 120 days of the receipt of your appeal.

APPENDIX B

Central City Medical Associates Office Procedure and Policy Manual

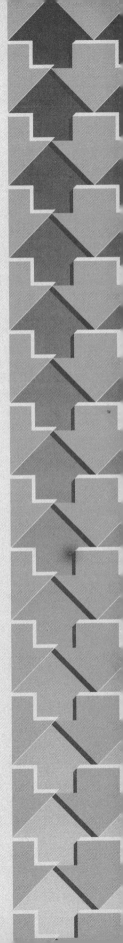

MISSION STATEMENT

Quality patient care and patient satisfaction are
the main goals of our practice. The enthusiasm and
efficiency of our staff are key segments in the
obtaining of these goals. Because of our commitment to
quality patient care, we hire staff who share in our
commitment by exhibiting motivation, cooperation,
productivity, and caring. This manual will help us
all to understand that commitment and reflects the
philosophy and direction of our practice.

ABOUT THE PRACTICE

Our practice is an academic-based practice with two
offices in the Central City area. We have a group
practice of four physicians who specialize in
cardiology. Our doctors are affiliated with the
following hospitals:

> **Medical College of Any State**
> **Community General Hospital**

Our offices are located at:

Suite One   **111 Central Avenue**
100 ''A'' Street   **Central City, USA 22222**
Central City, USA 11111

CONDUCT AND APPEARANCE

Our aim is to provide quality medical care to the patients we serve. What you say, what you do, and how you say and do it will either contribute substantially to the care of the patient or keep us from doing the best possible job. We strive for a continuously cooperative and friendly office environment, with the importance of personal growth recognized. Openness and support for co-workers are critical factors in our practice.

Many patients come to the office in less than a good mood. They are worried about their condition or depressed because their recovery might be slow. It's part of your job to be cheerful, tactful, and patient with our patients, even if their disposition sometimes causes them to be impatient with you.

Your personal appearance is important, too. It can inspire confidence in you and the entire practice. Neatness and cleanliness are, of course, particularly important in a doctor's office. We ask that our personnel wear clean, neat clothing and go light on the makeup and perfume.

GOOD EMPLOYEE MANNERS

Patients form quick and lasting impressions of all of us as we conduct our daily business on the telephone, in writing, or in person. Always be courteous. When answering the telephone, always give your name, so that the person on the other end will know who he or she is talking to. Remember, it's nice to be nice.

CONFIDENTIALITY

As an employee of this office, you're bound by medical ethics. This means that you must keep confidential any information entrusted to you regarding patients, doctors, your fellow employees, or any office matter. You should never mention a patient's name outside the office. All of us are legally responsible for guarding privileged information and can be subject to legal action if we divulge it. We are all professionals.

DISCIPLINE

Discipline is important to ensure that we meet our goal of quality patient care. Time at the office is for office-related work. A nonsmoking office is what we prefer; if you find it necessary to smoke, we ask that you do it outside the office building. Some buildings have designated areas for nonsmokers. Personal calls should be kept to a minimum, and incoming calls should be discouraged.

EMPLOYEE WARNING NOTICE

Notice will be given to employees who have not acted within the guidelines of our practice. After the second warning, the employee will be placed on probation. After the third warning, the employee's employment with our practice will be terminated. A copy of this form can be found at the end of this manual.

GOSSIP

Gossip can be poisonous, and we sincerely hope that no employee will ever be guilty of repeating any gossip concerning a fellow employee, a patient, a physician, or any other person associated with our office. Any violation can be grounds for dismissal.

TRAINING PERIOD

Your first 3 months of employment are considered to be a learning period. Your response to training, your ability to do the job assigned, your general attitude, and your ability to work with other people will be evaluated, and continued employment will be based on this evaluation.

If it is determined that your performance at any time during this 3-month period does not meet the established standards of the office, you may be dismissed. At the end of the learning period, if it is determined that your progress has been satisfactory, you will be considered for permanent employment.

JOB DESCRIPTION AND TEAMWORK

Each employee has been given a written job description for which he or she is responsible. Each position is given a job level that reflects the knowledge and responsibility required of the position. This in no way reflects the philosophy that teamwork is not important. We expect all employees to work together with initiative and cooperation. We ask that teamwork be recognized and used by all employees.

EMPLOYEE EVALUATIONS

Employee evaluations aid the office manager in determining the periodic adjustments in each employee's salary. A copy of the employee evaluation form is presented at the end of this manual for your review. Employee evaluations take place on a yearly basis before the end of the year. At this time, each employee meets with the practice manager to discuss the duties and responsibilities of each job and the key results anticipated. The purpose of this evaluation is to assist the employee in meeting the expectations of the practice, the practice manager, and the physicians. Each employee is rated on a set of factors that our medical practice believes to be critical to overall performance of the group.

BREAKS

All full-time employees are entitled to a 15-minute break in the morning, a half-hour lunch, and a 15-minute break in the afternoon. The lunch period is paid.

HOURS

All employees are expected to be in the office at their designated times. To ensure quality flow of patients in the office, it is necessary for personnel to work on their designated days. Any changes must be approved by the practice manager. If the occasion arises that a part-time employee needs a different day off, it is best to use vacation time for this, so as not to interrupt the general flow of the office. Employee hours may sometimes be staggered to accommodate the needs of the office. The office has the right to change an employee's work schedule and assignment when it is in the best interests of patient flow and quality of care.

PART-TIME EMPLOYEES

A part-time employee is one who works fewer than 30 hours per week. Part-time employees are paid hourly. Part-time employees are eligible for sick leave in proportion to the hours that they work. If a part-time employee works 16 hours a week, this employee would be eligible for 16 hours of sick leave per year. Part-time employees are eligible to take paid vacation time after 1 full year of employment that is also in proportion to the amount of hours they work. A part-time employee who works 16 hours per week is eligible, after 1 year's employment, to 4 days of paid vacation time per year. Because of the guidelines of the insurance company, part-time employees are not eligible for health insurance benefits if they work fewer than 30 hours per week. There will not be an increase in eligible vacation days for part-time employees.

PERSONAL TIME AND EMERGENCIES

Each full-time employee is given 2 personal days. Part-time employees are not given personal days. If a family emergency requires additional personal time, the matter will have to be discussed with the office manager. It is customary for employees to use vacation time for this.

TERMINATION

If it becomes necessary for a staff member's employment to be terminated, he or she will be given 2 weeks' notice. We expect that employees who end their employment with the office will provide the same courtesy, giving 2 weeks' notice in writing to the office manager.

SALARY/PAYROLL

Your salary is a confidential matter and should never be discussed with other employees. If you have a question regarding your salary, you should speak directly with the practice manager. Your salary will be reviewed when an employee evaluation takes place. At this time, adjustments will be granted or denied on the basis of the quality and quantity of work performed, progress, attitude, attendance, and the general state of the office economy. Payroll is biweekly and is distributed on Thursdays for your banking convenience.

SCHEDULING OF PATIENTS

Patients who call our office are ill and generally need to be seen quickly. If there is a difficulty in giving them an appointment quickly, the doctor in the office should be asked when he or she feels the patient should be scheduled.

Of course, we should always be scheduling **all** emergency patients immediately. With the medical-legal situation the way it is today, we cannot take the risk of making an emergency patient wait. Always advise the doctor of any conversation that you have with a patient who feels he or she is having an emergency. If there is no doctor in the office at the time of the call, tell the patient you need to review the schedule and will call him or her back in a few minutes. Immediately beep or page the doctor nearest your vicinity to advise him or her of the situation so that he or she can decide when and where to see the patient. Always advise the physician when he or she gets behind in this office schedule. No one likes to wait an excessive amount of time, and the doctors certainly do not want to keep their patients waiting. This situation causes everyone—patient, doctor, and office staff—to become anxious. If the physicians are made aware of the situation, they will try their best to catch up.

TELEPHONE TIPS

If patients call for the results of their tests, always pull their chart to make sure you have the results, and then tell them you will have the physician call them. If the result is not in the chart and you think that it has been a reasonable amount of time in which to receive a report, you should call the appropriate place and obtain the report for the physician. Do not give the results over the phone unless you have been instructed to do so by the physician.

DOCTOR'S PHONE CALLS

When physicians call the office to speak with one of our physicians, put them through to our physician immediately. If there is no physician in the office, ask callers for their name and number and tell them you will gladly contact the doctor for them.

Regarding calls from patients, check with each doctor at the beginning of hours to see whether he or she wants to return some calls during hours or wishes to wait until the end of hours. Remember, doctors have their own style; we must respect that and be flexible.

BILLING

Refer all billing questions to the billing manager at the Central City office. Do not attempt to answer these questions yourself. There are many insurance carriers today, and each offers several plans. It is impossible for the front-desk staff to be knowledgeable about all these different plans. It is better to let the billing manager at the Central City office answer all billing questions.

RELEASE OF RECORDS

If patients call and request that their records be sent to another physician, you must pull their chart and give it to the the physician in our office who treated them. The physician will instruct you on what to copy and send to the new physician. This, of course, requires the patient's signature on a Records Release Form. If we are sending records to a specialist to whom we referred the patient, we do not require the patient's signature; however, you must still pull the chart and ask what records the doctor would like to have sent.

HOLIDAYS

New Year's Day
Good Friday
Memorial Day
Fourth of July
Labor Day
Thanksgiving Day
Christmas Day

SICK LEAVE

Sick leave with pay is granted to employees who have an illness that keeps them from doing their job. It is not to be considered something to which one is entitled for any other reason. The number of sick days allotted to a full-time employee is 5. Any day beyond this number will be considered a vacation day or will be deducted from that week's salary.

VACATION

Upon completion of 1 year of full-time continuous service, you will be eligible for 2 weeks of vacation with full pay. Persons with 5 consecutive years of full-time service will receive 3 weeks of vacation with full pay. Vacation will be arranged as nearly as possible to the employee's satisfaction, subject to the best interests of the office.

PENSION/PROFIT SHARING

At the present time, each employee is automatically enrolled in the program after 1,100 hours of service. After the first year, the employee is 20% vested. After the second year, the employee is 40% vested, and so on. At the end of 5 years, the employee is 100% vested. Any other questions regarding these plans should be directed to the practice manager. Contributions to the plan are made each year by the physician officers of the practice and are in addition to the employee's salary. The plan is intended to reward devoted employees for their service.

MEDICAL CARE

One of the benefits of working in a medical office is that all employees receive free medical care from our staff of physicians. This benefit covers the immediate families of our employees also. It does not extend to hospital, drug expense, or medical equipment.

HEALTH INSURANCE

Health insurance through the practice is offered to all full-time employees after a 3-month waiting period, full-time being defined as 30 hours per week or more. This insurance benefit will be continued as long as it is financially feasible for the corporation to do so. Employees have arranged for additional coverage on their own for a prescription plan. The amount for this coverage may be deducted once a month from employees' checks, if they request it.

PREGNANCY

Maternity benefits will be handled on an individual basis. Length of service and potential for return to work will be considered. If complications dictate a longer leave, the situation will have to be discussed with the practice manager.

COMPASSION LEAVE

Each full-time employee is entitled to 3 paid days of leave for the death of an immediate family member. Immediate family members are mother, father, sister, brother, child, and spouse. One day of leave is permitted for the death of a more distant relative. Employees become eligible for this leave after 1 year of employment.

GENERAL QUESTIONS

If you ever have any questions or problems, please feel free to contact the practice manager.

APPENDIX C

Patient Information Handbook for Central City Gastroenterology Associates

<u>To Our Patients</u>

We appreciate your selection of this office to serve your health care needs.

Our office will do everything possible to provide you with the very best care.

In order to do so, we have prepared this patient information handbook to acquaint you with the office and its policies. We believe that the more you know about our policies and methods of practice, the more we can be of service to you, and thus annoyances and frustrations arising from misunderstandings can be avoided.

Welcome to our practice!

What Is a Gastroenterologist?

A gastroenterologist is a physician who specializes in the evaluation and treatment of problems of the digestive tract, including the stomach, intestine, colon, liver, and pancreas. Procedures sometimes performed by the gastroenterologist are sigmoidoscopy, colonoscopy, gastroscopy, and biopsy.

Our Vision

Quality patient care and patient satisfaction are the two main goals of our practice. The enthusiasm and efficiency of our staff are key elements in obtaining these goals. Because of our commitment to quality patient care, our staff exhibits motivation, cooperation, productivity, and caring. The physicians and staff at Central City Gastroenterology Associates share in that total commitment, exemplifying the philosophy and direction of our practice.

About Our Practice

Our practice is an academic-based practice with three offices in the Nice Town area. We are a group practice of three physicians who specialize in gastroenterology. The physicians in our group are:

- Joseph Kramer, M.D.
- Maureen Smith, M.D.
- Lawrence Williams, M.D.

All of our physicians are board certified in both internal medicine and gastroenterology. They regularly attend medical conferences and workshops designed to provide them with the latest in current therapies, practices, and procedures. Our physicians participate in lectures and courses for other physicians and actively teach interns, residents, and staff physicians.

Our physicians are affiliated with the following hospitals:

- Suburban Hospital, Anytown
- Community General Hospital, Anytown
- Medical College of Anytown, Anytown

Our offices are located at:

Plaza Office:	Office Hours:
Two Plaza Place	Monday: 9:00 AM to 4:00 PM
Suite One	Tuesday: 9:00 AM to 3:00 PM
AnyCity, USA	Wednesday: 8:30 AM to 6:00 PM
(555) 111-1234	Thursday: 12:00 PM to 4:00 PM

Hills Office
Woody Hills Complex
Suite 110
Nice Town, USA
(610) 888-2222

Office Hours:
Monday: 12:00 PM to 5:00 PM
Thursday: 8:30 AM to 2:00 PM

About Appointments

Our offices are open during the hours listed above. We are closed
on the following holidays:

- New Year's Day
- Good Friday
- Memorial Day
- Fourth of July
- Labor Day
- Thanksgiving Day
- day after Thanksgiving
- Christmas

Office visits at either of our offices are by appointment only.
We urge that you call as far in advance as possible for your
appointments. If you must cancel an appointment, please give us
as much notice as possible so that we may offer your appointment
time to another patient. We will be happy to reschedule your
appointment at a time that is convenient for everyone. If you
have a problem and do not have a scheduled appointment, we will
attempt to see you as quickly as possible, with proper respect
to other patients. We ask that our patients do their best to be
on time for their appointments. Lateness is unfair to other
patients who are being seen that day. Occasionally, our
physicians will have emergencies that will delay their arrival
at the office. We ask your patience and understanding at times
like this.

Office Telephones

Normally, our office telephones are open during our office hours. When you call any of our offices, kindly explain your problem to our receptionists. We have instructed them how to handle all incoming calls and to refer your call to the appropriate person. If there is an emergency, they will contact a physician immediately. If the doctor cannot speak with you at the time of your call for routine questions, our staff will take your number and have the doctor call you at some point during office hours. Our trained staff will efficiently gather the information to expedite the return call. Please cooperate with our staff by providing them with all the information necessary.

When calling the office for a prescription renewal, kindly have the following information available:

- name of medicine needed
- strength of medicine and dosage
- your telephone number
- your pharmacy's name and telephone number

This information will allow our office to process your request in a timely manner. If there is a holiday approaching, please check your medicine in advance so that if you require a renewal, it can be handled before that holiday.

Your First Visit to the Office

When you arrive at our office for the first time, you will be asked to fill out a Patient Registration Form. We would appreciate it if you would complete both sides of this standard form as thoroughly as possible. This information will aid our staff in processing your bills and insurance forms efficiently.

Please bring your insurance cards to the office, so that we can make copies of them. The information you provide on the Patient Registration Form will also help us contact you when necessary.

If you have recently had x-ray studies, lab work, or any other testing done, please obtain copies of these tests and bring them with you to our office. This will prevent the needless repetition of tests that have already been done.

You and Your Doctor

During the evenings, on weekends, and on holidays, one of our physicians is always on call and available to handle emergencies. The physician on call is the physician who will treat you if you call during off hours. If you need urgent care, arrangements will be made for you to see a physician. If your physician is away at a medical conference or unavailable for any reason, you will be notified either by phone or by mail that your appointment needs to be changed. There is always a physician in our group who is ready to take care of any of your medical needs. Our physicians always work closely with your referring physician.

Release of Medical Information

Should you require the release of any of your medical records, it is our office policy that you submit, in writing with your signature, a request that your records be forwarded. If you are near any of our offices, we have a Records Release Form that you may come in and fill out. Either method is satisfactory in obtaining a release.

Test Results

When inquiring about recent test results, please help our staff by telling them the type of test that was done, the date it was done, and where it was done. Our staff will obtain the results and have your physician return your call. Some tests may take a few days for us to obtain the results, so please be patient. Unfortunately, this delay is out of our control.

Note: Please call the office in which you were seen to obtain your test results. Your results will be sent to that particular office when completed.

Payment for Services

At the end of your visit, your physician will fill out a fee slip that will contain your diagnosis and your charges for the visit. Give this slip to the receptionist at the front desk for processing. If you need to have laboratory tests done, our medical assistants will show you to our laboratory, where your blood will be drawn for the testing that the physician ordered. After completion of the laboratory work, you will be guided to our front desk. The receptionist will then schedule your next appointment with the physician. Our policy is that payment for services be made at the time of the office visit. If you have Medicare or a managed care policy that covers office visits, we will submit the entire bill to that insurance company. Any testing or procedure done during the office visit will be automatically billed to your insurance company as a courtesy to you. We do ask that you pay the office visit portion of your bill at the time of the visit. You will be given a receipt that you can submit to any major medical plan to which you may belong. These plans generally reimburse patients a portion of the office visit fee. Our fee for the office visit varies, depending on the length of the visit and the complexity of the diagnosis and treatment procedures. These fees are established by the physicians and not by the staff.

If your account becomes past due, our billing manager will contact you regarding setting up a workable payment plan. If we do not hear from you, our policy dictates that legal collection proceedings will be initiated. It is important to remember that if you are having a problem paying your account, call the office and speak with the billing manager. This will prevent further action on our part and save you needless worry.

Insurance Payments

The insurance contract is ultimately between you and your insurance company. Our office participates in many insurance plans that allow us to complete the insurance form for you. We will complete insurance forms for any testing done in the office and for hospital care. The office visit is paid for at the time of service. It is important for you to provide our staff with correct and complete insurance information. After we submit your insurance form, the payment generally comes directly to the office. In the event that the insurance company sends the payment to you, please call our office for directions on how to handle this situation. Your insurance company will not always cover the entire fee for service, because of the nature of the plan or the deductible. Thus sometimes you are responsible for an unpaid balance. Our office will send a statement to you showing the amount due.

Patients Who Belong to Managed Care Plans (Health Maintenance Organizations/Preferred Provider Organizations)

Managed Care Patients (HMOs,/PPOs)

Managed care patients must obtain a referral from their primary physician before coming to our office. Your insurance company will not pay for services at our office without a referral. Your insurance company has instructed us to reschedule any patient who arrives without a referral, until a referral can be obtained. These regulations are specified by your insurance company and not by our office. Your insurance manual explains the importance of this referral. It is important for you to remember that if you carry this type of insurance, you cannot be seen anywhere without a referral.

Glossary

account balance   The difference between the total charges and the total payments

accounts payable   The amount that has been charged but not yet paid

accounts receivable ratio   The ratio that measures the amount of time it takes for accounts to be paid

administrative   Dealing with managerial duties

admissions   The number of patients accepted for hospital inpatient service in a period of time

advance directive   A statement in which a patient either expresses her or his choices about medical treatment or names the person who should make treatment choices if she or he becomes unable to do so

against medical advice (AMA)   When a patient in a hospital signs out against the advice of her or his physician

AGPA   American Group Practice Association

AHA   American Hospital Association

allied health   Health-related functions necessary for assisting physicians

alphabetic filing system   A filing system in which entries are organized from A to Z

alphanumeric   Consisting of both letters and numbers

AMA   American Medical Association

ambulatory care   Care given to patients at medical offices, outpatient departments, and free-standing health care centers

analysis by aging   An analysis that classifies accounts by their age

ancillary   Supplementary; for example, x-ray technicians are ancillary staff

AOA   American Osteopathic Association

ART   Accredited record technician

assignment of benefits   A signature that authorizes the insurance company to pay the fee directly to the patient's physician

average length of stay (ALOS)   The average stay, in days, of inpatients in a given time period

BC   Blue Cross

beneficiary   The person who receives the benefits from the insurance policy

BS   Blue Shield

capital purchase   The purchase of a major piece of office equipment or furniture (for example, a photocopier)

capitation payment   A fixed monthly fee that an insurance company pays to the physician on behalf of its members whether they received services or not

CCU   Coronary care unit

CDC   Centers for Disease Control

CEO   Chief executive officer

census   The number of inpatients receiving care on an average day in a hospital

CHAMPUS   Civilian Health and Medical Program of the Veterans Administration

chronological file   A filing system in which items are filed by date

claim   A request by the physician or patient for services to be paid by the insurance company to either the physician or patient

co-insurance   A specific ratio of the expenses due that are shared by the patient and the insurance company for services rendered

collection ratio   A ratio used to measure the billing and collection activities

CON   Certificate of Need

contamination   The introduction of infectious or hazardous materials

continuing education units (CEUs)   Units applied to individuals attending approved educational seminars and workshops

cross-reference   The specification in a file of another file in which the record may be found

CT   Computed tomography

daisy wheel   The printing wheel of a printer or typewriter; the daisy wheel is removable, and different daisy wheels have different fonts

DC   Doctor of chiropractic

deductible   The amount that an insurance company expects the patient to pay in a calendar year for medical services

dictation   The process whereby physicians record patient records and letters into a recording device (dictating unit)

direct filing system   A system based on itself, whereby an individual can locate information without having to check an alternate source

disability   A condition that prevents a person from working

disbursements   Any type of money that is paid out

DMD   Doctor of dental medicine

DO   Doctor of osteopathy

Drug Enforcement Agency (DEA)   A federal agency under the Department of Justice that controls narcotics and other abuse drugs

dual pitch   The capability of a typewriter to switch from pica to elite type

ED   Emergency department

EEG   Electroencephalogram

effective date   The date the patient's insurance becomes effective and can be used

elective admission   A patient who can be admitted to the hospital on any day and whose delayed admission will not cause harm to the patient

elite type   A type that generates 12 characters per inch

emergency admission   A patient who must be admitted and treated immediately

endorser   The person who signs over a check made out to her or him to another person

ER   Emergency room

EW   Emergency ward

exclusions   The specifics of a patient's insurance policy that exclude certain conditions not covered by the patient's plan

expendable   Office supplies that are used up on a daily basis (pencils, stamps, etc.)

externship   An individual allowed to gain experience in a medical office as part of an educational program

FDA   Food and Drug Administration

fee schedule   A list of procedures and visits from an insurance company that states the specific amount it will pay for each

fee slip   A document generally printed by a computer, that specifies the patient's demographics and lists the codes and fees for the medical services provided to the patient

filing system   Organization of records to ensure easy access at a later date

FP   Family practice

free-standing emergency center (FEC)   A facility equipped to handle medical emergencies that is not a hospital

ghost surgery   A situation in which a patient consents to surgery by one surgeon and later discovers that the surgery was performed by another surgeon

GME   Graduate medical education

GP   General practitioner

group practice   A medical practice consisting of three or more physicians

Health Care Financing Administration (HCFA)   The federal agency responsible for the administration of the Medicare and Medicaid programs

health maintenance organization (HMO)   A membership insurance company that provides payment for services at a fixed dollar amount

ICU   Intensive care unit

intermediate care facility (ICF)   A facility that provides nursing care and must have a supervising registered nurse or licensed practical nurse on each day shift

invasion of privacy   Unauthorized disclosure of information about a patient

invoice   A statement received with delivered goods that describes the goods and specifies the amount due

jargon   A specific vocabulary used by a specific group of people

JCAHO   Joint Commission on Accreditation of Health Care Organizations

liability   A situation in which an individual is responsible, as in a bill for services

LOS   Length of stay

LPN   Licensed practical nurse

MD   Doctor of medicine

medically indigent   A patient who is unable to afford basic medical care

member physician   A physician who has signed a contract with an insurance company to participate in that company's insurance plan and accept its reimbursements

microfilming   A procedure in which records are reduced in size and stored on film

MICU   Mobile intensive care unit

MT   Medical technologist

negligence   Failure to do what a reasonably prudent person would do under the same circumstances

numeric filing   A filing system in which records are filed by number

occupancy   The ratio of census beds to the number of beds in use

Occupational Safety and Health Administration (OSHA)   The federal agency under the Department of Labor that is responsible for industrial health and safety and the enforcement of related regulations

OD   Doctor of optometry

OR   Operating room

orientation   A period of time in which a new employee is trained in the methods of operation of a specific medical office

OTC   Over the counter

PA   Physician's assistant

packing slip   A slip enclosed in a supply carton that lists the items contained in that carton

payable   Any amount that one individual owes to another

payee   The person to whom a check is written

payer   The person who writes the check

patient demographics   The patient's name, address, date of birth, Social Security number, telephone number, sex, employer, etc.

patient statement   A document sent to patients requesting payment for services

PDR   *Physician's Desk Reference*

pica type   A type that generates 10 characters per inch

posting   Transferring information from one record to another

power of attorney   A legal document authorizing an individual to act in the place of another individual

PPC   Progressive patient care

preexisting condition   A condition that existed before the patient obtained a particular insurance policy

preferred provider organization (PPO)   An insurance company much like a health maintenance, with the exceptions that doctors are paid fees for service and patients may use nonnetwork physicians

PRO   Peer Review Organization

professional courtesy   A reduction in fee that a physician gives to colleagues

prognosis   A prediction of what course the patient's condition will take

prudent   Careful, foresighted

PT   Physical therapy

purging   The process of removing inactive files from active files and placing them in a separate but accessible area

reasonable prudence   The legal specification that a professional must act in the manner of the average professional

respondeat superior   "Let the master answer"; a legal term meaning that employers are legally responsible for the consequences of their employees' actions when they are acting within the scope of their employment

résumé   The listing of a person's education and work history that the person provides to a prospective employer

RN   Registered nurse

RPh   Registered pharmacist

RVS   Relative Value Scale

self-pay   Payment made by the patient

seminar   A gathering of individuals for the purpose of education

skilled nursing facility (SNF)   A facility that provides 24-hour nursing care and has at least one registered nurse on each dayshift

SMA   Sequential multiple analyzer

solo practice   A physician who practices medicine alone

SSA   Social Security Administration

standard of care   A description of the conduct that is expected of an individual in a given situation; a measure against which a defendant's conduct is compared

stat   Immediately

subscriber   The person who is named by the insurance company as the person holding the contract

superbill   A document that contains the information needed for payment of medical services

third-party check   A check made out by one party to a second party, who offers it as payment to a third party

third-party payer   A party other than the patient who is responsible for paying the patient's medical fees (for example, a lawyer or insurance company)

tickler file   A file in chronological order used for recalling patients at certain times of the year

transcription   Translation of dictation into written form

UR   Utilization Review

usual, customary and   The system used for determining payment of insurance benefits

VA   Veterans Administration

VNA   Visiting Nurse Association

Abbreviations and Symbols Used in the Medical Office

a̅a̅	of each	L&A	light and accommodation
A&W	alive and well	lat	lateral
abd	abdomen	LL	left lower
ac	before meals	LLQ	left lower quadrant
ad	right ear	LU	left upper
ant	anterior	LUQ	left upper quadrant
ad	left ear	m	mother
ASA	aspirin	M	heart murmur
au	both ears	med	medial, medication
b	brother	meds	medications
bid	twice a day	mEq	milliequivalents
BP	blood pressure	mg	milligram
BS	breath sounds	mm	millimeter
c̄	with	N&V	nausea and vomiting
Ca	carcinoma	neg	negative
cap	capsule	neuro	neurological
cath	catheter	NR	no repeat, no refill
CBC	complete blood count	occ	occasional
CCU	coronary care unit	OD	right eye
Chemo	chemotherapy	OS	left eye
cm	centimeter	OU	both eyes
c/o	complains of	p	palmar surface, palm
CPR	cardiopulmonary resuscitation	P	pulse
CXR	chest x-ray	pc	after meals
d	daughter, died, dorsal	PE	physical examination
dev	deviated	PERRLA	pupils equal, round, reactive to light and accommodation
dexter	right		
diff dx	differential diagnosis	pes	foot
dx	diagnosis	po	by mouth
ECG, EKG	electrocardiogram	pos	positive
ENT	ears, nose, and throat	post	posterior
et	and	PP	postprandial
ext	extremities	prn	as needed
f	father	pt	patient
FH	family history	PT	physical therapy
FU	follow-up	q6h	every 6 hours (can be any number)
FUO	fever of unknown origin	qd	every day
g, gm	gram	qid	four times a day
GI	gastrointestinal	qod	every other day
gtt(s)	drop(s)	qs	as much as necessary
h	hour	ret	return
Hct	hematocrit	r/o	rule out
Hgb	hemaglobin	rt	right
h/o	history of	RL	right lower
HR	heart rate	RLQ	right lower quadrant
h.s.	at bedtime	RU	right upper
Ht	height	RUQ	right upper quadrant
hx	medical history	Rx	treatment, prescription
ICU	intensive care unit	s	sister
IM	intramuscular	s̄	without
IV	intravenous	Sib	sibling

sig	directions for a prescription	Wt, W	weight
sm	small	WNL	within normal limits
SOB	shortness of breath	↓	low, decreased
stat	immediately	↑	high, increased
sub Q	subcutaneous	1^0	primary
Sx	symptoms	2^0	secondary
T	temperature	3^0	tertiary
tab	tablet	II	two
tid	three times a day	I	one
UA	urinalysis	l/d	once a day
ut dict	as directed	$\overline{ss}$	one half
VS	vital signs		

Index

Index

Note: Page numbers in *italics* refer to illustrations; page numbers followed by b refer to boxed material.